Regulation of Target Cell Responsiveness
Volume 1

BIOCHEMICAL ENDOCRINOLOGY

Series Editor: Kenneth W. McKerns

STRUCTURE AND FUNCTION OF THE GONADOTROPINS
Edited by Kenneth W. McKerns

SYNTHESIS AND RELEASE OF ADENOHYPOPHYSEAL
HORMONES
Edited by Marian Jutisz and Kenneth W. McKerns

REPRODUCTIVE PROCESSES AND CONTRACEPTION
Edited by KennethW. McKerns

HORMONALLY ACTIVE BRAIN PEPTIDES: Structure and Function
Edited by Kenneth W. McKerns and Vladimir Pantić

REGULATION OF GENE EXPRESSION BY HORMONES
Edited by Kenneth W. McKerns

REGULATION OF TARGET CELL RESPONSIVENESS, Volumes 1 and 2
Edited by Kenneth W. McKerns, Asbjørn Aakvaag, and Vidar Hansson

Regulation of Target Cell Responsiveness

Volume 1

Edited by

Kenneth W. McKerns

International Foundation for Biochemical Endocrinology
Blue Hill Falls, Maine

Asbjørn Aakvaag

Aker Hospital
Oslo, Norway

and

Vidar Hansson

Institute of Pathology
Oslo, Norway

PLENUM PRESS • NEW YORK AND LONDON

Library of Congress Cataloging in Publication Data

Main entry under title:

Regulation of target cell responsiveness.

(Biochemical endocrinology)
Proceedings from the tenth meeting of the International Foundation for Biochemical
Endocrinology, held in Geilo, Norway in Sept. 1982.
Bibliography: p.
Includes index.
1. Hormones — Physiological effect — Congresses. 2. Cellular control mechanisms —
Congresses. 3. Hormone receptors — Congresses. I. McKerns, Kenneth W. II. Aakvaag,
Asbjørn. III. Hansson, Vidar. IV. International Foundation for Biochemical En-
docrinology. V. Series. [DNLM: 1. Hormones — Physiology — Congresses. 2. Peptides
— Physiology — Congresses. WK 102 R3437 1982]
QP187.3.C44R44   1984   599′.0142   83-24773
ISBN 978-1-4684-4636-4   ISBN 978-1-4684-4634-0 (eBook)
DOI 10.1007/ 978-1-4684-4634-0

Preface

The tenth meeting of the International Foundation for Biochemical Endocrinology was held in Geilo, Norway near the end of September, 1982. The subject matter of the conference and the monograph was on "Regulation of Target Cell Responsiveness." The local organizing committee was Asbjørn Aakvaag and Vidar Hansson.

The scientific sessions covered a wide range of hormone action and cell response, including: peptide hormones and target cell response, regulation of insulin responsiveness, intracellular modulation of peptide hormone response, gonadotropins and target cell responses, hypothalamic hormones - effects and regulation, steroid receptors and cellular control, hormones and growth regulation, and hormones and gene regulation. The chairpersons for the sessions were L. Birnbauer - A. Aakvaag, S. Taylor - R. S. Horn, F. Labrie - F. Rommerts, A. R. Means - K. W. McKerns, P. F. Hall - V. Hansson K. Griffiths - K. M. Gautvik, E. J. Peck, Jr. - E. Haug, F. S. French - W. T. Schrader, and E. M. Ritzén - B. Jegou.

In addition to the scientific sessions in Geilo we were all delighted to sample some of the cultural and artistic attractions of Oslo, and to travel by train from Oslo via Geilo to Bergen. The scenery and hospitality were magnificant.

The Foundation thanks the many people who assisted at the meeting and in the preparation of the monograph. These include Mrs. Kjersti Gunneng who served as general secretary for the organization in Norway; Mrs. James Gilmore who acted as secretary for the Foundation in Maine and who assisted in the preparation of the index. Mrs. Francine Hood was in charge of the monumental job of retyping all of the manuscripts into the memory bank of a computer for the preparation of photo-ready copy. Mrs. Valerie McCadden acted as adviser to this preparation.

The 1983 meeting and monograph of the Foundation will be held in early October in Rehovot, Israel. This will deal broadly with the topic, "Hormonal Control of Hypothalamo-Pituitary-Gonadal Axis." The local organizing committee consists of Zvi Naor, Chairman, Nava Dekel, Yitzhak Koch, Fortune Kohen and Uriel Zor.

Kenneth W. McKerns

Blue Hill Falls, Maine

Acknowledgments

The following public organizations and private contributors have given financial assistance to support this colloque. The organizing committee and the Foundation members are grateful for this generous support:

Norwegian Agency for International Development (NORAD)

Norwegian Medical Research Council (NAVF)

Norwegian Society for Fighting Cancer

The Norwegian Cancer Society

The Royal Norwegian Ministry of Culture and Science

Bergman Instrumentering A/S

Heigar & Co. A/S

F. Hoffman - La Roche & Co. AG

Nyegaard & Co. A/S (NYCO)

Organon International bv

Ria-Data A/S

Schering AG, Berlin

Contents of Volume 1

Peptide Hormones and Target Cell Response

Contents of Volume 2

Hypothalamic Hormones - Effects and Regulation

Steroid Receptors and Cellular Control

Hormones and Growth Regulation

Hormones and Gene Regulation

Antiandrogens and Androgen Insensitivity

CONTENTS OF VOLUME 2A

Peptide Hormones and Target Cell Response

Peptide Hormones and Trophic Cell Responses

REGULATION OF SERTOLI CELL RESPONSIVENESS: DESENSITIZATION OF ADENYLYL CYCLASE BY FSH, ISOPROTERENOL AND GLUCAGON

H. Attramadal[a], T. Jahnsen[a], F. Le Gac[a], and
V. Hansson[a,b]

[a]Institute of Pathology, Rikshospitalet
[b]Institute of Medical Biochemistry
University of Oslo, Norway

1. Introduction

The function of the Sertoli cell is to provide a milieu in which germ cell proliferation and differentiation can take place. It is now believed that hormones regulating spermato-genesis are mediating their effects via the Sertoli cell (Hansson et al., 1976). The Sertoli cell is a target cell for both FSH (Hansson et al., 1973; Hansson et al., 1974b), and androgens (Hansson et al., 1974a; Hansson et al., 1975; Mulder et al., 1975; Sanborn et al., 1977). Furthermore, cAMP formation in cultured immature Sertoli cells is stimu-lated by β_1-andrenergic agonists (Verhoeven et al., 1979, 1981) and glucagon (Attramadal, H., Jahnsen, T., and Hansson, V., unpublished). However, neither β_1-adrenergic hormones nor glucagon have yet been ascribed any role in the regulation of spermatogenesis _in vivo_. However, it provides a system in which three agonists are acting on the same adenylyl cyclase system and facilitates studies on hormone-specific densensi-tization in living cells and in membrane particles.

The adenylyl cyclase complex comprises at least three distinct protein components; the receptor, with the hormone discriminating function, the guanine nucleotide regulatory unit (N or G/F component), and the catalytic subunit (C) which converts Mg^{2+}-ATP to cAMP. The N component is composed of subunits with different molecular weights, and possible different functions (for review see Kirchick et al., this volume). Well-defined effects of guanine nucleotides, Mg^{2+},

3

cholera toxin, and fluoride are mediated by the N component(s) of the adenylyl cyclase complex. The N component(s) are important for the functional "coupling" of the receptor to the catalytic subunit of the adenylyl cyclase.

The response of the Sertoli cell to hormones (FSH, iso-proterenol and glucagon) may be regulated at several different levels (Hansson et al., 1983). It is known for many systems that exposure of cells to a hormone may lead to a dramatic change in the number of available receptors at the cell membrane (Lefkowitz et al., 1980; Kirchick et al., this volume). Furthermore, frequently before any change in hormone receptors, one may observe a decrease in the responsiveness of the adenylyl cyclase due to deficient "coupling" between the hormone receptors and the catalytic subunit of the adenylyl cyclase (Bockaert et al., 1976). Finally, it has been demonstrated, at least in the Sertoli cell, that FSH, isoproterenol and cAMP cause a dramatic stimulation of high affinity cAMP phosphodiesterase activity, which would further tend to attenuate any cAMP-mediated signal (Conti et al., 1981; Verhoeven et al., 1981). In this chapter we will concentrate on how the Sertoli cell response may be regulated at the level of adenylyl cyclase, and we will describe some recent studies in our laboratories on the regulation of the responsiveness of the Sertoli cell adenylyl cyclase to FSH, isoproterenol and glucagon.

2.   FSH, Isoproterenol and Glucagon Responsive Adenylyl Cyclase in Cultured Sertoli Cells

Sertoli cell-enriched cultures (Dorrington et al., 1975) from the testis of 20 day old Sprague Dawley rats were preincubated for 3-4 days in the presence of 10% fetal calf serum, and the activity of the adenylyl cyclase and response to hormones were analyzed in membrane particles (Jahnsen et al., 1980a), using $[\alpha-^{32}P]$-ATP as radioactive substrate and isolating $[^{32}P]$-cAMP by double chromatography on Dowex-50 and alumina (Salomon et al., 1974). As shown in Fig. 1, FSH, isoproterenol and glucagon cause a concentration-dependent stimulation of adenylyl cyclase activity, with a K_m of 300, 110, and 350 ng/ml, respectivley. The hormonal activation achieved by these three hormones was highest for glucagon, followed by isoproterenol, whereas the lowest activation was seen by FSH. Interestingly, glucagon and isoproter-enol responses in seminiferous tubules isolated from living

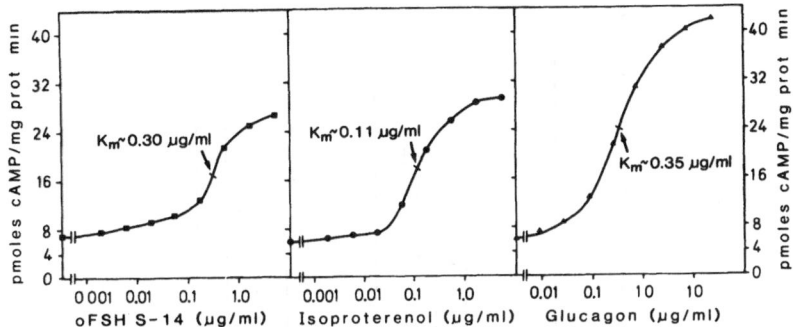

Figure 1. Stimulation of adenylyl cyclase activity in cultured immature Sertoli cells by FSH (A), isoproterenol (B) and glucagon (C).

animals, show a completely different picture; in this case very low response is seen both to glucagon and isoproterenol, whereas the FSH response is similar to that seen in the cultured cells. Thus, the responses to glucagon and iso-proterenol appear to increase during the four days culture period. This represents an example of how responsiveness of a cell may change during primary culture.

3.   Homologous Desensitization of Hormone Responsive
     Adenylyl Cyclases in Cultured Immature Sertoli Cells

We have examined how the adenylyl cyclase responses to FSH, isoproterenol and glucagon may be regulated in cultured immature Sertoli cells. To investigate whether the observed effects may be due to cAMP we have also examined to what extent the effects of hormones can be mimicked by dibutyryl cAMP.

As shown in Fig. 2, preincubation of Sertoli cell cultures with ovine FSH (0.5 µg NIH-FSH-S13) caused a hormone specific, homologous desensitization of the FSH responsive adenylyl cyclase, whereas the response to isoproterenol was unaffected. The function of the guanine nucleotide regulatory component of the adenylyl cyclase complex in hormonally desensitized Sertoli cells was normal, since activation of adenylyl cyclase by GTP, GMP-P(NH)P, fluoride and MG^{2+} was not affected by the hormone pretreatment.

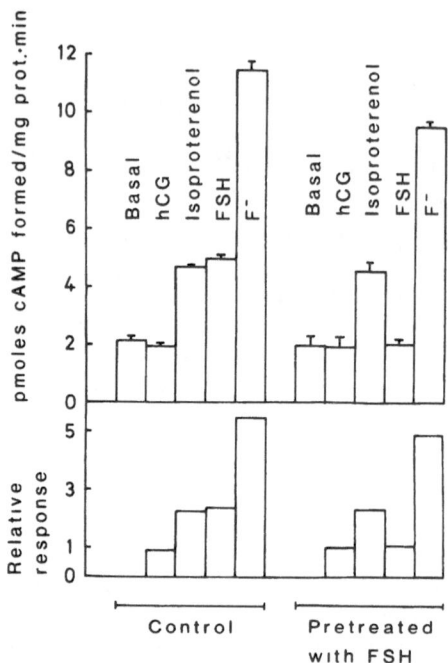

Figure 2. Hormone-stimulated adenylyl cyclase activity in membrane particle fraction from control Sertoli cell culture and from culture pretreated with FSH. The upper panel shows absolute activities in the presence of 0.04 mM GTP. The lower panel shows relative response (hormone stimulated adenylyl cyclase activity divided by basal adenylyl cyclase activity). The bars show mean values ± standard deviation of triplicate determinations (Jahnsen et al., 1982).

In Fig. 3 and 4 we have examined in more detail the time course of desensitization with either isoproterenol (Fig. 3) or FSH (Fig. 4). As can be seen from the figures, half maximal desensitization was achieved within one to two hr, after which a gradual loss in response was observed during the first 24 hr. Thus, the time course studies indicate that if sensitization of adenylyl cyclase may represent a mechanism of physiological response regulation, it may not be involved in the acute regulation of the response to hormones.

For this, the time required to achieve desensitization is far
too slow. Addition of glucagon to cultured immature Sertoli
cells for 24 hr also caused similar hormone-specific homologous desensitization in that the response was lost only for
glucagon, whereas responses for FSH and isoproerenol were
maintained. As yet, we have not examined the time kinetics
of glucagon-induced desensitization.

Figures 5, 6, and 7 demonstrate the concentration dependence of FSH (Fig. 5), isoproterenol (Fig. 6) and glucagon-
induced desensitization (Fig. 7). As seen from these figures,
the concentrations of hormones in the preincubation were
similar to those required for half maximal activation of the
adenylyl cyclase (Fig. 1). In all three experiments, the
addition of hormone was associated with loss of response for
the hormone added, whereas the other hormones as well as
fluoride-stimulated activities remained unaffected. The
studies reported above represent the first demonstration of
hormone specific homologous desensitization of the Sertoli
cell adenylyl cyclase in vitro.

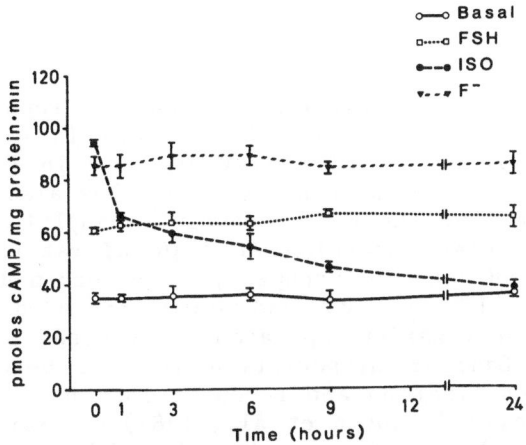

Figure 3. Homologous desensitization of isoproterenol responsive adenylyl cyclase in immature (20 days) Sertoli cell
cultures. Cultures were treated for varying time periods
with L-D-isoproterenol (5 μg/ml) and adenylyl cyclase activity
and response examined in membrane particles (Attramadal et
al., 1982, in press).

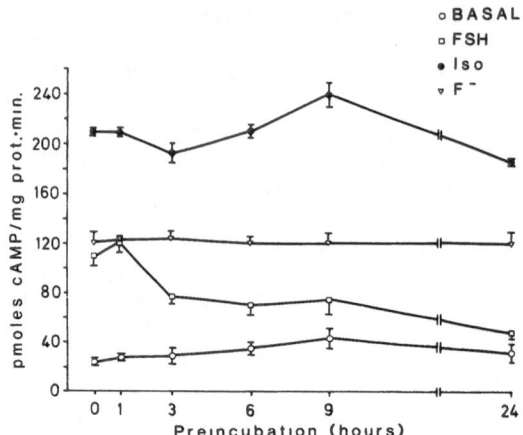

Figure 4. Homologous desensitization of FSH responsive adenylyl cyclase in immature (20 day) Sertoli cell cultures. Cultures were treated for varying time periods with NIH-FSH-S12 (10 μg/ml) and adenylyl cyclase activity and response examined in membrane particles (Le Gac et al., 1982, in press).

Jahnsen et al. (1980b) have, however, reported that the injection of high doses of FSH in rats in vivo, causes a transient decrease in FSH receptors and in FSH-responsive adenylyl cyclase. O'Shaughnessy (1980) has also demonstrated desensitization of the FSH-responsive adenylyl cyclase after an intratesticular injection of 1 μg of rat FSH. In these experiments FSH receptor occupancy was determined by injection of radioactive FSH in vivo, and it was concluded that adenylyl cyclase desensitization appeared to precede receptor down regulation. Similar dissociation in time between adenylyl cyclase desensitization and receptor loss has been described for Leydig cells (Jahnsen et al., 1981) and for corpus lutem (Bockaert et al., 1976). It is likely that desensitization is associated with a physical change in the hormone receptor which is associated with increased endocytosis and receptor loss (Kirchick et al., this volume).

We next examined whether the effects achieved by hormones could be mimicked by incubating the cultured Sertoli cells with dibutyryl cAMP. Preincubation of the Sertoli cell with a high concentration of dibutyryl cAMP (10^{-3}M) for 24 hr was associated with a 40 - 50% reduction in adenylyl cyclase activation both by FSH and by isoproterenol. However, fluoride-stimulated adenylyl cyclase activity as well as GTP-stimulated adenylyl cyclase activity were normal. Interestingly, dibutyryl cAMP induced desensitization of Sertoli cell adenylyl cyclase was associated with a significant (30 - 40%) loss of specific FSH binding sites as determined by ^{125}I-FSH. Thus, the decrease in hormone response can at least in part be accounted for by the reduction in specific FSH binding. At present we believe that desensitization achieved by dibutyryl cAMP may be different from that achieved by hormone. Figure 8 represents the time course of adenylyl cyclase desensitization in the presence of a high concentration of FSH (10 µg/ml NIHFSH-S12) or dibutyryl cAMP (1 mM).

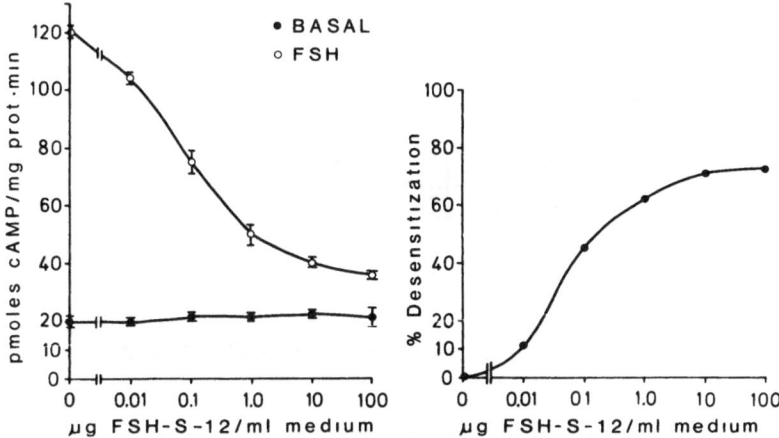

Figure 5. Desensitization of FSH responsive adenylyl cyclase in cultured immature (20 days) Sertoli cells. The cultures were preincubated with different concentrations of NIH-FSH-S12 and subsequently examined for adenylyl cyclase activity in the absence or presence of hormone. Left: Basal (closed circles) and FSH stimulated (open circles) activities. Right: Per cent desensitization as a function of FSH concentration during the preincubation (Le Gac et al., 1982, in press).

As seen from the figure, desensitization with dibutyryl cAMP
occurs much slower than that obtained with FSH.

The physiological significance of hormone-specific
homologous desensitization of the adenylyl cyclase is not
clear. However, the fact that loss of adenylyl cyclase
response occurs at hormone concentrations similar or lower
than that which regulate adenylyl cyclase activity in Sertoli
cell membrane, indicates that this may represent the mechanism
by which hormonal response of the Sertoli cell may be
regulated.

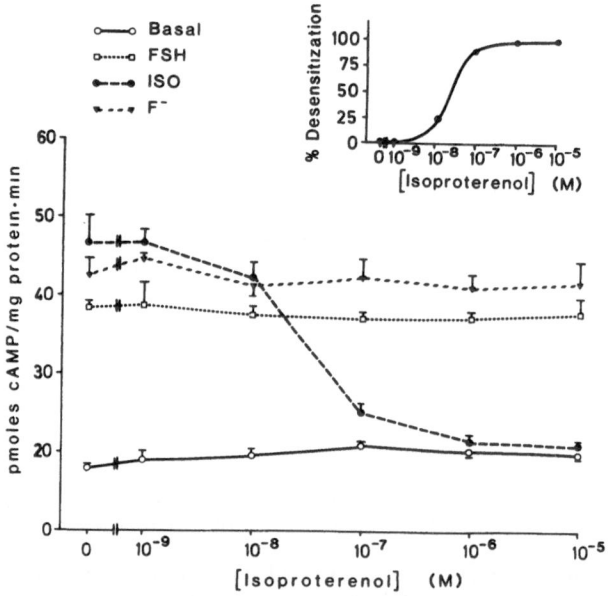

Figure 6. Homologous desensitization of isoproterenol responsive adenylyl cyclase in cultured immature Sertoli cells (20
days). Cultures were preincubated for 24 hr with different
concentration of L-D-isoproterenol and subsequently examined
for adenylyl cyclase activity and response to hormones and
fluoride (Attramadal et al., in press).

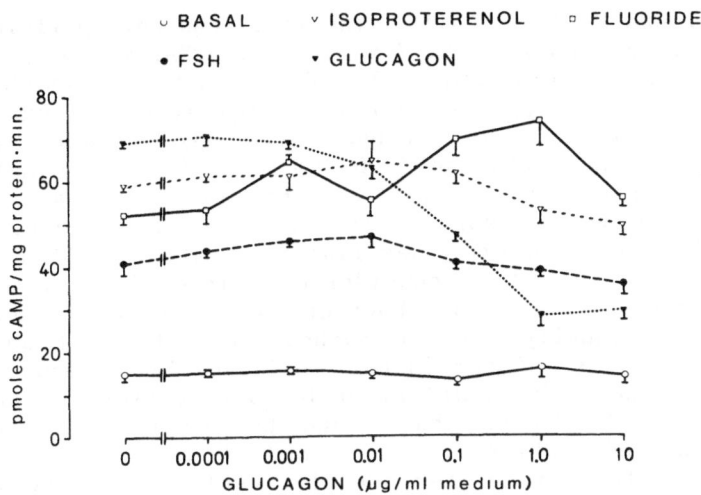

Figure 7. Desensitization of glucagon responsive adenylyl cyclase in immature cultured Sertoli cells pretreated for 24 hr with varying concentrations of homologous hormone.

4.   Homologous Desensitization of Hormone-Responsive Sertoli Adenylyl Cyclases in a Cell-Free System

In order to have a better understanding of the molecular mechanisms by which hormone-induced homologous desensitization occurs, we have examined this process in a cell-free system. Birnbaumer and collaborators (Iyengar et al., 1980) have previously shown that purified plasma membranes from liver cells, under defined conditions, may be desensitized, and that the desensitization was dependent on hormone, ATP and Mg^{2+}. For this type of studies the cultured Sertoli cell preparations may be advantageous since three different agonists regulate the activity of the same adenylyl cyclase. Thus, in such a system it would be easier to achieve indications whether or not hormone-induced desensitization in cell-free systems may be hormone specific. One typical experiment is shown in Fig. 9. Membrane particles from cultured immature Sertoli cells were incubated either in the presence of GTP (.02 mM) (basal) or GTP plus FSH (5 µg/ml of FSH-S14) (stimulated). In these experiments free magnesium concentrations were approximately 4.0 mM in excess of ATP

(1.0 mM) and EDTA (1.4 mM). The reactions were performed in
10 mM Tris-HCl buffer, pH 7.4 with 0.1% BSA, in the presence
of saturating concentration (1.0 mM) of cAMP to block phosphodiesterase activity, and with a ATP/GTP regenerating system
consisting of creatine phosphate (20 mM), creatine kinase
(0.2 mg/ml) and myokinase (0.02 mg/ml). A 50 µl sample was
withdrawn successively at varying time intervals, and
[α-^{32}P]-cAMP was measured. As shown in the figure, basal
adenylyl cyclase activity was linear for at least 90 min. In
the presence of FSH, a considerably higher initial rate of
cAMP formation was seen, however, the stimulated activity
decreased gradually and approached that of basal adenylyl
cyclase activity. After 45 min of incubation (arrow), a new
dose of either FSH (5 µl/ml) or D-L-isoproterenol (5 µg/ml)
was added both to the basal and to the tubes containing
FSH-stimulated membranes. The second addition of FSH was not
able to further stimulated adenylyl cyclase activity in the
previously FSH-treated membranes. This finding indicates
that the desensitization of the FSH-responsive adenylyl
cyclase during incubation was not due to breakdown and lack
of FSH during the first 45 min of incubation. Furthermore,
addition of isoproterenol after 45 min dramatically stimulated
adenylyl cyclase activity, indicating that hormone-specific

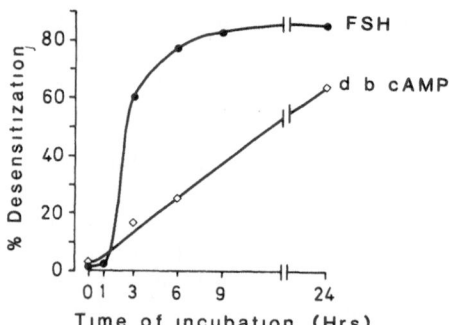

Figure 8. Time course of desensitization of FSH responsive
adenylyl cyclase in cultured immature Sertoli cells (20 days)
preincubated with maximal concentration of FSH (10 µg/ml,
NIH-FSH-S12) or dibutyryl-cyclic AMP (10^{-3}M). Desensitization
with dibutyryl-cyclic AMP is much slower and less complete
than that with FSH (Le Gac et al., 1982, in press).

desensitization had taken place. In addition, this non-stimulated membrane preparation (basal) responded normally to both
FSH and isoproterenol after 45 min of incubation, demonstrating that loss of responsiveness was not due to reduced
viability of the membranes. Identical experiments have also
been performed with both isoproterenol and with glucagon. In
these experiments again hormone-specific desensitization was
achieved, and the response was lost only for the hormone that
was present during the first 45 min of incubation (not shown).
The fact that the incubation procedures were performed in the
presence of saturating concentrations of cAMP (1 mM) indicates
that the refractoriness induced by the hormone was not mediated via cAMP. Furthermore, the observation that desensitized
follicular adenylyl cyclase can be resensitized by exogenous
addition of phospho-protein phosphatases (Hunzicker-Dunn et
al., 1979) strongly indicates that desensitization may be the
result of a protein (receptor)-phosphorylation.

Hormone-specific homologous desensitization in a
cell-free system allowed us to further examine the role of
Mg^{2+}, ATP and GTP for this process. In the experiments
depicted in Fig. 10, membrane particles from immature cultured
Sertoli cells were preincubated in the absence or presence of
hormones (in the figure shows FSH) and varying concentrations
of free Mg^{2+}. After this preincubation period the membranes
were sedimented by centrifugation and resuspended in a
standard assay mixture as described above. The hormone
response of the adenylyl cyclase after this preincubation was
now tested. As shown in the figure, Mg^{2+} in the presence of
hormone caused a dose-dependent loss in hormonal response,
and half maximal effect in the presence of hormone was
achieved at a concentration of 5 mM Mg^{2+}. Interestingly,
Mg^{2+} alone without hormones was able to induce hormonal
refractoriness, but at much higher concentrations ($K_m=30$
mM). Our results showing Mg^{2+}-induced desensitization of
Sertoli cell adenylyl cyclase are very similar to those
obtained by Iyengar et al. (1980) in the liver-glucagon
system. We have also examined the Mg^{2+} effects on isoproterenol and glucagon-induced desensitization with very similar
results (not shown).

Figure 11 shows the effect of ATP in a very similar
experimental design. In this case Sertoli cell membrane particles were preincubated for 45 min in the absence or presence
of hormone, and in the presence of varying concentrations of

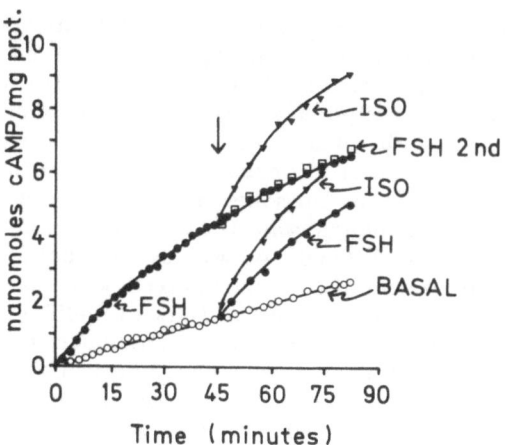

Figure 9. Homologous desensitization of FSH responsive
adenylyl cyclase in a cell-free system in membranes prepared
from cultured immature Sertoli cells. Sertoli cell membrane
particles (0.02 mg/ml of protein) were incubated at 32°C in
the absence (open circles) or presence (closed circles) of 5
μg NIH-FSH-S14. The incubation medium consisted of 10 mM
Tris-HCl buffer, pH 7.4, containing ATP (1 mM; ca 10^7 cpm of
[α-^{32}P]ATP/tube), GTP (0.02 mg/ml), creatine kinase (0.2
mg/ml), and creatine phosphate 20 mM. At varying time
intervals (2 min), 50 ul aliquots were withdrawn and assayed
for adenylyl cyclase activity. After 45 min of incubation
more FSH stimulated incubation. Note: Hormone specific loss
of FSH response whereas the isoproterenol responses are
maintained (Attramadal et al., 1982, in press).

ATP (0.1 - 2.0 mM). After this preincubation the membranes
were pelleted by centrifugation, resuspended, and adenylyl
cyclase activity and response to hormones examined in a
standard assay mixture. As shown in the figure, increasing
concentrations of ATP in the absence of hormone caused a
slight but significant reduction in subsequent FSH response.
Furthermore, preincubation in the presence of FSH, but in the
absence of ATP, also caused a small but significant loss in
response. However, increasing concentrations of ATP in the
presence of hormone caused a dramatic and dose-dependent

desensitization of the FSH-responsive adenylyl cyclase, with a half maximal effect at about .2 mM of ATP.

In all these experiments activation by guanine-nucleotides and fluoride was unaffected, indicating normal function of the N component. Furthermore, our results support the accumulating evidence that the lesion induced during homologous desensitization of the adenylyl cyclase is due to a phosphorylation reaction of some components proximal to the N component of the adenylyl cyclase system. This may probably involve a modification of the hormone receptor itself or of a receptor-associated protein. It is likely that such a modification may prevent the coupling of the receptor to the other components of the adenylyl cyclase system.

We have also examined the possible involvement of GTP. It has been reported by several authors that GTP is essential for hormone induced homologous desensitization. We have observed that when membrane particles from cultured Sertoli cells are exposed to either FSH or isoproterenol in the presence of GTP, a gradual desensitization occurs.

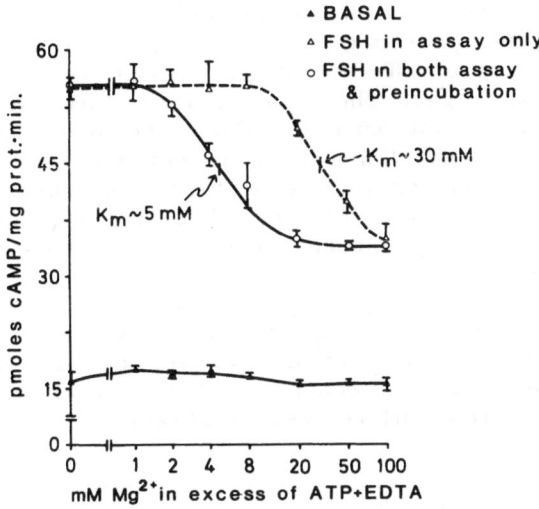

Figure 10. Effect of Mg^{2+} on hormone (FSH) induced desensitization in a cell free system.

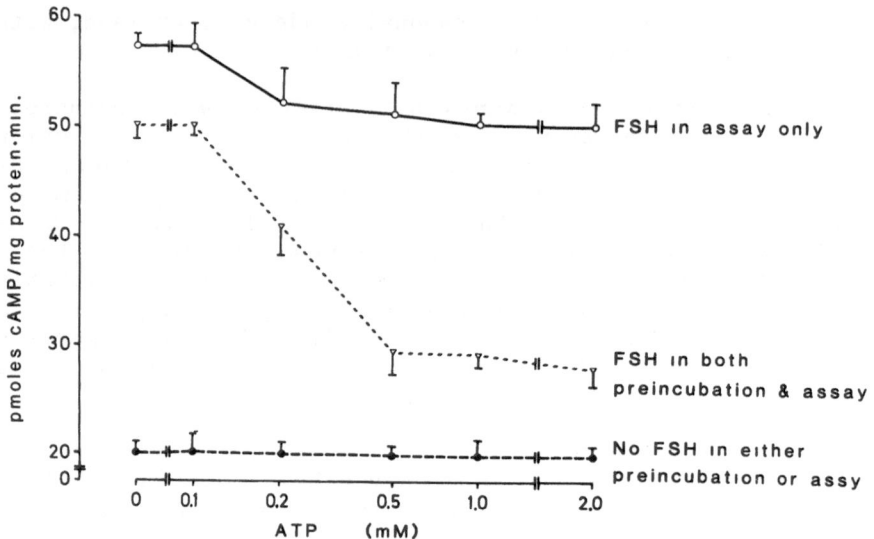

Figure 11. Effect of ATP on hormone (FSH) induced desensitization in a cell free system.

However, when the same membrane particles are exposed to hormones in the presence of the non-hydrolysable guanine nucleotide analogue GMP-P(NH)P, a hormone response is still seen, and in this case the rate of cAMP formation is linear for 60 - 90 min (not shown). One interpretation of these results could be that GMP-P(NH)P is not a suitable substrate for release of end-terminal phosphate. Another possibility is that GDP (which can be formed from GTP, but not from GMP-P(NH)P) plays an important role in the process of homologous desensitization.

Although the physiological implications of hormone-specific desensitization is not clear, our results clearly show that the responsiveness of the target cell may be modulated at the level of the cell membrane.

5.   Summary and Conclusions

Adenylyl cyclase (AC) activity in cultured Sertoli cells can be stimulated either by FSH, isoproterenol or glucagon.

When cultured Sertoli cells are exposed to any of these hormones, a time- and dose-dependent desensitization of the adenylyl cyclase was observed. This desensitization is hormone specific and the concentrations of hormones required to achieve desensitization are in the same order of magnitude as those required to stimulate adenylyl cyclase activity.

To pursue the molecular mechanism of hormone induced refractoriness in cultured Sertoli cells, we have investigated FSH, isoproterenol and glucagon regulation of the responsiveness of Sertoli cell adenylyl cyclase in a cell-free system. We demonstrate hormone-specific desensitization for all three hormones by the addition of the hormones directly to Sertoli cell membrane particles. The desensitization of the hormone-responsive adenylyl cyclases was dependent on the concentration of ATP (K_m = 0.2 mM) and Mg^{2+} ($K_m \sim$ 5 mM). Higher concentrations of Mg^{2+} caused, in the absence of hormone, desensitization of both the FSH- and isoproterenol-responsive adenylyl cyclases (glucagon not yet examined) with K_m of approximately 30 mM. Thus, while hormone-induced desensitization was specific and only involved the hormone used, Mg^{2+} induced desensitization (10 - 50 mM) reduced the responsiveness of the FSH- and isoproterenol-responsive adenylyl cyclases to the same extent. Hormone-induced desensitization may also require the presence of GTP. When substituting GTP with a non-hydrolysable analogue GMP-P(NH)P, hormone-induced desensitization did not occur. These results show an obligatory role of ATP, Mg^{2+}, and GTP for hormone-induced desensitization in cultured immature Sertoli cell membranes. This also indicates that the loss of response induced by homologous hormone may involve a phosphorylation reaction. Furthermore, hormone appears to accelerate desensitization of the adenylyl cyclase by increasing the sensitivity of the system to the actions of Mg^{2+}.

ACKNOWLEDGMENTS: The work presented in this chapter was supported by the Rockefeller Foundation, the Norwegian Research Council for Science and the Humanities (NAVF) and the Norwegian Cancer Society, (LMK).

REFERENCES

Bockaert, I., Hünzicker-Dunn, M., and Birnbaumer, L., 1976, Hormone stimulated desensitization of hormone-dependent adenylyl cyclase, J. Biol. Chem., 251:2653.

Conti, M., Geremia, R., Adams, S., and Stefanini, M., 1981, Regulation of Sertoli cell adenosine 3'5' monophosphate phosphodiesterase activity by follicle stimulating hormone and dibutyryl cyclic AMP, Biochem. Biophys. Res. Comm., 98:1044.

Hansson, V., Reusch, E., Trygstad, O., Torgersen, O., Ritzén, E. M., and French, F. S., 1973, FSH stimulation of testicular androgen binding protein (ABP), Nature, New Biol., 246:_.

Hansson, V., McLean, W. S., Smith, A. A., Tindall, D. J., Weddington, S. C., Nayfeh, S. N., French, F. S., and Ritzén, E. M., 1974, Androgen receptors in rat testis, Steroids, 23:823.

Hansson, V., Trygstad, O., French, F. S., MacLean, W. S., Smith, H. H., Tindall, D. J., Weddington, S. C., Pertrusz, P., Nayfeh, S. N., and Ritzén, E. M., 1974b, Androgen transport and receptor mechanisms in the testis and epididymis, Nature, 250:387.

Hansson, V., Ritzén, E. M., French, F. S., and Nayfeh, S. N., 1975, Androgen transport and receptor mechanisms in the testis and epididymis, in: "Handbook of Physiology," Section 7, Vol. 5, D. W. Hamilton, R. O. Greep, eds., pp. 173-202, American Physiology Society, USA.

Hansson, V., Calandra, R., Purvis, K., Ritzén, E. M., and French, F. S., 1976, Hormonal regulation of spermatogenesis Vitam. Horm., 34:187.

Hansson, V., Jegou, B., Attramadal, H., Jahnsen, T., Le Gac, F., Tvermyr, M., Frøysa, A., and Horn, R., 1983, Regultion of Sertoli cell secretion and response, in: "Recent Advances of Male Reproduction," d'Agata, ed., Raven Press, USA (in press).

Hunzicker-Dunn, M., Derda, D., Jungmann, R. A., and Birnbaumer, L., 1979, Resensitization of the desensitized follicular adenylyl cyclase system to luteinizing hormone, Endocrinology, 104:1785.

Iyengar, R., Mintz, P. W., Swartz, T. L., and Birnbaumer, L., 1980, Divalent cation-induced desensitization of glucagon stimulable adenylyl cyclase in rat liver plasma membranes: GTP dependent stimulation by glucagon, J. Biol. Chem., 255:11875.

Jahnsen, T., and Purvis, K., Birnbaumer, L., and Hansson, V., 1980, FSH and LH/hCG responsive adenylyl cyclases in adult rat testis: Methodology and assay conditions, Int. J. Androl., 3:396.

Jahnsen, T., Gordeladze, J. O., Torjesen, P. A., and Hansson, V., 1980b, FSH responsive adenylyl cyclase in rat testis:

Desensitization by homologous hormone, Arch. Androl.,
    5:169.
Jahnsen, T., Purvis, K., Torjesen, P. A., and Hansson, V., 1981,
    Temporal relationship between hCG induced desensitization
    of LH/hCG responsive adenylyl cyclase and down-regulation
    of LH/hCG receptors in the rat testis, Arch. Androl. 6:155.
Jahnsen, T., Verhoeven, G., Purvis, K., Cusan, L., and Hansson,
    V., 1982, Desensitization of FSH responsive adenylyl
    cyclase in cultured immature Sertoli cells by homologous
    hormone, Arch. Androl. 8:205.
Lefkowitz, R. J., Wessels, M. R., and Stadel, J. M., 1980,
    Hormone receptors, and cyclic AMP: Their role in target
    cell refractoriness, Curr. Top. Cell. Reg., 17:205.
Mulder, E., Peters, M. J., de Vries, J., and van der Melen,
    H. J., 1975, Characterization of anuclear receptor for
    testosterone in seminiferous tubules of mature rat testes,
    Mol. Cell. Endocrinol., 2:171.
O'Shaughnessy, P. J., 1980, FSH receptor autoregulation and
    cyclic AMP production in immature rat testis, Biol. Repro.,
    23:810.
Salomon, Y., Londos, C., and Rodbell, M., 1974, A highly sensi-
    tive adenylate cyclase assay, Analyt. Biochem., 58:541.
Sanborn, B. M., Steinberger, A., Tcholakian, R. K., and Stein-
    berger, E., 1977, Direct measurement of androgen receptors
    in cultured Sertoli cells, Steroids, 29:493.
Verhoeven, G., Dierick, P., and de Moor, P., 1979, Stimulation
    effect of neurotransmitters on the aromatization of testos-
    terone by Sertoli cell enriched cultures, Mol. Cell.
    Endocrinol., 13:241.
Verhoeven, G., Cailleau, J., and de Moor, F., 1981, Hormonal
    control of phosphodiesterase activity in cultured rat
    Sertoli cells, Mol. Cell. Endocrinol., 24:41.

DISCUSSION

RAO: Were you able to obtain more than 30% decrease in
labelled FSH binding to Sertoli cells as with other systems
like hCG or LH a more dramatic decrease in binding occurs
during desensitization?

ATTRAMADAL: In our studies we repeatedly get some 30% loss
in specific FSH binding, after 24 hr. It is possible, but we
have not done these studies, that a greater loss of receptors
may occur after a longer time of cAMP exposure.

MEANS: If homologous desensitization involves cAMP-independent phosphorylation of receptor, it seems possible that the
phosphorylation that occurs on receptors that do not stimulate
cyclase, such as EGF and insulin, may not be involved in the
positive cascade of the mechanism of action. Rather phosphorylation could be a mechanism to prevent the EGF or insulin
receptor from interacting with the component of adenylyl
cyclase.

ATTRAMADAL: That is possible. We have not done any work
with either EGF or insulin.

SELSTAM: In luteal membranes we have seen a spontaneous
decrease in sensitivity to LH but not to catecholamines when
the membranes were pre-incubated in plain buffer. Are your
membranes stable during the pretreatment period?

ATTRAMADAL: Yes. We have tested the viability of the
membrane preparations and we maintain constant activity and
normal hormonal response for at least 90 min. In order to
achieve this, protein content preparations must be very low
(20 - 50 µg/ml). At higher protein concentrations of your
membranes, the activity and hormonal responses are rapidly
declining, probably due to proteolytic activity in the
preparation.

STAGE-DEPENDENT DIFFERENCES IN FSH BINDING AND CYCLIC

NUCLEOTIDE SECRETION AND METABOLISM DURING THE CYCLE

OF THE RAT SEMINIFEROUS TUBULE

K. Purvis[a], M. Parvinen[b], K. Gautvik[c], and
V. Hansson[a]

[a]Institute of Pathology, Rikshospitalet, Oslo, Norway
[b]Institute of Biomedicine, Department of Anatomy,
University of Turku, SF-20520, Turku 52, Finland
[c]Institute of Physiology, University of Oslo,
Oslo, Norway

ABSTRACT

In living, freshly isolated rat seminiferous tubules, cyclic changes in FSH binding, cAMP secretion (basal and FSH stimulated) and the activities of cAMP and cGMP phosphodiesterases could be detected which were related to specific stages of spermatogenesis. FSH binding (per cm stage) increased gradually between stages VII and IX and then, after remaining relatively constant, was elevated further in stages XIV-I. Thereafter, binding fell to a nadir stage VIIa-b. FSH stimulated cAMP secretion was at its lowest in stage VIIa-b and maximal between stages XIV-V. The greatest specific activities of the cAMP and cGMP phosphodiesterases were detected in stages VII-VIII which are associated with spermiation in the rat. A degree of dissociation was found to exist in the cAMP and cGMP hydrolysing capacities at certain stages (IX-XII), suggesting the existence of different isoforms of the enzyme which may be differentially controlled. Exposure of the various stages to FSH or dibutyryl cAMP for 4 hr in vitro did not alter the profiles of phosphodiesterase activity.

The phosphodiesterase profiles were inversely related to the quantity of cAMP produced by the tubular segments after stimulation with FSH, both in the presence and absence of the

phosphodiesterase inhibitor, methyl isobutyl xanthine (MIX).
However, MIX elicited the greatest effect from the tubular
segments, in terms of FSH stimulated cAMP production, in
stages XIV-V, where direct measurements of phosphodiesterase
indicate the enzyme activity is relatively low. The reasons
for this apparent contradiction are discussed in relation to
previous findings on stage-dependent alterations in various
aspects of tubular function.

1.   Introduction

        Previous work from our laboratories have demonstrated
cyclic variations in certain parameters of Sertoli cell
(Ritzén et al., 1980; Parvinen et al., 1980) and germ cell
(Cusan et al., 1981; Gordeladze et al., 1981) function during
the spermatogenic cycle. Maximum secretion of androgen
binding protein (Ritzén et al., 1980) and plasminogen activator (Lacroix et al., 1981) occur in stages VII and VIII and
yet this is the region of the tubule which is associated with
the lowest binding of FSH (Parvinen et al., 1980) and the
smallest activation of the FSH-responsive adenylyl cyclase
(Gordeladze et al., 1981). Furthermore, in these preliminary
studies, where the various stages were assayed in four pools
(Parvinen et al., 1980), the profile of FSH binding did not
closely correspond to the pattern of FSH-stimulated cAMP
secretion. Whereas the highest FSH binding was detected in
stages XIII-I the tubules retained a high capacity for cAMP
secretion beyond these stages (II-VI). The reasons for this
discordance between these various parameters of Sertoli cell
function is unclear. One of the purposes of the present
study was to confirm the apparant dissociation between FSH
binding and FSH-stimulated cAMP secretion but in more finely-
dissected material where the 14 stages of spermatogenesis
could be divided into 10 pools instead of the previous four.

        In view of the important role played by the cyclic
nucleotide phosphodiesterases in the expression of trophic
hormone effects, we also decided to examine the distribution
of these enzymes in the various tubular segments to ascertain
whether their activity could be related to specific stages of
the spermatogenic cycle. In addition, and for comparison,
the quantitites of endogenous cAMP secreted by each stage in
vitro under basal conditions and after maximum stimulation
with FSH were measured in the absence/presence of the
phosphodiesterase inhibitor methyl isobutyl xanthine (MIX).

Finally, in view of the large volume of literature describing the hormonal responsiveness of the phosphodiesterase in other organs (Loren and Sneyd, 1973; Thompson and Williams, 1974; Gardner et al., 1976) a parallel series of tubular fragments at defined stages were exposed in vitro to high doses of FSH or dibutyryl cAMP to ascertain whether the enzyme profiles along the seminiferous tubule could be altered by acute stimulation with trophic hormone.

2.   Materials and Methods

2.1. Preparation of Tubular Segments

The details of the transillumination technique for recognizing and dissecting the various stages of the spermato-genic cycle have been described elsewhere (Parvinen and Ruokonen, 1982). Previously with this technique, pools of four segments could be isolated corresponding to stages VII-VIII, IX-XII, XIII-I and II-VI (e.g. Parvinen et al., 1980). Further refinements of the method now facilitate the preparation of ten pools corresponding to VIIa,b, VIIc,d, VIII, IX-XI, XII, XIII, XIV-I, II-III, IV-V and VI. Briefly, seminiferous tubules from 90 day old rats were isolated by wet dissection in a Petri dish cntaining Dulbecco's medium (Flow Laboratories, U.K.) at room temperature. Two mm segments, representing the above spermatogenic stages were measured and isolated by reference to 1 mm squared graph paper located under the Petri dish. Forty mm of each segment were pooled (equivalent to approximately 4 mg wet weight), washed once in fresh medium and then subjected to the various treatments.

2.2. FSH Binding in Membrane Particles

In two series of experiments, segments of seminiferous tubules from the different stages (80 mm each) were trans-ferred to tubes containing phosphate-buffered saline, pH 7.4 (800 µl) containing 0.1% BSA and 0.05% Neomycin, and sonicated on ice for 5 sec (MSE 100-watt ultrasonic disintegrator). The sonicates were centrifuged for 30 min at 27,000 xg (Sorvall SS-34 rotor) at 4°C. The pellets were washed once in buffer, recentrifuged and finally resuspended in 500 µl of the same buffer. Aliquots of the resulting membrane particles

(100 µl) were then subjected to an FSH binding assay which
has been described previously (Hansson et al., 1978; Parvinen
et al., 1980). The assay involved triplicate measurements at
a single concentration (25,000 cpm, 80 µCi/ug) of ^{125}I-hFSH
(hFSH-P_2; 15,000 IU/mg by RIA) in a total volume of 200 µl.
An excess of non-radioactive FSH (10 µg NIH-FSH-S12) was
added to parallel tubes for the assessment of non-specific
binding. Incubation was overnight (16 hr) at 30°C. Specific
binding was expressed as cpm per cm segment (equivalent to
approximately 1 mg wet weight).

2.3. Release of cAMP from Seminiferous Tubules In Vitro

Ten pools of intact seminiferous tubules associated wtih
the different stages were incubated in Medium 199 (300 µl,
modified with Earle's salts and 2.2 g/l sodium bicarbonate,
Flow Laboratories, U.K.) containing 2 mM methyl isobutyl
xanthine (Aldrich-Europe, Jansson Pharmaceuticals) with or
without 10 µg FSH (NIH-FSH-S12). Samples were incubated at
32°C for 4 hr, by which time cAMP secretion had become maximal
(unpublished observations). They were then heated at 80°C
for 8 min, centrifuged (5,000 xg for 10 min) and the clear
supernatant was transferred to storage tubes which were then
kept at -20°C until the day of assay. The study was then
repeated but in the absence of MIX.

Two assay methods for cAMP were used: a protein binding
technique for measuring the large quantities of cAMP when
stages were incubated in the presence of MIX and a radioimmunoassay method, which was necessary to detect the small
amounts of cyclic nucleotide produced in the absence of the
phosphodiesterase inhibitor. Details of the protein binding
assay, which utilizes a commercially available binding protein
(BDH Chemicals, England) have been described elsewhere (Tovey
et al., 1974).

For studies without MIX, cAMP was measured in the
incubation solution (50 µl in duplicate) by radioimmunoassay
using a kit from Becton Dickinson Immundiagnostics,
Orangeburg, New York, USA. Within assay variation of 10
replicate samples is less than 8% and interassay variation is
less than 20%. Increasing volumes gave a displacement curve
which was parallel to the standard curve.

2.4. Phosphodiesterase Assay

Two series of stages were dissected. In one case the ten pools were incubated in the absence or presence of 50 µg FSH (NIH-FSH-S12) in 500 µl Medium 199, for 4 hr at 34°C. Each pool contained the equivalent of 40 mm of tubule corresponding to a specific stage of spermatogenesis as designated earlier. In a second study corresponding segments were incubated under similar conditions with and without dibutyryl cAMP (1 mM). In both studies, after incubation the tubular segments were gently washed once with fresh medium and stored frozen at -70°C. On the day of assay the tubules were resuspended in 10 mM Tris-HCl buffer, pH 7.1 (500 µl) and sonicated for 10 sec. Aliquots of the sonicate were then assayed for high affinity cAMP and cGMP phosphodiesterases using 1 µM substrate. This assay has been described in detail elsewhere (Purvis et al., 1981) and was used without further modification.

3.   Results

3.1. Release of cAMP from Different Segments of Seminiferous Tubules

The quantity of cAMP released by the various tubular segments under basal conditions and after FSH (10 µg) stimulation in the presence (upper panel) and absence (lower panel) of MIX is shown in Fig. 1. The greatest effects of MIX on cAMP secretion was observed in stages XIII-V. In the presence of MIX, maximal stimulation of cAMP secretion was obtained in tubular segments corresponding to stages XIV-V and the smallest effects were elicited from stages VII-VIII. Without MIX the profile was very similar although the absolute levels of cAMP secreted were only 1/15 of that obtained in the presence of the enzyme inhibitor.

In the presence of MIX the ratio of FSH-stimulated to basal levels of cAMP gradually increased up to stage XII (VIIa,b: 3; VIIc,d: 7; VII: 8; IX-XI: 11; XII: 25). Thereafter this ratio remained relatively constant (XIII-V: 8-9) until it became reduced in stage VI (4). In contrast, in the absence of MIX this trend between stages VII and XII was reversed (stimulated: basal ratio gradually declined from 2.0 to 1.0).

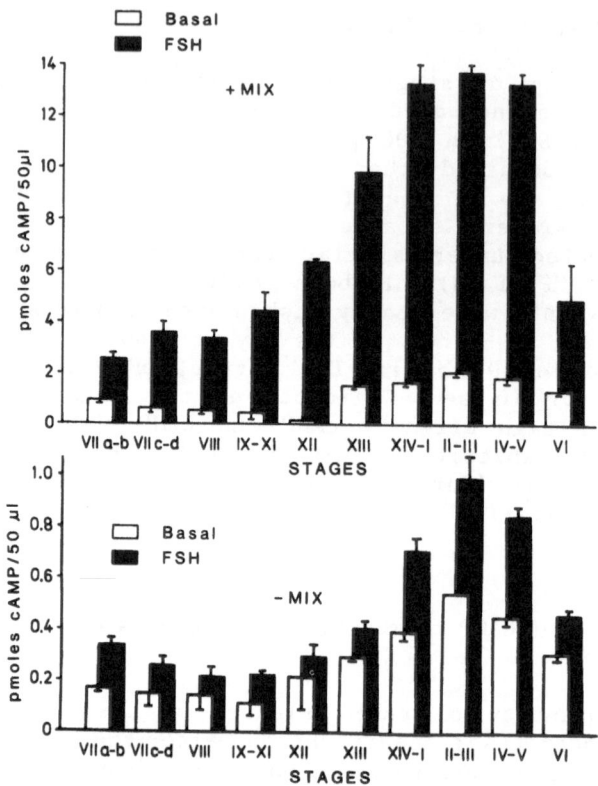

Figure 1. Secretion of cAMP by pools of ten tubular segments corresponding to the 14 stages of spermatogenesis in the rat, under basal conditions (open columns) and after FSH (10 µg NIH:FSH S 12) stimulation (stippled columns) for 4 hr. The segments were incubated in the presence (upper panel) and absence (lower panel) of methyl-isobutyl-xanthine (MIX). Vertical bars represent sd. of duplicate determinations.

3.2. Binding of ^{125}I-FSH to Segments of Seminferous Tubules

Figure 2 presents two profiles of ^{125}I-FSH binding obtained from two separate studies, to tubular segments corresponding to the stages assayed above. All segments bound ^{125}I-FSH and in general the binding profile reflected the alterations in cAMP caused by MIX and FSH, especially between

stages VII and XIV. Specific binding was at its lowest
between stages VI-VIIa,b and gradually increased thereafter
to peak values between stages XIII and I. Subsequently, the
binding capacity gradually fell in those stages where the
greatest FSH stimulated cAMP secretion was still being maintained at high levels.

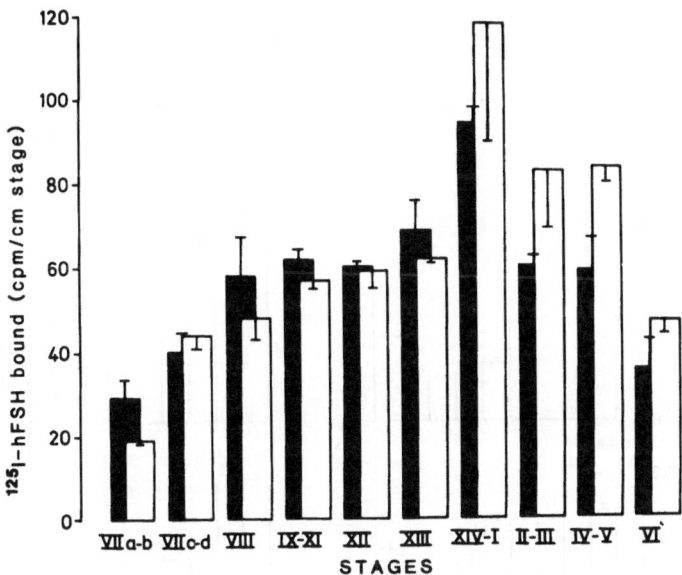

Figure 2. Specific binding of ^{125}I-hFSH to membrane particles
from tubular segments. The two profiles (stippled and open
columns) are derived from two separate studies. Vertical
bars represent sd. of triplicate determinations. See text
for details.

3.3. Cyclic Nucleotide Phosphodiesterase Activity in Segments of Seminiferous Tubules

Figure 3 shows the pattern of both cGMP (upper panel)
and cAMP (lower panel) phosphodiesterase activity in homogenates of various segments of rat seminiferous tubules
defined by stage in the absence and presence of FSH (10 µg).
Using low substrate conditions (1 µM) these enzyme activity
profiles and the previously described assay conditions

(Purvis et al., 1980) apply to the high affinity enzymes. It is apparent that cyclic fluctuations of activity do exist between the different segments, with the greatest specific activities associated with stages VII-VIII and a nadir around stages I-III. At stages IX-XII, when cGMP hydrolysing capacity was falling, cAMP hydrolysing capacity was maintained suggesting different roles for the two cyclic nucleotide phosphodiesterases.

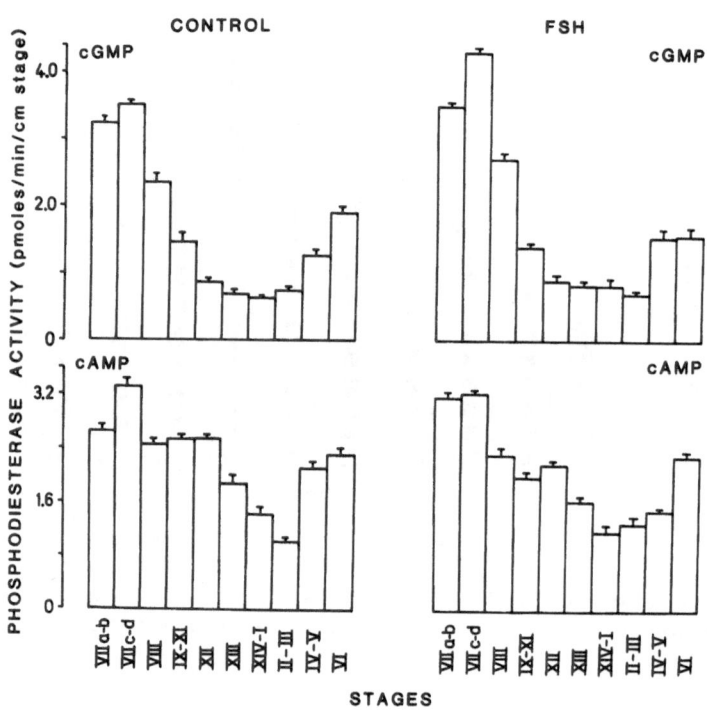

Figure 3. High affinity (measured with 1 µM substrate) phosphodiesterase activity in sonicates of tubular segments. Alterations in the profile of cGMP (upper panel) and cAMP (lower panel) hydrolysis are shown in control segments (left side) and segments exposed for 4 hr to FSH (50 µg NIH-FSH-S12: right side). Vertical bars represent sd. of triplicate determinations.

Figure 3 also presents the activity profiles in the presence (right side) or absence (left side 1) of FSH (10 µg). As indicated, after 4 hr of exposure to the hormone in vitro, no significant alteration in the profile could be detected. A similar result was obtained after exposure of intact segments to high levels of dibutyryl cAMP (data not shown). There is an indication of an inverse relationship between cAMP release under basal conditions and the activity of the cAMP phosphodiesterase.

4.   Discussion

In confirmation of earlier findings (Parvinen et al., 1980), the present study indicates that the quantity of cAMP secreted by segments of the seminiferous tubule in vitro is not constant, but changes according to the stage of the spermatogenic cycle. In both the presence and absence of MIX, the quantity of cAMP secreted by the segments after exposure to FSH, is generally low between stages VII and IX and gradually increases to a maximum between XIV and V. As noted previously (Parvinen et al., 1980) this profile is not identical to the pattern of FSH binding and FSH-stimulated cAMP production generally increases between stages VII and I. However, in segments II-V when cAMP secretion is at its highest, FSH binding already begins to decline. Since the number of Sertoli cells per µm seminiferous tubule appears to be relatively constant regardless of spermatogenic stage (Ulvik and Dahl, personal communication), alterations in FSH binding presumeably reflect differences in the number of receptors per cell. One would anticipate, if all FSH receptors were functionally coupled to the adenylyl cyclase, that a greater correlation would be obtained between their concentration and the quantity of cAMP produced after stimulation, especially after stage XIV-I, than was obtained in the present study. The discrepancy between the pattern of FSH binding and cAMP secretion in stages II-V has been suggested by Gordeladze et al. (1981) to be due to an increasing contribution from the germ cell adenylyl cyclase. Certainly the activity of the specific germ cell enzymes such as the Mn^{2+}-dependent adenylyl cyclase and protein carboxyl methylase are maximal in stages II-III (Cusan et al., 1981) and this elevation in germ cell adenylyl cyclase in stages II-III may in part explain the higher basal and stimulated levels of cAMP in these segments. Such an explanation, however, also assumes that FSH can indirectly stimulate the germ cell adenylyl cyclase via the Sertoli cells.

Cyclic nucleotide phosphodiesterases potentially have a pivotal role to play in controlling the expression of trophic hormone effects in target tissue. Indeed, it has been suggested that the relative lack of response of the adult rat Sertoli cell to FSH, which can be reversed by MIX, may be due to an increase in the activity of this enzyme with development (Means et al., 1978). The finding of such clear cyclic variations in both cAMP and cGMP phosphodiesterase activities along the length of the seminiferous tubule implies that these enzymes may also be important for local regulation of tubular function. Of particular interest is the observation that there appears to be a degree of dissociation between cAMP and cGMP hydrolysing capacity in specific segments of the tubule (IX-XII) suggesting the existance of different isoforms of the enzyme which may be differentially controlled.

In general, the stages containing the greatest phosphodiesterase activity (VII-VIII) correspond to those exhibiting the lowest capacity for cAMP secretion (in the presence of MIX) and the lowest binding of ^{125}I-FSH (Parvinen et al., 1980). Moreover, germ cell-specific enzymes such as the soluble Mn^{2+}-dependent adenylyl cyclase (Gordeladze et al., 1981) and protein carboxyl methylase (Cusan et al., 1981) are also minimal in stages VII-VIII and show maximal activities in the tubular segments corresponding to stages II-III. Thus these latter enzymes exhibit activities which are almost the mirror image of the profile of phosphodiesterase activity. It is tempting to speculate that those stages associated with the greatest responsiveness of the receptor-cyclase system (Sertoli cells or germ cells) are generally those in which the activities of the phosphodiesterases appear to be attenuated. However, this may be an oversimplification, at least in the case of the Sertoli cells response to FSH, for two reasons. MIX has its greatest effect on FSH-stimulated cAMP secretion between stages XIII and V, implying that under normal conditions and particularly in these stages, phosphodiesterases are attenuating the FSH signal. Secondly, in the absence of MIX, the Sertoli cells should have responded poorly to FSH in those stages exhibiting the greatest phosphodiesterase activity (VII-VIII) and to a greater degree when the cAMP hydrolysing capacity is at its lowest (XII-V). In fact, relative to basal secretion, the degree of stimulation of cAMP secretion by FSH is gradually reduced between stages VII and XII, although the absolute levels of cAMP secreted follow a similar profile to that obtained in the presence of MIX (possibly reflecting the stage-dependent differences in adenylyl cyclase activity). Both of these observations imply that the assessment of total phosphodiesterase activity in the different tubular segments does little to clarify the degree of involvement of these enzymes at the level of the individual Sertoli cells, at least in relation to FSH responsiveness. Nevertheless, the great difference in magnitude of the cAMP response after the addition of MIX emphasizes that this relatively low level of phosphodiesterase activity may have an important role to play in the expression of the FSH response.

Why are both the cGMP and cAMP hydrolysing capacities so high at stages VII-VIII? Stages VII-VIII are associated with spermiation. It has been demonstrated that high doses of dibutyryl cAMP injected intraperitoneally into Syrian hamsters inhibit spermiation (Gravis, 1978) and spermatozoa are retained in stage X. Does this indicate that low cAMP levels are a prerequisite for normal spermiation to occur and that the high levels of phosphodiesterase, in combination with the low levels of adenylyl cyclase (Gordeladze et al., 1981), serve to guarantee that this is achieved? Germ cells possess at least two isoforms of cyclic nucleotide phosphodiesterase (Stephens et al., 1979) and it is likely that these isoforms contribute to the total phosphodiesterase activity in the tubular segments. Stages VII-VIII contain the most advanced germ cells preparing for spermiation and it may be that the elevated phosphodiesterase activity observed in these stages reflects the activation of these enzymes in the mature cells.

The heterogeneity of cell types in the seminiferous tubule, combined with the ubiquitous nature of the phosphodiesterases, frustrate to a large extent a detailed interpretation of the cyclic changes in total activity which occur along the length of the rat seminiferous tubule. However, in this regard it is of great interest that such clear cut changes can be recorded, and that in certain tubular segments, despite the large number of varied cells present, phosphodiesterase activity is reduced to such relatively low levels. The obvious interpretation is that these enzymes are locally regulated, and the mechanisms of this regulation and their cellular localization will be the subject of further investigations.

5.   Summary and Conclusions

In living, freshly isolated rat seminiferous tubules, cyclic changes in FSH binding, cAMP secretion (basal and FSH stimulated) and the activities of cAMP and cGMP phosphodi- esterases could be detected which were related to specific stages of spermatogenesis. FSH binding (per cm stage) increased gradually between stages VII and IX and then, after remaining relatively constant, was elevated further in stages XIV-I. Thereafter, binding fell to a nadir in stage VIIa-b. FSH stimulated cAMP secretion was as its lowest in stage VIIa-b and maximal between stages XIV-V. The greatest spec- ific activities of the cAMP and cGMP phosphodiesterases were detected in stages VII-VIII which are associated with spermiation in the rat. A degree of dissociation was found to exist in the cAMP and cGMP hydrolysing capacities at certain stages (IX-XII), suggesting the existence of different isoforms of the enzyme which may be differentially controlled. Exposure of the various stages to FSH or dibutyryl cAMP for 4 hr in vitro did not alter the profiles of phosphodiesterase activity.

The phosphodiesterase profiles were inversely related to the quantity of cAMP produced by the tubular segments after stimulation with FSH, both in the presence and absence of the phosphodiesterase inhibitor, methyl isobutyl xanthine (MIX). However, MIX elicited the greatest effect from the tubular segments, in terms of FSH stimulated cAMP production, in stages XIV-V, where direct measurements of phosphodiesterase indicate the enzyme activity is relatively low. The reasons for this apparent contradiction are discussed in relation to previous findings on stage-dependent alterations in various aspects of tubular function.

ACKNOWLEDGMENTS. This investigation was supported by grants from the Rockefeller Foundation (New York), World Health Organization, the Norwegian Council for Science and the Humanities (NAVF), the Norwegian Cancer Society, the Academy of Finald (project #200 at the Medical Research Council) and by the organization "Nordiska Forskerkurser."

REFERENCES

Cusan, L., Gordeladze, J. O., Parvinen, M., Clausen, O. P. F., and Hansson, V., 1981, Protein carboxyl-methylase and germ cell adenylyl cyclase at specific stages of the spermatogenic cycle of the rat, Biol. Reprod., 25:915.

Gardner, E. A., Thompson, W. J., and Stancel, G. M., 1976, Characterization of uterine phosphodiesterase and effects of estrogen on enzyme activity, Fed. Proc., 35 Abstr. 2224.

Gordeladze, J. O., Parvinen, M., Clausen, O. P. F., and Hansson, V., 1981, Stage-dependent variation in Mn^{2+}-sensitive adenylyl cyclase (AC) activity in spermatids and FSH-sensitive AC in Sertoli cells, Arch. Andrology, 8:43.

Garvis, C. J., 1978, Inhibition of spermiation in the Syrian hamster using debutyryl cyclic-AMP, Cell. Tiss. Res., 192: 241.

Hansson, V., Purvis, K., Attramadal, A., Torjesen, P., Andersen, D., and Ritzen, E. M., 1978, Sertoli cell function in the androgen insensitive (Tfm) rat, Int. J. Androl., 1:96.

Lacroix, M., Parvinen, M., and Fritz, I. B., 1981, Localization of testicular plasminogen activator in discrete portions (stages VII and VIII) of the seminiferous tubule, Biol. Reprod., 25:143.

Loten, E. G., and Sneyd, J. G. T., 1973, Evidence for separate sites of action for the antilipolytic effects of insulin and prostaglandin E_1, Endocrinology, 93:1315.

Means, A. R., Dedman, J. R., Fakunding, J. L., and Tindall, D. J., 1978, Mechanism of action of FSH in the male rat, in: "Receptors and Hormone Action," Vol. III, pp. 363-392, L. Birnbaumer, B. W. O'Malley, eds., Academic Press, New York.

Parvinen, M., Marana, R., Robertson, D. M., Hansson, V., and Ritzén, E. M., 1980, Functional cycle of the rat Sertoli cells: Differential binding and action of follicle-stimulating hormone at various stages of the spermatogenic cycle, in: "Testicular Development, Structure, and Function," pp. 425-432, A. Steinberger, E. Steinberger, eds., Raven Press, New York.

Parvinen, M., and Ruokonen, A., 1982, Endogenous steroids in rat seminiferous tubules. Comparison of different spermatogenic stages isolated by transillumination-assisted microdissection, J. Androl., in press.

Purvis, K., Olsen, A., Barry, M., and Hansson, V., 1981, Testicular cyclic nucleotide phosphodiesterase in the rat. Kinetic properties and changes with age, Arch. Andrology, 6:327.

Ritzén, E. M., Parvinen, M., Hansson, V., French, F. S., and
    Feldman, M., 1980, Role of Sertoli cell in spermatogenesis,
    in: "Proc. VI Int. Congr. Endocrinol.," pp. 159-161,
    Australian Academy of Science, Canberra.
Stephens, D. T., Wang, J. -L., and Hoskins, D. D., 1979, The
    cyclic AMP phosphodiesterase of bovine spermatozoa:
    Multiple forms, kinetic properties and changes during
    development, Biol. Reprod., 20:483.
Thompson, W. J., and Williams, R. H., 1974, Effect of adrenal-
    ectomy on cyclic 3',5'-guanosine monophosphate metabolism
    of rat liver and other tissues, Arch. Biochem. Biophys.,
    165:468.
Tovey, K. C., Oldham, K. G., and Whelan, J. A. M., 1974, A
    simple direct assay for cyclic AMP in plasma and other
    biological samples using an improved competitive protein
    binding technique, Clin. Chim. Acta 56:221.

DISCUSSION

HALL: Why can't one study binding of radioactive FSH by
autoradiography which would give a measure of binding and
clear evidence of spermatogenic stage?

HANSSON: We have tried both autoradiography and immunocytochemistry in this respect but without success.

ROMMERTS: As you know, the stage-dependent activity of the
tubules depends on the normalization procedure. So you
should either normalize on the number of Sertoli cells if
Sertoli cell properties are investigated, or normalize on the
number of specific germ cells when germ cell activities are
investigated. Can you comment on this?

HANSSON: I agree. As far as Sertoli cell parameters are
concerned, morphometric analyses have revealed that the
number (and volume) of Sertoli cells per unit tubular length
is constant. Furthermore, when expressing activities of germ
cell specific enzymes (adenylyl cyclase, protein carboxyl-
methylase), we have assessed the relative number of various
germ cells by micro-flow-cytophometry.

FRENCH: Evidence has been presented by your laboratory and
others that Sertoli cell secretory functions are highest in
stage VII of the spermatogenic cycle. How do you explain

this finding in view of the finding that FSH-binding and adenylyl cyclase activity are lowest at this stage?

HANSSON: FSH in the adult rat is probably not the major stimulus for Sertoli cell secretion. For that reason it is not surprising that secretory activity is dissociated from FSH binding and FSH response. Another possibility is that stages showing maximal secretion has a way of protecting themselves from further FSH stimulation.

CHRISTOFFERSEN: Just a question about negative controls: Have you looked at any enzyme activities that do not show this typical stage-dependent pattern, i.e. that do not correlate so closely with the adenylate cyclase?

HANSSON: Other general parameters of metabolic activity in germ cells like protein synthesis, RNA and DNA synthesis, show a completely different picture.

DEVELOPMENT OF SENSITIVITY TO CATECHOLAMINES IN GRANULOSA

AND LUTEAL CELLS

Gunnar Selstam, Sheela Rani, Knut Nordenström,
Ensio Norjavaara, Sten Rosberg and Kurt Ahrén

Departments of Physiology
Universities of Umeå and Gothenburg
Sweden

1.   Introduction

Catecholamines have a wide variety of physiological effects on a number of organ systems, including the nervous system, the circulation and the metabolism. The first indications that catecholamines could influence gonadal function was probably the observation that stress can depress the androgen blood level in the male (Levin et al., 1967) and the observation that the fibromuscular layer surrounding the mature follicle can increase the intrafollicular pressure and possibly promote the ovulatory process (Walles et al., 1976). The role of these effects are, however, still under debate. Catecholamines also have effects on the blood vessels of the gonads resulting in changes in blood flow (e.g. Damber et al., 1982; Selstam, 1975). The arteries are innervated (Burder, 1978), but the role of catecholamines on gonadal blood flow also remains to be investigated.

Effects of catecholamines on corpus luteum. Studies of metabolic effects of catecholamines on the ovary have mainly been focused on effects on the corpus luteum. It was first reported by Marsh (1970) that catecholamines can stimulate luteal adenylate cyclase and by Condon and Black (1976) that progesterone production could be increased. Increased cyclic AMP accumulation together with increased progesterone production has been shown for whole corpora lutea from the cow (Godkin et al., 1977) and the rat (Norjavaara et al., 1982) and dispersed ovine luteal cells (Jordan et al., 1978). In order to test whether these effects were mediated via

37

β-receptors, receptor antagonists have been used (Godkin et
al., 1977; Jordan et al., 1978; Norjavaara et al., 1982).
With low doses only inhibition of catecholamine effects
were seen. High doses exert unspecific inhibitory effects
independent of the use of d- or l-form of the antagonist
(Norjavaara et al., 1982). Furthermore, the high doses
inhibit the release of cyclic AMP into incubation media
(Norjavaara and Selstam, unpublished). Other evidence
that catecholamines have receptors on luteal cells is the
specific binding of β-agonists that have been shown to bind
specifically to ovaries with luteal tissue (Coleman et al.,
1979; Jordan, 1981) and to corpora lutea (Abramowitz et al.,
1982).

The adrenergic innervation of the follicle. For the
ovary, catecholamines have been implicated to play a role in
the process of ovulation. Presumably catecholamines would be
released from adrenergic nerve terminals. As first shown for
the rabbit (Owman and Sjöberg, 1966) and later for a large
number of species (for ref. see Bahr et al., 1974; Burden,
1978), adrenergic nerve terminals have a close relation to
the follicular wall. Since the theca layer contains, and
probably to a large extent constitues of muscle elements,
the functional nature of this fibromuscular unit based on
different types of experiments, implies a role for the ovulatory process (Owman et al., 1979). There are many events
leading to ovulation and activation of adrenergic nerves may
not be a necessary condition, since ovulations can occur in
in vitro perfusion systems (Janson et al., 1982). However,
no measurements of catecholamine content have been made in
these systems.

Effects of catecholamines on follicles and stromal
tissue. Few studies have been published concerning metabolic
effects of catecholamine on the follicle. There are, to
our knowledge, no studies where metabolic effects of catecholamines on isolated small follicles have been performed.
Adrenaline can act on ovaries that contain only small follicles by stimulating glycogen phosphorylase enzyme (Ahrén and
Selstam, 1971). It may be an effect on small follicles since
granulosa cells from immature rats respond to isoproterenol
with a 2-fold increase in cyclic AMP accumulation (Kliachko
and Zor, 1981). Effect of catecholamines on adenylate cyclase
of the rabbit interstitium has, however, been reported to be
minimal (Hunzicker-Dunn, 1982). Effects of catecholamines on
larger follicles have been performed before the endogenous

gonadotropin surge. Adenylate cyclase activity of membranes from whole isolated follicles was slightly stimulable by catecholamines (Birnbaumer et al., 1976). The response to catecholamines on adenylate cyclase activity of young corpora lutea are much larger than by follicles (Hunzicker-Dunn, 1982). Granulosa cells taken from mature follicles of Pregnant Mare Serum Gonadotropin (PMSG) primed rats before the endogenous gonadotropin surge showed a small response to catecholamines (Kliachko and Zor, 1981). When the granulosa cells were cultured up to 48 hr without addition of gonadotropins, a marked response in both cyclic AMP and progesterone production developed (Kliachko and Zor, 1981). In hypophysectomized and diethylstilbestrol treated rats no such response developed over the same time period unless FSH was supplied in vivo or in vitro (Adashi and Hsueh, 1981).

It is thus evident that the corpus luteum or luteal tissue can respond to catecholamines with an increased steroidogenesis that apparently is mediated via the cAMP system. The response of follicular tissue taken before the ovulation is, however, small or absent and hormonal and other treatment conditions has been necessary to induce a significant catecholamine response. The aim of our studies has been to further characterize the development of the catecholamine response and test the gonadotropin dependency.

2.   Methodological Considerations

In all experiments PMSG rat ovulatory models were used. PMSG (490 IU) were injected (0800-0930) to 26 day-old rats. This treatment results in an endogenous LH and FSH surge in the afternoon (1500-1900) of day 28 and a subsequent ovulation (0200-0500) the next morning. When adenylate cyclase activity was studied rats were housed with inverted light setting. PMSG was then injected in the evening (2000-2130) of day 26 and ovulations occurred at 1400 ± 1 hr of day 29. Corpora lutea have a lifespan of approximately 10 days (Herlitz et al., 1974). In some experiments the gonadotropin surge was blocked by nembutal anesthezia (4 mg/100 g b.w.) or injection of specific antisera.

When follicles or corpora lutea were incubated, they were preincubated for 30 min and then incubated for indicated times in modified Krebs bicarbonate buffer with glucose and 0.1% 1-ascorbic acid. Granulosa cells were isolated from

preovulatory follicles either before (AM) or after (PM) the
endogenous gonadotropin surge and cultured (10^6 cells per
dish) in Eagles-MEM with Hepes buffer (25 mM). After the
culture period the medium was changed to Krebs buffer and
cells (10^6 per tube) incubated for 30 min. Cyclic AMP was
determined by the protein binding technique described by
Gilman (1970). Progesterone was determined with RIA-tech-
nique. Adenylate cyclase activity of membrane fractions of
follicles and corpora lutea was determined according to the
method described by Birnbaumer et al., 1976) using 3 mM ATP
and 10 mM Mg^{2+} (other conditions see Khan and Rosberg, 1979).
Gpp(NH)p (10 μm) was added to all tubes. Protein content was
determined according to the Lowry method.

In the _in vivo_ experiments hormones were infused or
injected via the tail artery to rats anesthetized with
Nembutal. The abdomen was opened through a midline incision
and ovaries excised at 2 min after injection (LH) or start of
infusion (noradrenaline). After excision one ovary was
directly homogenized for cyclic AMP content and the other was
dissected into luteal and non-luteal compartments before
homogenization. Values are given as mean ± SEM of at least 4
rats in each group.

3.   Results and Comments

3.1. Effects of Catecholamines on the Preovulatory Follicle
     and the Corpus Luteum.

Effects of noradrenaline and LH on adenylate cyclase
activity was studied on preovulatory follicles and young
corpora lutea before and after the ovulation. The effect of
noradrenaline undergoes a dramatic increase over this time
period (Fig. 1). The effect of noradrenaline on adenylate
cyclase activity of membranes prepared from whole preovulatory
follicles isolated before the gonadotropin surge is small but
significant. This finding thus confirms earlier studies by
Birnbaumer et al. (1976), where likewise the effect of
catecholamines on the follicles was smaller than those of LH
or FSH. Where in the follicle the effect of catecholamines
is exerted is at present difficult to say. It could be on
vascular or endocrine cell compartments. When noradrenaline
is tested _in vitro_ on isolated preovulatory follicles (Fig.
2), no effect was seen on cAMP accumulation. In comprison
the effect on young corpora lutea as well as the effect of LH

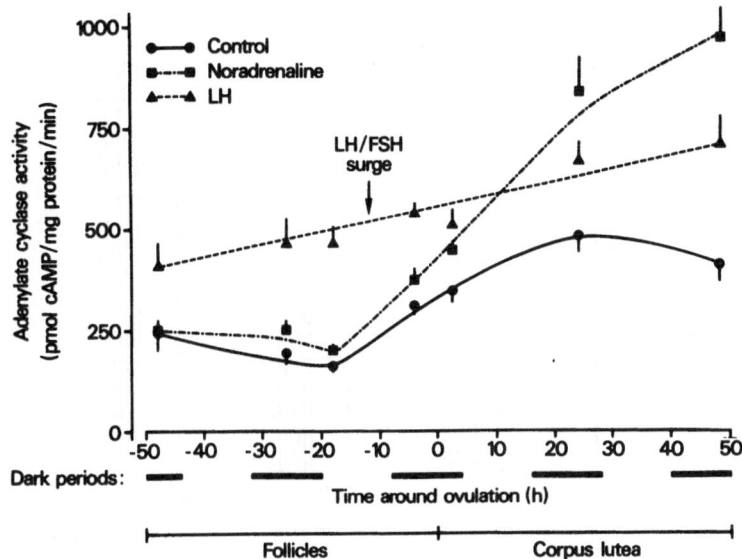

Figure 1. Adenylate cyclase activity of membrane fractions from follicles and corpora lutea isolated during the pre-ovulatory period. The effects of noradrenaline (5μg/ml) and LH (1 μg/NIH-LH-B9 ml) in vitro were tested. (Data from Selstam, Norjavaara, Rosberg, Damber and Cajander; to be published.)

is shown. The effect of LH on preovulatory follicles is also seen in Fig. 1. The relative effect decreases after the endogenous gonadotropin surge and it is usually assumed that this decrease is due to a refractory state after the endogenous surge (e.g., Ahrén et al., 1979). Concomitant with the activation of adenylate cyclase an increase in the cAMP level and an increased steroidogenesis are seen, which are all well established effects of LH on the mature follicle.

The effect of noradrenaline on adenylate cyclase was larger than for LH up to the third day of luteal age (Fig. 1). This effect has been compared also at later ages in the PMSG model (Selstam et al., to be published). The effects of catecholamines were maximal on the third day of luteal age whereafter a slow decline was seen. The effect of LH increased steadily with luteal age and at five days or later the effect of LH was the same or larger than catecholamines.

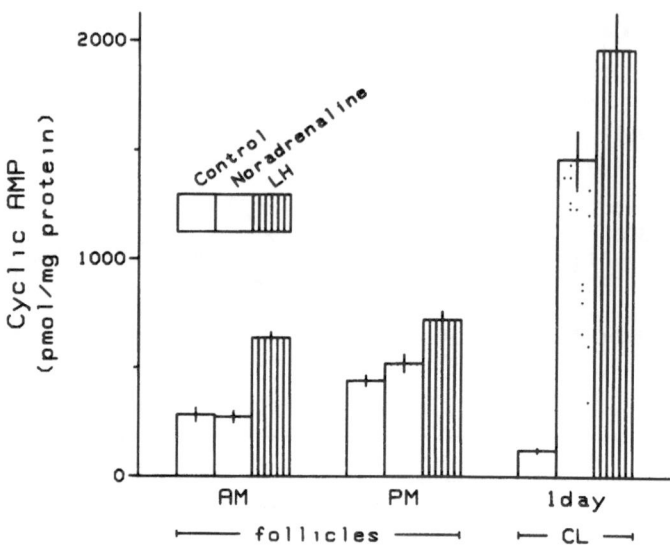

Figure 2. Effect of noradrenaline (10 μM) and LH (1 μg/ml) on cAMP formation in preovulatory follicles or newly formed corpora lutea. Preovulatory follicles isolated in the morning (AM) or evening (PM) of the preovulatory day and corpora lutea were incubated for 20 min at 37°C and the cAMP content of the tissue determined. (Data from Rani, Nordenström, Norjavaara and Ahrén; to be published.)

The effects of catecholamines in vitro on the corpus luteum in terms of cAMP and progesterone production are seen in Fig. 3 and are very similar to those of LH (Hertlitz et al., 1974; Ahrén et al., to be published). The effects of catecholamines and LH are of the same magnitude, but there is a difference in time-relationships for cAMP production. The effect of adrenaline on the cAMP content is much more rapid, but with a shorter duration (Norjavaara et al., 1982). There could be many explanations to the differences between catecholamines and LH on the cAMP system. But the easiest explanation is that this is an effect of different diffusion properties.

All studies so far of catecholamines on the corpus luteum have been performed in vitro. It was therefore considered important to test whether catecholamines have effects in vivo.

A two min infusion of noradrenaline increased the luteal content of cAMP, without changing the interstitial content (stroma), Fig. 4. The effect on the ovary of noradrenaline was different from that of LH, since LH also increases stromal content. The difference in effect between catecholamines and LH on the ovary may at least partly be explained by their action on different receptors. This lack of effect of noradrenaline on the stroma is in accordance with studies by Hunzicker-Dunn (1982) on adenylate cyclase activity. Whether this lack of effect is due to absence of receptors is at present unknown.

3.2. Dependency of the Endogenous Gonadotropin Surge for the Luteal Response to Catecholamines

In granulosa cells that were isolated after the endogenous gonadotropin surge (PM-GC) were cultured for 12 hr, a considerable effect of noradrenaline on cAMP formation was

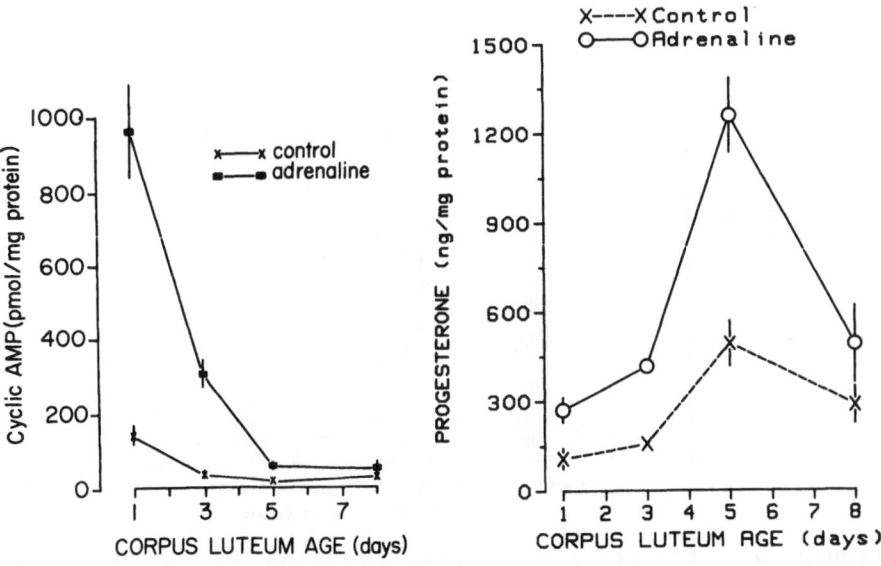

Figure 3. Effect of adrenaline (5 µg/ml) on tissue cAMP content and progesterone accumulation in incubation medium of 1-8 days old corpora lutea. Corpora lutea were incubated for 30 min at 37°C and tissue content of cAMP and medium content of progesterone was measured. (From Norjavaara, Selstam and Ahrén, 1982).

seen (Fig. 5). Granulosa cells taken before the gonadotropin surge did not develop such a sensitivity for noradrenaline when cultured up to 24 hr. The effect of LH was of the same magnitude for both AM and PM granulosa cells. Several experimental conditions were used to investigate the importance of the gonadotropin surge (Fig. 6). When the surge was blocked by Nembutal anesthesia, PM-granulosa cells did not develop a catecholamine sensitivity. When LH (10 µg) was substituted, the catecholamine response developed. Specific rat gonadotropic antisera, described in detail earlier (Rani and Moudgal, 1977), were used to demonstrate that the development of catecholamine responsiveness was dependent on the LH moiety of the endogenous surge. The catecholamine sensitivity did not develop when LH antiserum was injected, while the FSH antiserum had no effect (Fig. 6).

In order to search for how LH in our system can mediate the appearance of catecholamine responsiveness in granulosa cells at 12 hr of culture, the granulosa cells were cultured with a protein synthesis inhibitor in a concentration which

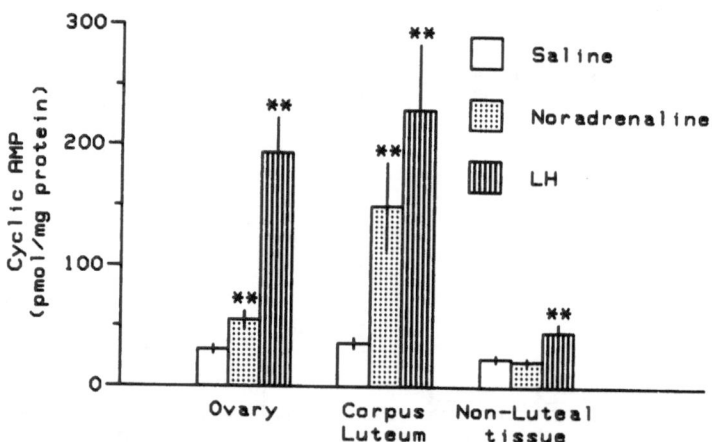

Figure 4. Effect of in vivo infusion of noradrenaline (0.4 µg/min) or in vivo injection of LH (5 µg) on cAMP accumulation of rat ovaries bearing 2 day-old corpora lutea. Whole ovaries, corpora lutea or non-luteal ovarian tissue were analysed for cAMP after 2 min. (Data from Norjavaara, Selstam, Damber and Johansson; to be published).

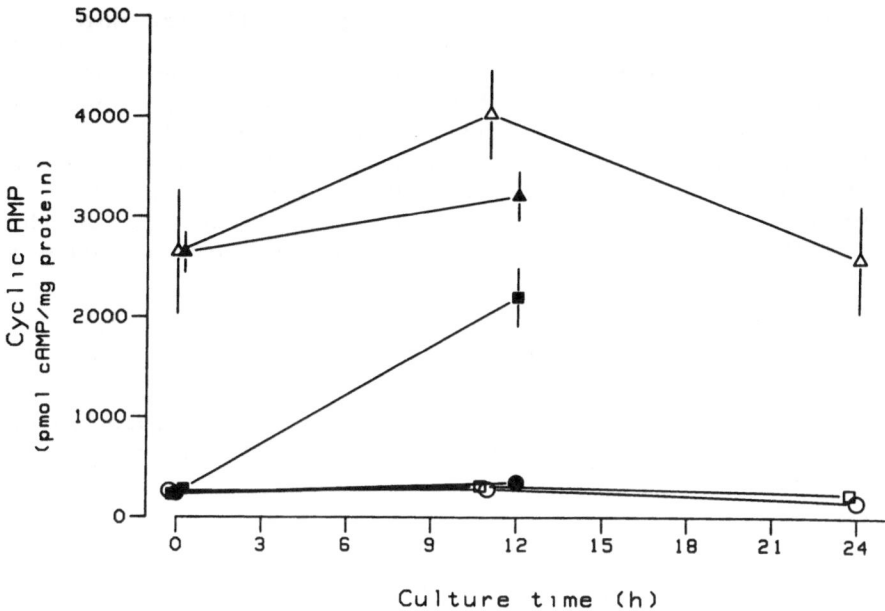

Figure 5. Effect of noradrenaline (10 μM) on cAMP formation
of granulosa cells cultured for various periods. The granulosa cells were isolated from preovulatory follicles in the
morning (AM-CG, open symbols) or in the evening (PM-CG,
closed symbols). After culture granulosa cells were incubated
for 30 min in control medium (open circles, closed circles),
noradrenaline (open squares, closed squares), or LH (open
triangles, closed triangles). (Data from Rani, Nordenström,
Norjavaara and Ahren, to be published).

inhibits the protein synthesis of the ovary. The catecholamine response did never develop and the protein synthesis may
play a role (Rani et al., to be published).

    When the development of the catecholamine response was
studied on adenylate cyclase activity, the same LH dependency
was seen (Fig. 7 and 8). Luteal membranes from rats anesthetized with Nembutal and substituted with LH showed the same
response to noradrenaline on adenylate cyclase compared to
control rats. Luteal membranes from anesthetized and LH
substituted rats on the third day after ovulation had the
same response of adenylate cyclase to noradrenaline and LH

compared to control rats, indicating that the FSH moiety of
the endogenous gonadotropin surge is not necessary. That LH
can induce catecholamine response was shown by injecting
10 µg LH to 27 day-old PMSG rats and measuring adenylate
cyclase activity of the follicles 16 hr later (Fig. 8). It
should, however, be remembered that membranes were prepared
from whole isolated follicles and a further separation of
follicular compartments is needed to test whether at this
preovulatory time LH could induce catecholamine response in
the granulosa cells.

4.   Discussion and Conclusions

The effects of catecholamines on the corpus luteum
reported so far are stimulation of the cAMP system and

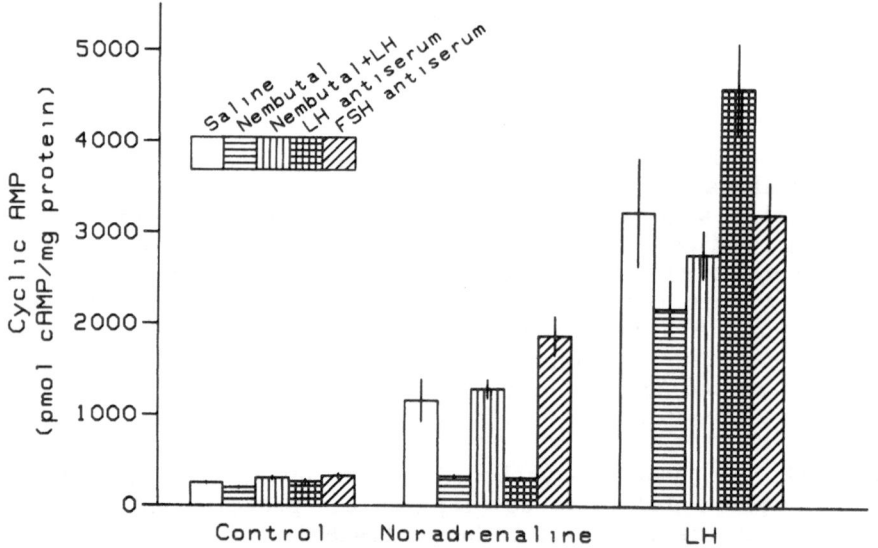

Figure 6. Effective of selective blockade of the preovulatory
gonadotropin surge on the development of noradrenaline responsiveness in cultured granulosa cells. The cells were isolated
in the evening of- the preovulatory day (PM-GC) and cultured
for 12 hr and then incubated for 30 min with nonadrenaline
(10 µM) or LH (0.1 µg/ml). Total cAMP (tissue and medium)
was measured. Nembutal anesthesia was used to block endogenous gonadotropin surge. 10 µg LH was used for substitution.
Antisera were given i.v. (data from Rani, Nordenström,
Norjavaara and Ahrén; to be published).

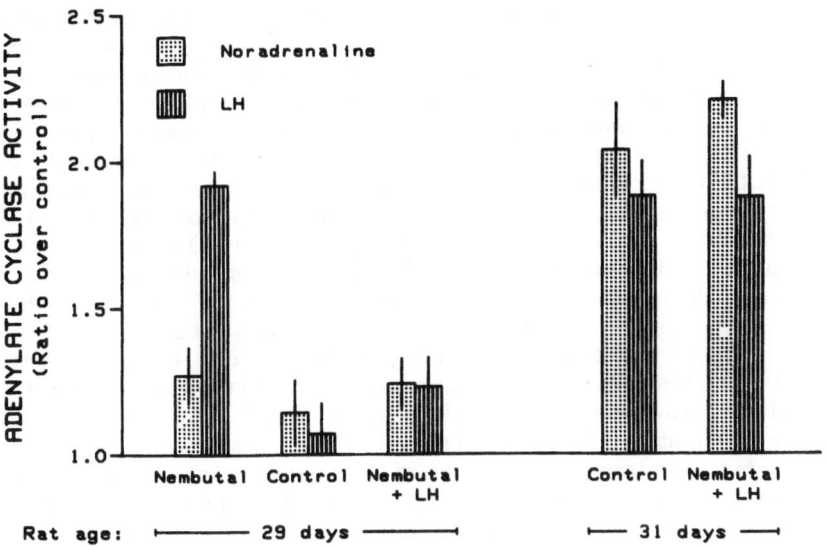

Figure 7. Effect of nembutal blockade and substitution of LH (10 µg) on adenylate cyclase activity. Tissues were taken out 4 or 49 hr on days 29 and 31, respectively, after ovulation. Effect of noradrenaline (5µg/ml) or LH (1 µg/ml) was tested (data from Selstam, Norjavaara, Rosberg, Damber and Cajander; to be published).

progesterone production. In this respect the catecholamines have a luteotropic activity and have effects similar to that of LH.

There are, however, differences: Catecholamines have a more rapid effect, are more effective on adenylate cyclase in young corpora lutea and in vivo effects are seen exclusively in the corpus luteum. β-Receptors have been described in the corpus luteum and they seem to have special characteristics (Coleman et al., 1979; Abramowitz et al., 1982). The β-receptors seem to be discrete from the gonadotorpin receptors, since LH-specific loss of responsiveness can be induced without affecting the adrenaline response (Rosberg et al., 1981).

The main effects of catecholamines seem to be on the corpus luteum and developed shortly after ovulation (Fig. 7),

that is during luteinization. Our studies with interference
of the endogenous gonadotropin surge clearly indicate that
the development is dependent on LH during the gonadotropin
surge. We found no spontaneous development of catecholamine
response before the surge. In the study by Adashi and Hsueh
(1981) where granulosa cells from hypophysectomized and
diethylstilbertrol-stimulated rats were cultured, no spontaneous development of catecholamine response occurred. When
FSH was added in vivo or in vitro, a catecholamine response
developed. LH was not tested. In the study by Kliachko
and Zor (1981) a spontaneous development of the catecholamine response of granulosa cells was found as well
as in hypophysectomized diethylstilbestrol treated rats.
There were, however, differences in the culture and incubation
conditions, including the addition of fetal calf serum to the
culture medium. In all studies the relatively long time
period for maximum induction of catecholamine response and
the obvious importance of experimental conditions make it
likely that the gonadotropic induced catecholamine responsiveness requires one or several intermediates. It is therefore

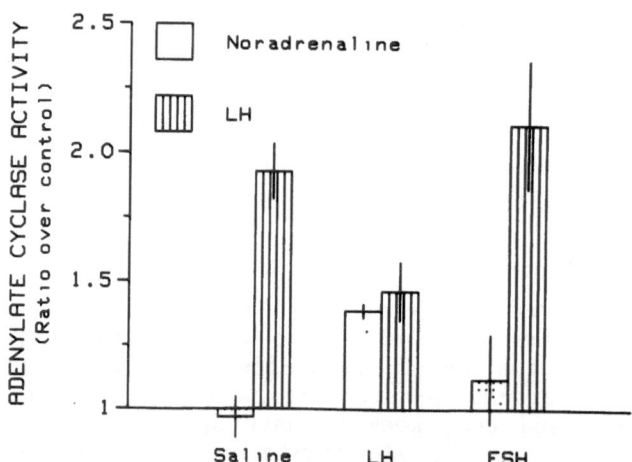

Figure 8. Effect of LH on the development of catecholamine
response of membranes from ovulatory follicles. LH or FSH
(10 µg) was given i.p. 48 hr before expected ovulation time
and follicles were isolated 16 hr later for adenylate cyclase
activity in presence of noradrenaline (5 µg/ml) or LH
(1 µg/ml) (data from Selstam, Norjavaara, Rosberg, Damber and
Cajander; to be published).

difficult to evaluate the FSH dependency as found by Adashi and Hsueh (1981) in relation to our studies. FSH in the study by Adashi and Hsueh may be needed by the follicles which have been deprived for several days of endogenous gonadotropins and/or FSH may have induced similar favorable conditions for development of catecholamine responsiveness in their model as endogenous LH does in PMSG primed rats.

Whether catecholamines have a physiological role in luteal function is an open question. If one considers the metabolic effects of catecholamines, the development of catecholamine response in the preovulatory period and the rich adrenergic nerve supply providing a source for endogenous noradrenaline, it is tempting to assume that a physiological role exists.

ACKNOWLEDGMENTS. This study was supported by the Swedish Medical Research Council (04X-05653; 04X-00027), the Medical Faculties, and Gunvor and Josef Anérs Research Foundation.

REFERENCES

Abramowitz, J., Iyengar, R., and Birnbaumer, L., 1982, Guanine nucleotide and magnesium ion regulation of the interaction of gonadotropic and β-adrenergic receptors with their hormones: A comparative study using a single membrane system, Endocrinology, 110:336.

Adashi, E. Y., and Hsueh, A. J. W., 1981, Stimulation of β-adrenergic responsiveness by follicle stimulating hormone in rat granulosa cells in vitro and in vivo, Endocrinology, 108:2170.

Ahrén, K., and Selstam, G., 1971, Hormonal regulation of ovarian phosphorylase activity, Acta Physiol. Scand., 82:31.

Ahrén, K., Norjavaara, E., Rosberg, S., and Selstam, G., Development of prostaglandin F2α-inhibition of epinephrine stimulated cyclic AMP and progesterone production by rat corpora lutea, Manuscript in preparation.

Ahrén, K., Bergh, C., Ekholm, C., Hamberger, L., Hillensjö, T., Khan, I., Nilsson, L., Nordenström, K., Rosberg, S., and Selstam, G., 1979, Development of refractoriness of the ovarian cyclic AMP system to gonadotropins, in: "Advances in the Biosciences: Development of Responsiveness to Steroid Hormones, A. M. Kaye and M. Kaye, eds., pp. 319-341, Pergamon Press, Oxford.

Bahr, J., Kao, L., and Nalbandov, A. W., 1974, The role of cate
    cholamines and nerves in ovulation, Biol. Reprod., 10:273.
Ben-Jonathan, N., Baw, R. H., Laufer, N., Reich, R., Bahr, J.
    M., and Tsafriri, A., 1982, Norephinephrine in Graafian
    follicles is depleted by follicle stimulating follicle
    stimulating hormone, Endocrinology, 110:457.
Birnbaumer, L., Yang, P. C., Hunzicker-Dunn, M., Bockaert, J.,
    and Duran, J. M., 1976, Adenylyl cyclase activities in
    ovarian tissues. I. Homogenization and conditions of
    assay in Graafian follicles and corpora lutea of rabbits,
    rats and pigs: Regulation of ATP, and some comparative
    properties, Endocrinology, 99:163.
Burden, H. W., 1978, Ovarian innervation, in: "The Vertebrate
    Ovary", R. E. Jones, ed., pp. 615-638, Plenum Press, New
    York.
Coleman, A. J., Paterson, D. S., and Somerville, A. R., 1979,
    the β-adrenergic receptor of rat corpus luteum membranes,
    Biochem. Pharmacol., 28:1003.
Condon, W. A., and Black, D. L., 1976, Catecholamine induced
    stimulation of progesterone by the bovine corpus luteum
    in vitro, Biol. Reprod., 15:573.
Damber, J. -E., Lindahl, O., Selstam, G., and Tenland, T.,
    1982, Testicular blood flow measured with a laser doppler
    flow meter: Acute effects of catecholamines, Acta.
    Physiol. Scand., 115:209.
Gilman, A. G., 1970, A protein binding assay for adenosine
    3',5' cyclic monophosphate, Proc. Natl. Acad. Sci. USA,
    67:305.
Godkin, J. D., Black, D. L., and Dudy, R. T., 1977, Stimulation
    of cyclic AMP and progesterone synthesis by LH, PGE_2 and
    isoprotereol in bovine corpus luteum in vitro, Biol.
    Reprod., 17:514.
Herlitz, H., Hamberger, L., Rosberg, S., and Ahrén, K., 1974,
    Cyclic AMP in isolated corpora lutea of the rat: Influ-
    ences of gonadotropins and prostaglandins, Acta Endocrinol
    (Copenh.), 77:737.
Herlitz, H., Koch, Y., and Khan, I., and Ahrén, K., 1976, Effec
    of follicle stimulating hormone on cyclic AMP levels in
    young corpora lutea of rat, Eur. J. Obstet. Gyn. Reprod.
    Biol., 6:175.
Hunzicker-Dunn, M., 1982, Epinephrine-sensitive adenylyl cyclas
    activity in rabbit ovarian tissues, Endocrinology, 110:233
Janson, P. -O., LeMaire, W. J., Källfeldt, B., Holmes, P. V.,
    Cajander, S., Bjersing, L., Wigvist, N., and Ahrén, K.,
    1982, The study of ovulation in the isolated perfused
    rabbit ovary. I. Methodology and pattern of steroido-
    genesis, Biol. Reprod., 26:456.

Jordan, A. W., 1981, Changes in ovarian β-adrenergic receptors
     during the estrous cycle of the rat, Biol. Reprod.,
     24:245.
Jordan, A. W., Caffrey, J. L., and Niswender, G. D., 1978,
     Catecholamine-induced stimulation of progesterone and
     adenosine 3',5'-monophosphate production by dispersed
     ovine luteal cells, Endocrinology, 103:385.
Kahn, I., and Rosberg, S., 1979, Acute suppression by PGF on LH,
     epinephrine and fluoride stimulation of adenylate cyclase
     in rat luteal tissue, J. Cycl. Nuc. Res., 5:55.
Kliachoko, S., and Zor, U., 1981, Increase in catecholamine-
     stimulated cyclic AMP and progesterone synthesis in rat
     granulosa cells during culture, Mol. Cell. Endocrinol.,
     23:23.
Levin, J., Lloyd, C. W., Lobotski, J., and Friedrich, E. H.,
     1967, The effect of epinephrine on testosterone production,
     Acta Endocrinol. (Copenh.), 55:187.
Marsh, J. M., 1970, The stimulatory effect of luteinizing hor-
     mone on adenyl cyclase in bovine corpus luteum, J. Biol.
     Chem., 245:1596.
Norjavaara, E., Selstam, G., Damber, J. -E., and Johansson,
     B. -M., Stimulatory effect of noradrenaline in vivo on the
     cyclic AMP level in rat corpora lutea. (Manuscript in prep).
Norjavaara, E., Selstam, G., and Ahrén, K., 1982, Catecholamine
     stimulation of cyclic AMP and progesterone production in
     rat corpora lutea of different ages, Acta Endocrinol.
     (Copenh.), 100:613.
Owman, C., and Sjöberg, N. -O., 1966, Adrenergic nerves in the
     female genital tract of the rabbit with remarks on cholin-
     esterase containing-structures, Z. Zell forsch,
     74:182.
Owman, C., Sjöberg, N. -O., Wallach, E. E., Walles, E., and
     Wright, K. H., 1979, Neuromuscular mechanisms of ovulation,
     in: "Human Ovulation: Mechanisms, Prediction, Detection
     and Induction", E. S. E. Haez, ed., pp. 57-100, North
     Holland, Amsterdam.
Rani, S., and Moudgal, N. R., 1977, Examination of the role of
     FSH in preovulatory events in the hamster, J. Reprod.
     Fertil., 50:37.
Rani, S., Nordenström, K., Norjavaara, E., and Ahrén, K., Devel-
     opment of catecholamine responsiveness in granulosa cells
     from preovulatory rat follicles - dependence on preovula-
     tory LH surge. (Manuscript in preparation.)
Rosberg, S., Khan, I., Selstam, G., and Ahrén, K., 1981,
     LH-induced desensitization of adenylate cyclase in
     membranes of rat corpora lutea, Acta Endocrinol. (Copenh.),
     suppl. 243, 97:68.

Selstam, G., 1975, Studies on regulatory mechanisms of the
    cyclic AMP system in the ovary. Thesis, University of
    Gothemburg, Sweden, p. 15.
Selstam, G., Norjavaara, E., Rosberg, S., Damber, J. -E., and
    Cajander, S., Studies of the luteinization process: Induc-
    tion of catecholamine response on adenylate cyclase activ-
    ity by LH. (Manuscript in preparation.)
Selstam, G., Norjavaara, E., Rosberg, S., Khan, I., Hamberger,
    B., and Hamberger, L., 1982, Catecholamine content and
    effects of luteinizing hormone and catecholamines on
    adenylate cyclase activity in rat corpora lutea on differ-
    ent ages. (Manuscript in preparation.)
Walles, B., Edvinsson, L., Owman, C., Sjoberg, N. -O., and
    Sporrong, B., 1976, Cholinergic nerves and receptors
    mediating contraction of the Graafian follicle, Biol.
    Reprod., 17:423.

DISCUSSION

BIRNBAUMER: Do you have a hypothesis as to why granulosa
cells respond only to LH and not to FSH by developing a
catecholamine response even though these cells are responsive
to both FSH and LH in terms of cAMP production?

SELSTAM: If this development of catecholamine responsiveness
involves cAMP production we have no good explanation.
However, LH and FSH have different effects of e.g. protein
synthesis and steroidogenesis and the development of the
response may involve specific mediators. The long delay of
the appearance of the catecholamine response suggests one or
several intermediates.

BIRNBAUMER: I should like to caution researchers in the
field not to label all loss of hormonal responsiveness that
may occur upon membrane incubation as "desensitization".
Many factors may cause loss of hormonal responsiveness, some
are meaningful and others less so (e.g. proteolysis, heat-
denaturation). Thus, their possible relation to what I would
call "true" desensitization, as it occurs in intact cells
after hormonal stimulation, as to be evaluated very carefully
before it can be claimed that a given cell free effect is
indeed a desensitization. This, of course, should not detract
interest from Dr. Selstam's finding that membrane incubation
in the absence of ATP leads to a loss of LH response which
can be reversed by postincubation with ATP.

LABRIE: When you infused adrenaline, were the animals hypophysectomized or treated with gonadotropin antisera in order to determine if the effect was direct on the ovary? Secondly, were the changes in cAMP levels accompanied by changes of serum steroid levels?

SELSTAM: The animals were not hyophysectomized or treated with antisera. The effect is, however, very rapid (30 sec) and systemic administration of catecholamines does not increase plasma levels of gonadotropins. We therefore consider it likely that it is a direct effect. Steroid levels were not measured.

CHRISTOFFERSEN: One of the most striking results you showed was that whereas $PGF_{2\alpha}$ did not affect catecholamine-induced cAMP generation in 1-day old corpora lutea it was strongly inhibitory at 3 days. Do you have any explanations, or physiological correlates, for that phenomenon?

SELSTAM: The same inhibitory pattern is also seen when LH effect on cAMP accumulation is inhibited by $PGF_{2\alpha}$. It is not only cAMP accumulation that shows a changed response to $PGF_{2\alpha}$ with luteal age, but also the progesterone production. It is known that hCG for some time can prevent the inhibitory action of $PGF_{2\alpha}$ and the ovulatory gonadotropin surge may perhaps prevent the action of $PGF_{2\alpha}$. A more likely explanation is that $PGF_{2\alpha}$ cannot act on young corpora lutea since they have few $PGF_{2\alpha}$ receptors.

EFFECTS OF PROSTAGLANDIN $F_{2\alpha}$ ON ADENYLYL CYCLASE ACTIVITY AND STEROID SECRETION IN THE SUPERLUTEINIZED RAT OVARY

Peter A. Torjesen and Asbjørn Aakvaag

University of Oslo Hospitals
Hormone Laboratory, Aker Hospital
Oslo 5, Norway

1.   Introduction

The corpus luteum (CL) is necessary for the maintenance of early pregnancy in all mammals, and for some species, luteal function is required throughout pregnancy. By interfering with the function of the CL, possible means of controlling fertility may be obtained.

Luteolysis has two aspects, anatomical-structural and functional. The functional luteolysis of the rat is characterized by the following phenomena: (1) A fall in progesterone production; (2) Increased 20α-dihydroprogesterone (20α-DHP) production; and (3) Loss of luteinizing hormone (LH) receptor in the CL.

It is firmly established that prostaglandin $F_{2\alpha}$ ($PGF_{2\alpha}$) is the luteolysin from the uterus in a number of animal species, including the rat (for a review, see Horton and Poyser, 1976). It has been reported that $PGF_{2\alpha}$ treatment decreases LH stimulated adenylyl cyclase in the CL of the rat (Thomas et al., 1978; Khan and Rosberg, 1979). On the other hand, human chorionic gonadotropin (hCG) injection prevents the luteolytic effect of subsequently administrated $PGF_{2\alpha}$ (Fuchs et al., 1974; Aakvaag and Torjesen, 1981). These seemingly conflicting observations moved us to study the changes in basal and stimulated adenylyl cyclase of ovarian homogenates as well as ovarian cAMP content in relation to steroidogenic activity during $PGF_{2\alpha}$ induced luteolysis, and how hCG pre-treatment modified these changes.

The importance of the association of the GTP activated
GTP binding unit to the hormone receptor complex and the
catalytic unit of the adenylyl cyclase for maximal production
of cAMP has in recent years been revealed (for a review, see
Spiegel et al., 1981). As the underlying mechanisms for
attenuation of LH stimulated adenylyl cyclase activity during
PG induced luteolysis is still unknown, we studied whether
the association of the activated GTP binding unit to the
catalytic unit might be involved. The effects of $PGF_{2\alpha}$ were
evaluated in this context by measuring the possible effects
on (1) GTP turnover by substituting GTP with Gpp(NH)p, the
more stable analogue, (2) the coupling between the hormone
receptor complex and the rest of the adenylyl cyclase system
by using three different activators, and (3) the direct
activation of the GTP binding unit using fluoride.

2.   Animal Model

Superluteinization was induced in 25 day-old rats by sc
injection of 50 IU pregnant mare serum gonadotropin (pmSG)
followed by 25 IU hCG 65 hr later (Parlow, 1961). The superluteinized ovary contains 95% luteal tissue and the ovarian
function can be monitored by measuring the serum levels of
progesterone and 20α-DHP. Seven days after the hCG administration, luteolysis was induced by sc injection of 5 µg of
the $PGF_{2\alpha}$ analogue cloprostenol (Torjesen and Aakvaag, 1977).

3.   Adenylyl Cyclase Activity in Ovarian Homogenates
      During PG Induced Luteolysis

We have previously reported several aspects of the PG
induced luteolysis of rats with superluteinized ovaries
(Aakvaag and Torjesen, 1981). The functional luteolysis
occurs within 15 min after the treatment, as can be seen from
decreased serum levels of progesterone. This takes place
several hours before any changes in the number of binding
sites for LH can be detected while the LH stimulated adenylyl
cyclase of the plasma membrane of the CL was decreased within
one hour after PG injection. These observations suggest that
PG affects the adenylyl cyclase via a mechanism that is not
related to the binding of LH to its receptor. In this
connection it should be pointed out that Khan and Rosberg
(1979) reported that a membrane fraction of CL showed
decreased LH as well as epinephrine stimulated adenylyl
cyclase activity within 15 min after $PGF_{2\alpha}$ injection into
pmSG treated rats.

We have performed a study on the temporal aspects of adenylyl cyclase activity of CL during PG induced luteolysis. The adenylyl cyclase activities were correlated to the serum levels and ovarian content of progesterone and 20α-DHP as indicators of luteal function. The ovarian content of cAMP was measured to detect possible changes in cAMP production and metabolism in vivo during PG induced luteolysis.

3.1. Serum Levels of Progesterone and 20α-DHP

The serum levels of progesterone decreased from 1700 ± 300 nM (mean ± SEM) to 810 ± 170 nM within 15 min of cloprostenol administration (Fig. 1). A further decline to 71 ± 3 nM was observed during the next 4 hr. After the PG injection the 20α-DHP levels also declined, but less pronounced, and at 12 hr the levels has increased and surpassed control levels in agreement with previous observations (Torjesen et al., 1978). The increased production of 20α-DHP reflects the induction of the enzyme 20α-hydroxysteroid dehydrogenase (Aakvaag and Torjesen, 1981) which is a typical feature of the luteolysis in the rat (Wiest et al., 1968).

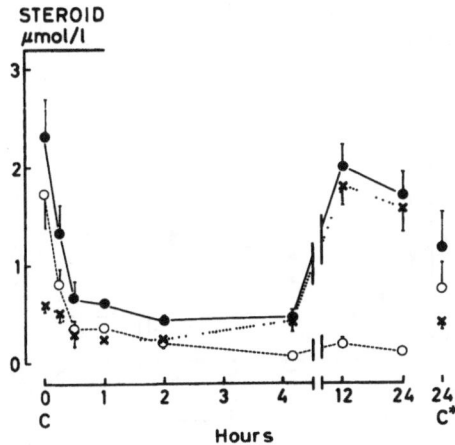

Figure 1. Serum progesterone (open circles), 20α-DHP (x···x) and progesterone plus 20α-DHP (closed circles) levels before and after cloprostenol treatment. Mean ± SEM, n = 4. *C - Control sample obtained 24 hr after saline injection.

3.2. Ovarian Content of Progesterone and 20α-DHP

The ovarian contents of progesterone and 20α-DHP (Fig. 2) were rather closely related to the serum levels during PG induced luteolysis. However, the change in ovarian concentrations of steroids seemed to precede the corresponding changes in the serum levels. This suggests that during luteolysis the serum levels of progesterone and 20α-DHP are regulated by the ovarian steroid production capacity.

3.3. Ovarian Content of cAMP

Ovarian cAMP content was measured in individual ovaries by competitive protein binding assay after homogenization in ethanol (Gilman, 1970). During the initial 3 hr after PG treatment the ovarian cAMP content remained close to control levels (Fig. 3). The early phase of luteolysis with the sharp drop in the progesterone level in serum was not related to the tissue concentration of cAMP. Later on the cAMP content increased and was significantly (p < 0.008) elevated 12 hr after the PG injection. The rise in cAMP content corresponds to the increase in 20α-DHP production, suggesting that the resumed steroidogenesis may be due to increased adenylyl cyclase activity or reduced phosphodiesterase activity.

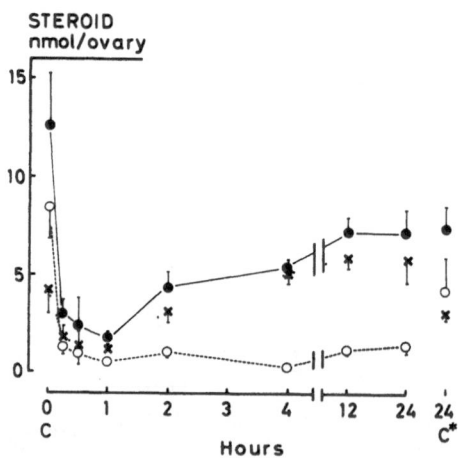

Figure 2. Ovarian progesterone (open circles), 20α-DHP (x···x) and progesterone plus 20α-DHP (closed circles) concentrations before and after cloprostenol treatment. Mean ± SEM, n = 4.
*C - Control sample obtained 24 hr after saline injection.

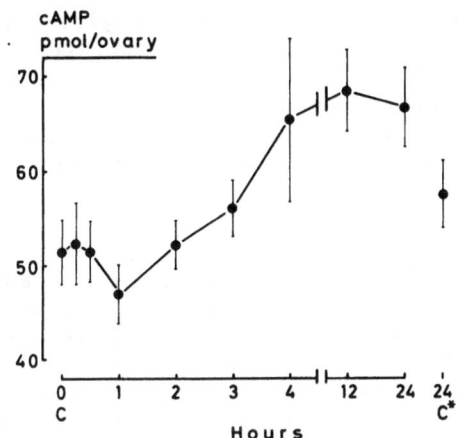

Figure 3. cAMP content in ovaries obtained from superluteinized rats before and after cloprostenol injection. Mean ±
SEM, n = 8 except for preparations obtained 3 and 4 hr after
treatment where n = 4.
*C - Control ovary obtained 24 hr after saline injection.

3.4. Adenylyl Cyclase Activity of Ovarian Homogenates

Adenylyl cyclase activity was determined in ovarian
homogenate according to Birnbaumer et al. (1976). The assay
buffer contained 3 mM ATP, 5 mM $MgCl_2$, 1.0 mM 3-isobutyl-1-
methylxanthine (MIX) and 10 µM GTP. The adenylyl cyclase was
stimulated with hCG (170 IU/ml), isoproterenol (0.1 mM), NaF
(25 mM) or PGE_1 (0.03 mM). After incubation, the samples
were treated with alumina (20 mg in 140 µl water) to remove
ATP, centrifuged and assayed for cAMP by competitive protein
binding assay.

Cloprostenol treatment decreased hCG stimulated adenylyl
cyclase activity from 20 ± 3 pmol/mg protein/min to 9 ± 1
pmol/mg protein/min within 15 min (Fig. 4). The stimulation
that could be achieved with fluoride and isoproterenol was
also reduced within 15 min while basal and PGE_1 stimulated
adenylyl adenylyl cyclase activity remained unchanged
(Fig. 5). In ovaries obtained 12 hr after the cloprostenol
administration hCG, isoproterenol and fluoride stimulated
adenylyl cyclase had returned to pretreatment levels whereas
basal and PGE_1 stimulated adenylyl cyclase activity were both

increased. The hCG stimulated adenylyl cyclase activity
observed in response to hCG 24 hr after the PG injection was
significantly (p = 0.032) lower than in controls in contrast
to the activation achieved with the other stimulating substances. Substituting GTP with Gpp(NH)p did not change the
pattern for hCG and isoproterenol stimulated adenylyl cyclase
(Fig. 5).

The acute suppression by $PGF_{2\alpha}$ administration on LH,
epinephrine and fluoride stimulation of adenylyl cyclase
activity in rat luteal cells has been reported by Khan and
Rosberg (1979) while the selective suppression of LH stimulated adenylyl cyclase at 21 hr after Estrumate injection was
reported by Wakelin and Green (1981) and Aakvaag and Torjesen
(1981). The selective decrease in hCG stimulated adenylyl
cyclase activity which occurred 24 hr after treatment might
be explained by the decreased number of LH receptors observed
at that time (Hichens et al., 1974; Torjesen et al., 1978).

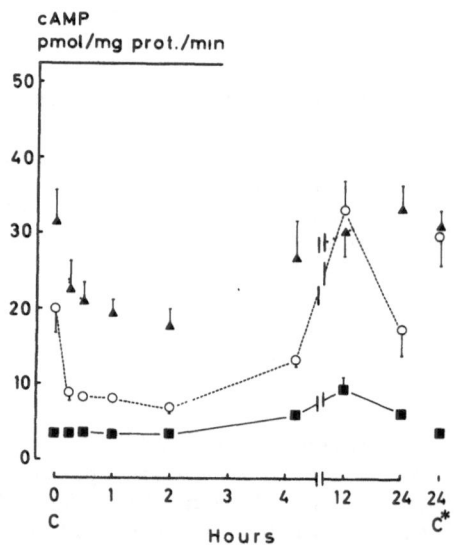

Figure 4. Adenylyl cyclase activity of ovaries obtained
before and 15 min to 24 hr after cloprostenol injection
assayed in the presence of $10^{-5}M$ GTP. Basal (closed squares),
hCG (open circles) and NaF (closed triangles) stimulated
activity. Control animals received saline only. Mean ± SEM,
n = 4.
*C - Control ovary obtained 24 hr after saline injection.

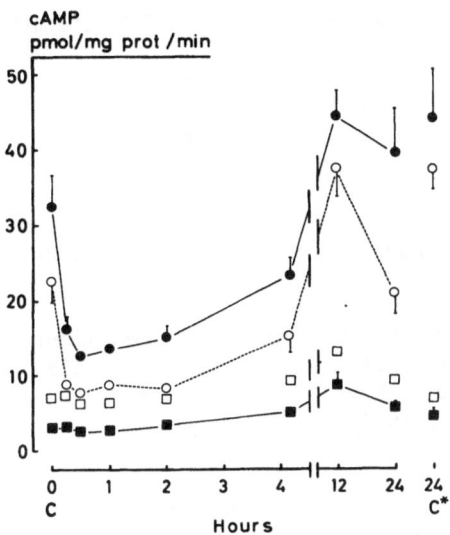

Figure 5. Adenylyl cyclase activity of ovaries obtained before and 15 min to 24 hr after cloprostenol injection assayed in the presence of $10^{-5}M$ Gpp(NH)p. Basal (closed squares), hCG (open circles), PGE_1 (open squares) and isoproterenol (closed circles) stimulated activity. Mean ± SEM, n = 4.
*C - Control ovary obtained 24 hr after saline injection.

During the initial phase of the induced luteolysis there was a close correlation between steroid production and loss of adenylyl cyclase response to several activators which indicates that the adenylyl cyclase is affected in a general way beyond the binding of a hormone to its receptor. The reduced response to stimulation was not due to deactivation of the GTP binding unit of the adenylyl cyclase complex via increased GTPase activity as fluoride stimulated adenylyl cyclase was decreased and the reduction was not modified when GTP was substituted with the more stable analogue Gpp(NH)p. Still, the GTP binding unit could have been modified in other ways to attenuate its stimulatory effects on the catalytic unit of the adenylyl cyclase. Also, the catalytic unit could have been modified directly. Possibly the activation of an inhibitory GTP binding unit (Rodbell, 1980), or association of $PGF_{2\alpha}$ receptors to GTP binding units rendering less GTP binding units available for stimulation (Spiegel and Downs, 1981) or phosphorylation of plasma membrane components (Hunzicker-Dunn et al., 1979) could be involved.

3.5. Dose-Response Relationship for hCG Stimulated Adenylyl Cyclase

The dose-response relationship for hCG stimulated adenylyl cyclase was assayed in homogenates obtained from animals 1 hr after PG injection (Fig. 6). Maximal stimulation was obtained with 30-160 IU hCG/ml. Again, the response was lower than in controls, but the dose required for maximal or half-maximal stimulation was not changed following PG treatment.

These observations further strengthen the concept that the immediate effects of PG administration are beyond the hormone receptor level in agreement with previous data (Torjesen et al., 1978).

4.   hCG Pre-treatment and Adenylyl Cyclase Activity During PG Induced Luteolysis

It has been reported (Fuchs et al., 1974; Aakvaag and Torjesen, 1981) that hCG injection protects the CL against

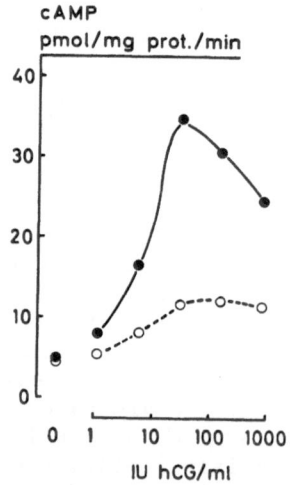

Figure 6. Dose response relationship for hCG stimulated adenylyl cyclase in ovaries obtained before (closed circles) and 1 hr after (open circles) cloprostenol injection.

the luteolytic effects of subsequent $PG_{H2\alpha}$ administration. This observation seemed difficult to explain in relation to a mechanism for PG induced luteolysis which suggested that the adenylyl cyclase was modified beyond the binding of LH to its receptor. Accordingly, it seemed interesting to study the effect of cloprostenol administration of the adenylyl cyclase activity of CL from rats that had been pre-treated with hCG.

4.1. Steroid Production

hCG injected alone or in combination with cloprostenol led to slightly elevated serum levels of progesterone as reported previously (Aakvaag and Torjesen, 1981). Thus, it was confirmed that hCG pre-treatment protected the CL against the luteolytic action of the $PGH_{2\alpha}$ analogue. The ovarian contents of progesterone and 20α-DHP did not change following hCG treatment alone or together with cloprostenol, that again led to decreased ovarian steroid content when given alone (data not shown).

4.2. Ovarian Content of cAMP

Ovarian cAMP content was increased 40-fold 90 min after sc injection of 25 IU hCG (Table 1). When the animals received cloprostenol 60 min after hCG, the ovaries still contained elevated cAMP levels, but only 4% of the cAMP levels of ovaries from animals that had received hCG only. These observations indicate that hCG administration leads to a production of cAMP in excess of what is needed for the maintenance of the luteal function and the elevated ovarian cAMP is insufficiently reduced by the $PGF_{2\alpha}$ treatment to cause luteolysis. Thus, hCG pretreatment protects the ovary against the luteolytic action of $PGF_{2\alpha}$ because of stimulated cAMP formation rather than by protecting against the action of the PG.

4.3. Adenylyl Cyclase Activity of Ovarian Homogenates

Administration of hCG in vivo gave rise to a 40-fold increase in the luteal content of cAMP (Table 1). This

increase was not associated by a measureable increase in the
adenylyl cyclase activity, when a homogenate of luteal tissue
was assayed for this enzyme activity after hCG injection in
vivo (Fig. 7) in agreement with Lee (1979). This apparent
discrepancy may principally have two different explanations.
The tissue concentration of cAMP may, to a large extent, be
controlled by breakdown rather than by synthesis which leads
to the proposal that hCG may inhibit phosphodiesterase
activity. The other possibility is that the measurement of
adenylyl cyclase in vitro does not fully reflect the activity
of this enzyme in vivo.

When cloprostenol was administered 1 hr after hCG, a 95%
reduction in the tissue concentration of cAMP was observed,
whereas no effect on adenylyl cyclase activity could be
detected (Fig. 7). The same effect on stimulated adenylyl
cyclase was induced by cloprostenol in hCG treated and
untreated animals. hCG treatment did not modify the effect
of cloprostenol on adenylyl cyclase activity in spite of the
fact that this treatment completely prevented luteolysis to
occur in response to cloprostenol. One is therefore tempted
to suggest that PG induces luteolysis by mechanisms other
than interfering with the adenylyl cyclase.

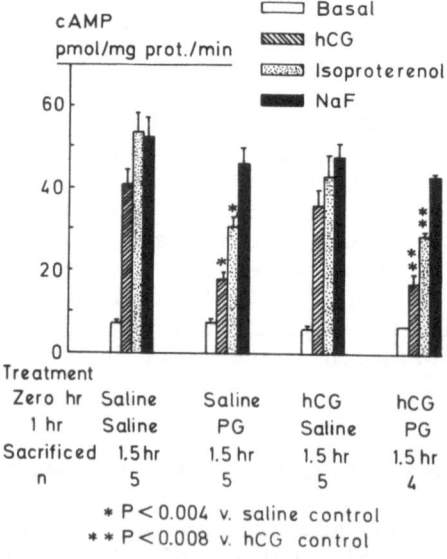

Figure 7. Effect of hCG pretreatment on ovarian adenylyl
cyclase activity following cloprostenol administration in
vivo. Mean ± SEM.

Table 1. Effect of hCG Pretreatment on cAMP
Content of Ovarian Tissue after Treatment with
Cloprostenol In Vivo (mean ± SEM)

| Treatment | | cAMP | |
hCG (25 IU - 0 hr)	Cloprostenol (5 µg - 1 hr)	(pmol/mg protein) (1½ hr)	n
-	-	17 ± 1	5
-	+	13 ± 1[c]	5
+	-	653 ± 75[b]	5
+	+	29 ± 4[a]	4

[a] p < 0.008 vs. control
[b] p < 0.004 vs. control
[c] Wilcoxon test not significant vs. control

hCG Injection induces loss of adenylyl cyclase
responsiveness, but this aspect of the hCG desensitization
process takes 6 hr or more to occur (for a review see Catt et
al., 1979). Our findings are in agreement with those results
as no effect was detected on the adenylyl cyclase activity 90
min after hCG injection. The loss of hCG responsiveness
following PG administration occurred much faster than seen
during hCG induced desensitization. Thus the mechanism by
which the two substances regulate the adenylyl cyclase
responsiveness has to be different, at least in the early
phase.

It has been suggested that the LH receptor was involved
in PG induced luteolysis since hCG injection protects the CL
against the luteolytic effects of subsequent $PGF_{2\alpha}$ administration (Fuchs et al., 1974; Aakvaag and Torjesen, 1981).
The model of Henderson and McNatty (1977) suggesting that the
binding of hCG to the LH receptor prevented the subsequent
binding of $PGF_{2\alpha}$ to its receptor provided an attractive
hypothesis for this protection. The present data show that
pretreatment with hCG does not prevent a $PGF_{2\alpha}$ analogue from
having an effect on the CL, in fact identical values were

observed for adenylyl cyclase activity after cloprostenol regardless of hCG pretreatment.

5.   General Discussion

PG induced luteolysis in the superluteinized rat seems to consist of three phases: (1) A period of rapid block of progesterone production which coincides with a decreased adenylyl cyclase response to activation. (2) A phase of resumed steroidogenesis from 4 to 12 hr after PG administration which is accompanied by reactivation of adenylyl cyclase response to stimulation and increasing basal adenylyl cyclase activity as well as ovarian cAMP content. (3) A phase of selectively decreased adenylyl cyclase response to hCG activation and loss of LH receptor.

During the initial phase of PG induced luteolysis the changes in hCG, isoproterenol and fluoride activated adenylyl cyclase correlated with steroid secretion. As no changes were observed in ovarian cAMP content or basal adenylyl cyclase activity, one may postulate a causal relationship between initiation of luteolysis and generally decreased adenylyl cyclase response to stimulation.

Our observations are in agreement with those of Thomas et al. (1978) who reported that $PGF_{2\alpha}$ blocked the LH activated production of cAMP in cultured luteal cells while $PGF_{2\alpha}$ alone had no effect on cellular cAMP accumulation or the adenylyl cyclase activity. Furthermore, the block could not be prevented by the addition of theophylline, indicating that phosphodiesterase was not involved. Khan and Rosberg (1979) reported the effect of $PGF_{2\alpha}$ treatment on epinephrine and fluoride as well as LH stimulated adenylyl cyclase in isolated CL from pmSG treated rats, thus emphasizing the general nature of the loss of adenylyl cyclase response to activation following administration of $PGF_{2\alpha}$.

We have previously reported the effect of a repeated cloprostenol treatment 24 hr after the first (Aakvaag and Torjesen, 1981), at a time of reduced LH receptor quantity and reduced adenylyl cyclase response to hCG activation. Nevertheless, the repeated PG treatment leads to a drop in the serum 20α-DHP levels which resembled that of progesterone after the first injection. Thus, the PG induced block of steroidogenesis was independent of LH receptor quantity and intact adenylyl cyclase response to hCG activation, again suggesting that PG modifies the adenylyl cyclase in a general way beyond the binding of LH to its receptor.

It is postulated that the initiation of luteolysis is in some way related to reduced adenylyl cyclase response to stimulation. The tissue content of cAMP did, however, remain constant after PG administration. One may postulate that the block in steroid production could be due to changes in tissue levels of cAMP that were too small to be detected. In this connection it may be of relevance that Mendelson et al. (1975) found that the testosterone production of isolated Leydig cells were maximally stimulated by LH before cellular cAMP levels were significantly increased.

Previously it was reported that hCG pretreatment protected the CL against the luteolytic effect of subsequent PG administration in vivo. As $PGF_{2\alpha}$ was shown to decrease the LH stimulated progesterone secretion in cultured luteal cells (Thomas et al., 1978), there seemed to be a difference between the effect of PG treatment in vitro and in vivo. In the present study we confirmed that hCG pretreatment protected the ovary against the luteolytic action of cloprostenol, although the $PGF_{2\alpha}$ analogue did have effects on adenylyl cyclase and the tissue cAMP concentration. The fact that the tissue concentration of cAMP was still above that seen in untreated animals, might suggest that there could be a critical concentration of cAMP under which luteolysis may occur.

Norjavaara et al. (1982) showed that adrenaline stimulated cAMP and progesterone production in isolated CL of pmSG treated rats vary with the age of the CL. We found a correlation between steroidogenesis and isoproterenol stimulated adenylyl cyclase activity during PG induced luteolysis. These observations suggest a functional role for catecholamines in the regulation of CL function. Further studies are needed to investigate possible sources for catecholamines in the ovary and how they vary with CL function.

During the phase of resumed steroidogenesis a close correlation was found between steroid production and all measured aspects of cAMP production, i.e. ovarian cAMP content, basal, hCG, isoproterenol, fluoride and PGE_1 stimulated adenylyl cyclase. The mechanism for this general activation of adenylyl cyclase activity could involve prolactin as the serum levels of prolactin were increased 5- to 10-fold between 3 and 9 hr after cloprostenol injection (Torjesen et al., 1978).

The third phase of cloprostenol induced luteolysis seems to be the only part of the luteolytic process that involves the LH receptor. A selective loss of hCG responsive adenylyl cyclase was measured, which could be related to the loss of LH receptor.

In conclusion, the initial effect of PG induced luteolysis seemed to involve a decreased adenylyl cyclase response to stimulation by several activators. This general modification of the adenylyl cyclase activity did not involve increased GTPase activity, but the GTP binding unit might be affected in other ways. The data are also compatible with a direct effect on the catalytic unit of the adenylyl cyclase complex.

ACKNOWLEDGMENTS. Cloprostenol (ICI 80996) was kindly supplied by Dr. Bolton of the Imperial Chemical Industries Limited, England. We are grateful to Ms. Sidsel Bugge for expert technical help and to Ms. Kjersti Gunneng for secretarial help.

REFERENCES

Aakvaag, A., and Torjesen, P. A., 1981, Prostaglandin-induced luteolysis in the superluteinized rat ovary, in: "Reproductive Processes and Contraception," K. W. McKerns, ed., pp. 677-690, Plenum Publishing Corp., New York.

Birnbaumer, L., Yang, P.-C., Hunzicker-Dunn, M., Bockaert, J., and Duran, J. M., 1976, Adenylyl cyclase activities in ovarian tissues. I. Homogenization and condition of assay in graafian follicles and corpora lutea of rabbits, rats, and pigs: Regulation by ATP, and some comparative properties, Endocrinology, 99:163.

Catt, K. J., Harwood, J. P., Richert, N. D., Conn, P. M., Conti, M., and Dufau, M. L., 1979, Luteal desensitization:

Hormonal regulation of LH receptors, adenylate cyclase and steroidogenesis in the luteal cell, in: "Ovarian Follicular and Corpus Luteum Function," C. P. Channing, J. Marsh, W. A. Sadler, eds., pp. 647-662, Plenum Press, New York.

Fuchs, A.-R., Mok, E., and Sundaram, K., 1974, Luteolytic effects of prostaglandins in rat pregnancy, and reversal by luteinizing hormone, Acta Endocrinol. Copenh., 76:583.

Gilman, A., 1970, A protein binding assay for adenosine 3',5'-cyclic monophosphate, Proc. Natl. Acad. Sci. USA, 67:305.

Henderson, K. M., and McNatty, K. P., 1977, A possible inter-relationship between gonadotrophin stimulation and prostaglandin $F_{2\alpha}$ inhibition of steroidogenesis by granulosa cells in vivo, J. Endocrinol., 73:71.

Hichens, M., Grinwich, D. L., and Behrman, H. R., 1974, $PGF_{2\alpha}$ induced loss of corpus luteum gonadotrophin receptors, Prostaglandins, 7:449.

Horton, E. W., and Poyser, N. L., 1976, Uterine luteolytic hormone: A physiological role for prostaglandin $F_{2\alpha}$. Physiol. Rev., 56:595.

Hunzicker-Dunn, M., Derda, D., Jungmann, R. A., and Birnbaumer, L., 1979, Resensitization of the desensitized follicular adenylyl cyclase system to luteinizing hormone, Endocrinology, 104:1785.

Kahn, M. I., and Rosberg, S., 1979, Acute suppression by $PGF_{2\alpha}$ on LH, epinephrine and fluoride stimulation of adenylate cyclase in rat luteal tissue, J. Cyclic Nucleotide Res., 5:55.

Lee, C. Y., 1979, hCG induced loss of LH-hCG receptor and desensitization of adenylate cyclase, in: "Ovarian Follicular and Corpus Luteum Function," C. P. Channing, J. Marsh, W. A. Sadler, eds., pp. 717-722, Plenum Press, New York.

Mendelson, C., Dufau, M., and Catt, K., 1975, Gonadotropin binding and stimulation of cyclic adenosine 3':5'-monophosphate and testosterone production in isolated Leydig cells, J. Biol. Chem., 250:8818.

Norjavaara, E., Selstam, G., and Ahrén, K., 1982, Catecholamine stimulation of cyclic AMP and progesterone production in rat corpora lutea of different ages, Acta Endocrinol. Copenh, 100:613.

Parlow, A. F., 1961, Bioassay of luteinizing hormone by ovarian ascorbic acid depletion, in: "Human Pituitary Gonadotrophins," A. Albert, ed., pp. 300-310, Charles C. Thomas, Springfield, Illinois.

Rodbell, M., 1980, The role of hormone receptors and GTP-regu-
    latory proteins in membrane transduction, Nature (London),
    284:17.
Spiegel, A. M., and Downs, R. W. Jr., 1981, Guanine nucleotides:
    Key regulators of hormone receptor-adenylate cyclase inter-
    action, Endocrine Rev., 2:275.
Thomas, J.-P., Dorflinger, L. J., and Behrman, H. R., 1978,
    Mechanism of the rapid antigonadotropic action of prosta-
    glandins in cultured luteal cells, Proc. Natl. Acad. Sci.
    USA, 75:1344.
Torjesen, P. A., and Aakvaag, A., 1977, The serum levels
    of progesterone and 20α-dihydroprogesterone, and the
    ovarian LH, FSH, and PRL binding during luteolysis of
    the superluteinized rat ovary, Acta Endocrinol. Copenh.,
    86:162.
Torjesen, P. A., Dahlin, R., Haug, E., and Aakvaag, A., 1978,
    The sequence of hormonal changes during prostaglandin
    induced luteolysis of the superluteinized rat ovary, Acta
    Endocrinol. Copenh., 87:617.
Wakeling, A. E., and Green, L. R., 1981, In vitro and in vivo
    effects of a luteolytic prostaglandin (Estrumate, I.C.I.
    80996) on rat ovarian adenylate cyclase activity, Biochem.
    Soc. Trans., 9:94.
Wiest, W. G., Kidwell, W. R., and Balogh, K. Jr., 1968,
    Progesterone catabolism in the rat ovary: A regulatory
    mechanism for progestational potency during pregnancy,
    Endocrinology, 82:844.

DISCUSSION

RAO: Is there a change in the sensitivity of the corpus
luteum to PGF as a function of age of corpus luteum?

TORJESEN: We have not studied that, but other investigators
have reported that $PGF_{2\alpha}$ does not induce luteolysis for the
first 2 days following ovulation.

BIRNBAUMER: In your studies, $PGF_{2\alpha}$-induced luteolysis is
associated with a decreased progesterone production but a
dramatic increase in 20α-DHP. According to my simplistic
view, luteolysis is associated with regression of the corpus
luteum and cell death. How can you then explain the dramatic
increase in steroidogenesis?

TORJESEN: The steroidogenesis is after a period of inhibition switched over to 20α-DHP, reflecting the induction of the enzyme 20α-hydroxysteroid dehydrogenase. The secretion of 20α-DHP continues for more than 2 days in our animal model.

ELECTROPHOSIOLOGICAL ASPECTS OF THE RESPONSE OF PITUITARY

CELLS TO STEROID AND PEPTIDE HORMONES

Bernard Dufy, Luce Dufy-Barbe, Evelyne Zyzek, Jean-Marc
Israel and Jean-Didier Vincent

Inserm - U.176 - Rue Camille Saint-Saëns
Bordeaux-Cedex 33077 (France)

1.   Introduction

The mechanism by which physiological secretagogues
control the release of anterior pituitary hormones has been
the subject of numerous studies over the past ten years. It
has been clearly demonstrated that the release of these
hormones is a calcium-dependent process (for review, see
Trifaro, 1977). However, the exact source of calcium is
still a matter of controversy since a number of reports
favor intracellular calcium sources (Moriarty, 1977; Hopkins
and Walker, 1978).

Recently, certain cells from the anterior pituitary have
been shown to be excitable and to exhibit action potentials
in response to physiological stimuli (for review, see Dufy
and Vincent, 1982). A similar phenomenon has been observed
in other endocrine cells secreting peptides, for example,
cells of the endocrine pancreas (Dean and Matthews, 1970;
Meissmer and Schmelz, 1974; Matthews and Sakamoto, 1975;
Atwater et al., 1979). The electrical excitability of endocrine cells which pairs them to neurons may arise from a
common enbryological origin (Pearse and Takor, 1976). Excitable endocrine cells belong to the Pearse's APUD (amine
precursor uptake and decarboxylase) system, they arise from
the neuroendocrine programmed ectoblast and constitute the
third endocrine division of the nervous system.

The ionic requirements for action potentials in endocrine
cells is different from those of neurons. They also differ
among the various types of endocrine cells: most pituitary

73

cells of the pars distalis only require calcium (Ca^{2+})
(Kidokoro, 1975; Dufy et al., 1979; Taraskevich and Douglas,
1980) whereas cells of the pars intermedia seem to require
both Na^+ and Ca^{2+} to substain spiking activity (Douglas and
Taraskevich, 1978). However, spiking activity always results
in an activation of Ca^{2+} channels and hence an increase in
intracellular Ca^{2+} concentration. Calcium ions which enter
the cells as a result of action potentials may then provide
the ionized calcium required for the process of exocytosis.
This hypothesis is consistent with observations that in
pituitary cells the response to a number of substances that
stimulate the release of prolactin (PRL) is associated with
an increase in the firing rate of action potentials and
conversely, the response to several substances known to
inhibit hormone release is a reduction or cessation of firing
(Dufy et al., 1979a,b). However, at the present time a
generalization of this hypothesis to all types of pituitary
cells is hazardous. Although the calcium requirement for the
action of several neuropeptides has been adequately demonstrated, it is not yet proven that a single mechanism controls
the membrane permeability to this ion (Dufy et al., 1982).
Using electrophysiological techniques we present evidence
that physiological stimuli for pituitary hormone release may
control membrane ionic permeabilities in different ways.

2.   Materials and Methods

The introduction of electrophysiological techniques to
the study of glandular cells, such as they were utilized on
the nerve or the neuron, has given results demonstrating the
ionic movements during the resting or activity phases and the
chronology of cellular activation evoqued by hormonal stimulation (Kidokoro, 1975; Taraskevich and Douglas, 1977, 1980;
Dufy et al., 1979a,b; Ozawa and Kimura, 1979; Sand et al.,
1980). Electrophysiological investigations do allow a very
precise temporal resolution for the measure of the electrical
phenomena and the possibility of studying single cells.
Moreover, individual properties of ionic channels can be
studied by voltage-clamp techniques and membrane noise
analysis, recently introduced (Dufy and Baker, 1982).

The first attempt to study electrophysiological properties of pituitary cells were done in vivo (York et al.,
1973). The difficulties of the approach, the impossibility

of characterizing the recording cells hindered the interpretation of the results obtained. With the aim of characterizing
the electrophysiological properties of pituitary cells, most
of the recent works have used pituitary cells in culture as
either primary cultures (Taraskevich and Douglas, 1977, 1978)
or permanent clonal cell lines (Dufy et al., 1982). Several
methods have been successfully used to enrich cell dissociates
to obtain a particular pituitary cell type. Velocity sedimentation of isolated pituitary cells at unit gravity has proved
to be a suitable method for obtaining fractions which are
enriched in somatotrophs, mammotrophs (Hymer et al., 1974,
1976), thyrotrophs (Leuschen et al., 1978), gonadotrophs
(Denef et al., 1976; Benoist et al., 1981). However, no
electrophysiological data has been obtained up to now from
these enriched cell populations. Reasonably homogeneous
populations of TSH, PRL, GH and ACTH-secreting human pituitary
cells can also be obtained following dissociation of corresponding human pituitary adenoma. Electrophysiological
recordings may be performed on cells 4 days to 3 months after
plating (Dufy et al., 1982).

The models extensively used for the study of pituitary
cellular functions are the continuous anterior pituitary
cell lines. At present, the GH3 clonal cell line and
its sub-clones, isolated from a rat anterior pituitary
tumor which is shown to secrete growth hormone (GH) and
prolactin (PRL), (Tashjian et al., 1970; Tixier-Vidal
et al., 1975) are the most extensively studied and are
considered as a reference. Morphology of the GH3 cells,
their secretory behavior to various drugs (Ostlund et al.,
1978; Gourdji, 1980) and their electrophysiological characteristics have been studied in detail (for review see references
above).

3.   The Electrically Operated Calcium Channel

It has been known for a long-time that high potassium
(K^+) stimultes anterior pituitary hormone release (Gautvik
and Tashjian, 1973; Milligan and Kraicer, 1974; Ostlund et
al., 1978). The effect of potassium on hormone release is
dependent upon extracellular calcium and the depolarization-
secretion coupling is thought to be mediated by the influx of
calcium ions from the extracellular fluid through voltage
sensitive Ca^{2+}-channels (Douglas, 1968).

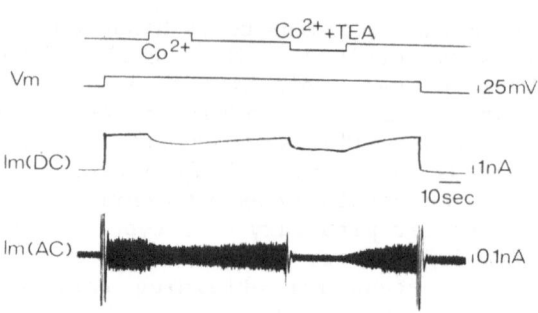

Figure 1. Effect of Co^{2+} (1 mM) and Co^{2+} (1 mM) and TEA (2 mM) on ionic channels activated by depolarization (GH3/B6 pituitary cell); Im (Dc) represents membrane current and Im (Ac) membrane current fluctuations. Membrane potential (Vm) was held under voltage clamp at -45 mV and stepped at -15 mV. Co^{2+} partially blocks the outward current response and associated increase in Im (Ac) activated at -15 mV. TEA applied in addition to Co^{2+} further attenuates the current response and associated variance (from Dufy and Barker, 1982).

Recent experiments have shown that there are at least two pharmacologically distinct K^+ permeabilities present in the membranes of GH3 cells (Dufy and Barker, 1982). The first one, P_K, is increased by membrane depolarization and is partially blocked by tetraethylammonium (TEA); the other, $P_{K[Ca^{2+}]_i}$ is activated by an increase in the level of intracellular Ca^{2+} and is blocked by cobalt (Co^{2+}) (Fig. 1). The effect of TEA both on P_K and as a stimulating agent of PRL release might be explained by that part of the K^+ permeability in GH3 cells which is sensitive to variation in the membrane potential. By depolarizing the cell and prolonging action potential duration, TEA may increase Ca^{2+} entry and thereby stimulate PRL increase. Similarly, thyroliberin (TRH) rapidly increases membrane resistance of human pituitary cells in culture; this effect is associated with a depolarization and a generation of Ca^{2+} dependent action potentials (Fig. 2).

Recent studies on the nature of this initial depolarization of the membrane of human pituitary cells suggest that this is due principally to a rapid reduction in K^+ permeability (Dufy et al., 1982).

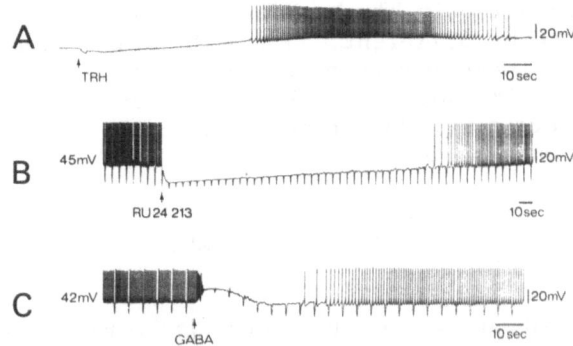

Figure 2. Effect of TRH (0.5×10^{-6}M), of a dopamine agonist from Roussel-UCLAF (RU 24213; 10^{-6}M) and GABA (10^{-4}M) on the electrical activity of 3 pituitary cells cultured from human pituitary fragments. The substances were administered through a micropipet by a pressure injection system. TRH induced a depolarization which triggered a burst of action potentials. Ejection of RU 24213 clearly induced a strong hyperpolarization associated with a decrease in the resistance of the membrane. Hyperpolarizing current pulses (downward deflection) of fixed amplitude (0.2 nA) were used to measure the membrane resistance. GABA induced a depolarizing response owing to a decrease of the membrane resistance. The results show that human pituitary cells are sensitive to GABA. The action of GABA is mediated by a strong decrease in the membrane input resistance and differs from the effect of DA and DA agonist.

Estrogen, which has been shown to rapidly increase PRL release (Zyzek et al., 1981) is also able to induce Ca^{2+} spikes in pituitary cells (Dufy et al., 1979); however, the mechanism of action of this steroid is not yet understood.

Conversely, depamine (DA) or the DA-agonist RU 24213 (Roussel UCLAF) hyperpolarize the cell through a rapid increase in membrane permeability. The reversal potential of this effect, which is close to -90 mV, suggests that DA inhibition of Ca^{2+} spikes is also achieved by way of a rapid change in K^+ permeability.

These few examples show that the membrane permeability of pituitary cells to K^+ ions is the key to the control of electrically operated Ca^{2+}-channels. The mechanism of action

of TEA, which directly blocks potassium channels, and that of
TRH is certainly different. The molecular understanding of
interaction between neuropeptides such as TRH and the potassium channel is not yet clear. However, like for the
muscarinic receptor, the effector molecule appears to be a
plasma membrane channel.

4.   Receptors Mediated Changes in Membrane Ionic
      Permeabilities

Recent advances in the techniques of pituitary cell
culture and in the assay of pituitary hormones have provided
considerable information on the intracellular processing and
the release mechanisms of adenohypophyseal hormones.

In most early studies, the cellular mechanisms leading
to increased hormone production were thought to be mediated
by interaction of the secretagogue with a receptor site,
activation of an adenylate cyclase molecule and subsequent
production of the second messenger cyclic-AMP (for review,
see Tixier-Vidal and Gourdji, 1981). Although the Ca^{2+}
requirement has been adequately demonstrated, its relation
with cyclic-AMP is less understood. It has been suggested
that cyclic-AMP may increase the intracellular ionized concentration of Ca^{2+} using a cyclic-AMP-mediated increase in cell
membrane permeability to Ca^{2+} or may mobilize Ca^{2+} from an
intracellular pool of stored Ca^{2+} (for review see Greengard,
1978).

Somatostatin (SRIF) which has been isolated for its
inhibitory effect on GH release from adeno-hypophyseal cells
has also been found to affect PRL release (Drouin et al.,
1976). Whereas SIRF does not seem to affect basal release of
PRL, the peptide blocks the stimulation of PRL release induced
by TRH (Enjalbert et al., 1982).

The mechanisms of such interactions have been analyzed
using electrophysiological techniques. Under conventional
recording conditions, SRIF does not modify membrane resistance of GH3 cells recorded at resting level and does not
affect action potentials, except in a few cases where action
potentials were reduced in amplitude. Under voltage clamp,
SRIF induced a slow and progressive decrease in membrane
conductance for depolarized levels (Fig. 3) with a slow and
progressive decrease of the calcium inward current. Therefore

cells treated by SRIF showed a reduced permeability of electrically operated Ca^{2+} channels. This reduced permeability developed over a 10 min period; this contrasts sharply with changes in K^+ conductance following RU 24213 which occured within seconds. Although the receptor coupling process of SRIF in GH and PRL secreting cells is still poorly understood, a number of studies have favored a possible involvement of adenylate cyclase (Borgeat et al., 1974). The finding that SIRF progressively reduces the conductance of electrically operated Ca^{2+} channels suggests the possibility of a receptor mediated control in Ca^{2+} permeability of pituitary cells.

5. Peptides That Do Not Affect Electrically Operated Ca^{2+} Channels

In contrast to peptides such as TRH or SRIF which operate directly or indirectly through voltage dependent Ca^{2+} channels, other peptidergic substances do not modify the electrophysiological properties of pituitary cells. This is the case for vasoactive intestinal peptide (VIP), a well known gut peptide, which has been shown to be a powerful stimulator of PRL release.

While the role of cyclic-AMP mediating the release of pituitary hormones remains controversial, a number of investigators have presented evidence that VIP stimulates the release

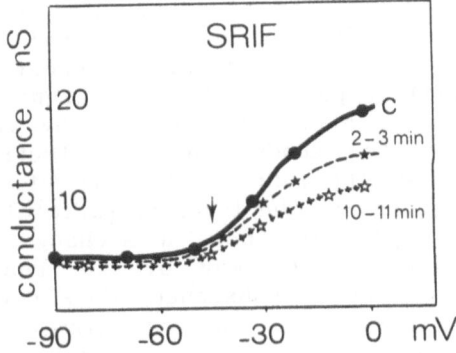

Figure 3. Progressive decrease in membrane conductance following administration of somatostatin (SRIF; 10^{-6}M).

of PRL by its ability to activate cyclic-AMP. Indeed, in a
number of systems, VIP has been shown to activate adenylate
cyclase; in PRL secreting cells, the peptide increases cyclic-
AMP production and is a real stimulator of PRL secretion
(Ruberg et al., 1978; Bataille et al., 1979; Gourdji et al.,
1979; Enjalbert et al., 1980; Rotsztejn et al., 1980). In
many tissues, cyclic-AMP plays a role as a modulator of
calcium homeostasis and may contribute to the mobilization of
intracellular sequestered Ca^{2+}. Therefore, it is conceivable
that stimulation of hormone release by activation of cyclic-
AMP and mobilization of intracellular stores of Ca^{2+} does not
have the same requirements for Ca^{2+} ions as a stimulation
which by-passes the cyclic-AMP system. Transmembrane influx
of Ca^{2+} such as those which may be predicted from the Ca^{2+}-
dependent action potentials induced by TRH, do not occur and
may not be necessary for stimulation of PRL release by VIP
(Dufy et al., 1982).

6.   Conclusion

Electrophysiological studies of pituitary cells in
culture have shown that these cells are excitable and able to
display Ca^{2+}-dependent action potentials generated via
electrically operated Ca^{2+} channels. There is a general
agreement that K^+, which passively depolarizes membranes,
stimulates the release of secretion products: this depolarization opens the voltage-dependent Ca^{2+} channels. In contrast
to this unspecific process, a number of substances stimulate
or inhibit hormonal release by interactions with specific
receptor sites and then by altering the electrical properties
of the cells (modification of K^+ or Cl^- conductance) lead to
activation or inactivation of electrically operated Ca^{2+}
channels. This process occurs with a short time course (in
terms of seconds) suggesting that few steps are involved. A
second mechanism of action is mediated by slowly developing
modifications of the conductance of electrically operated
Ca^{2+} channels. As the functional state of calcium channels
is probably dependent on the level of intracellular cyclic-AMP
metabolism, it is possible that these changes in Ca^{2+} permeabilities are mediated by way of one enzymatic process.
Finally, a third type of substances does not affect voltage
dependent Ca^{2+} conductance. The mechanism of action of these
substances appear to involve a receptor-mediated enzymatic
process which may lead to mobilization of intracellular Ca^{2+}
stores or ionic movements which we have not been able to
detect with our electrophysiological techniques.

REFERENCES

Atwater, I., Dawson, C. M., Ribalet, B., and Rojas, E., 1979,
    Potassium permeability activated by intracellular calcium
    in the pancreatic cell, J. Physiol. 288:575.
Bataille, D., Peillon, F., Besson, J., and Rosselin, G., 1979,
    Vasoactive intestinal peptide (VIP): recepteurs spécifi-
    ques et activation de l'adénylate cyclase dans une tumeur
    hypophysaire humaine à prolactine, C. R. Acad. Sci. D
    (Paris) 288:1315.
Borgeat, P., Labrie, F., Drouin, J., Belanger, A., Immer, I.,
    Seetany, K., Nelson, V., Grotz, M., Schally, A. V., Coy,
    D. H., and Coy, E. J., 1974, Inhibition of adenosine 3'-5'-
    monophosphate accumulation in anterior pituitary gland in
    vitro by growth hormone release inhibiting hormone,
    Biochem. Biophys. Res. Commun. 56:1052.
Benoist, L., Le Dafniet, M., Rotsztejn, W. H., Besson, J., and
    Duval, J., 1981, Gonadotrophin release by gonadotrophs
    incubated with gonadotrophin-releasing hormone is inde-
    pendent of intracellular c-AMP accumulation, Acta Endo.
    Kbh 97:329.
Dean, P. M., and Matthews, E. K., 1970, Glucose-induced elec-
    trical activity in pancreatic islet cells, J. Physiol.
    210:255.
Denef, C., Hautekee, E., and Rubin, L., 1976, A specific popu-
    lation of gonadotrophs purified from immature female rat
    pituitaries, Science 194:848.
Douglas, W. W., 1968, Stimulus-secretion coupling: the concept
    and clues from chromaffin and other cells, Br. J. Pharma-
    col. 34:451.
Douglas, W. W., and Taraskevich, P. S., 1978, Action potentials
    in gland cells in rat pituitary pars intermedia: inhibi-
    tion by dopamine, an inhibitor of MSH secretion, J.
    Physiol. 285:171.
Drouin, J., De Lean, A., Rainville, D., Lachance, R., and
    Labrie, F., 1976, Characteristics of the interaction
    between thyrotropin releasing hormone and somatostatin for
    thyrotropin and prolactin release, Endocrinology 98:514.
Dufy, B., and Barker, J. L., 1982, Calcium-activated and
    voltage-dependent potassium conductances in clonal pitui-
    tary cells, Life Sci. 30:1933.
Dufy, B., and Vincent, J. D., 1982, Electrophysiology of anter-
    ior pituitary cells, in: "Pituitary Hormones and Related
    Peptides", M. Motta, M. Zanisi and F. Piva, eds., pp. 89-
    99, Academic Press, London and New York.

Dufy, B., Vincent, J. D., Fleury, H., Du Pasquier, P., Gourdji, D., and Tixier-Vidal, A., 1979a, Membrane effects of thyrotropin-releasing hormone and estrogen shown by intracellular recording from pituitary cells, Science 204:509.

Dufy, B., Vincent, J. D., Fleury, H., Du Pasquier, P., Gourdji, D., and Tixier-Vidal, A., 1979b, Dopamine inhibition of action potentials in a prolactin secreting cell line is modulated by estrogen, Nature 282:855.

Dufy, B., Israël, J. M., Zyzek, E., Dufy-Barbe, L., Guerin, J., Fleury, H., and Vincent, J. D., 1982, An electrophysiological study of cultured human pituitary cells, Mol. Cell. Endocrinol. 27:179.

Dufy, B., Israël, J. M., Zyzek, E., and Gourdji, D., 1982, Differential effects of K^+, TRH and VIP on the electrophysiological properties of pituitary cells in culture, Neuroendocrinology Lett. 4:245.

Dufy, B., Zyzek, E., and Dufy-Barbe, L., 1982, Etude electrophysiologique des propriétés des canaux ioniques associés à la libération des hormones hypophysaires, in: "Multihormonal Regulations in Neuroendocrine Cells", Colloques Internationaux de l'INSERM (in press).

Enjalbert, A., Arancibia, S., Ruberg, M., Priam, M., Bluet-Pajot, M. T., Rotsztejn, W. H., and Kordon, C., 1980, Stimulation of in vitro prolactin release by vasoactive intestinal peptide (VIP), Neuroendocrinology 31:200.

Enjalbert, A., Epelbaum, J., Arancibia, S., Tapia-Arancibia, L., Bluet-Pajot, M. T., and Kordon, C., 1982, Reciprocal interactions of somatostatin with thyrotropin-releasing hormone and vasoactive peptide on prolactin and growth hormone secretion in vitro, Endocrinology 111:42.

Gautvik, K. M., and Tashjian, A. H., 1973, Effects of Ca^{++} and Mg^{++} on secretion and synthesis of growth hromone and prolactin by clonal strains of pituitary cells in culture, Endocrinology 92:573.

Gourdji, D., 1980, Characterization of thyroliberin, (TRH) binding sites and coupling with prolactin and growth hormone secretion in rat pituitary cell lines, in: "Synthesis and Release of Adenohypophyseal Hormones", M. Jutisz and K. W. McKerns, eds., pp. 463-493, Plenum Press, New York.

Gourdji, D., Bataille, D., Vauclin, N., Grouselle, D., Rosselin, G., and Tixier-Vidal, A., 1979, Vasoactive intestinal peptide (VIP) stimulates prolactin (PRL) release and c-AMP production in a rat pituitary cell line (GH3/B6). Additive effects of VIP and TRH on PRL release, FEBS Lett. 104:165.

Greengard, P., 1978, "Cyclic Nucleotides, Phosphorylated Pro-
    teins, and Neuronal Function", (Distinguished lecture
    series of the Society of General Physiologists, Vol. 1)
    Raven Press, New York.
Hopkins, C. R., and Walker, A. M., 1978, Calcium as a second
    messenger in the stimulation of luteinizing hormone secre-
    tion, Mol. Cell. Endocrinol. 12:189.
Hymer, W. C., Snyder, J., Wilfinger, W., Swanson, N., and Davis,
    J. A., 1974, Separation of pituitary mammotrophs from the
    female rat by velocity sedimentation at unit gravity,
    Endocrinology 95:107.
Hymer, W. C., Snyder, J., Wilfinger, W., Bergland, R., Fisher,
    B., and Pearson, O., 1976, Characterization of mammotrophs
    separated from the human pituitary gland, J. Nat. Cancer
    Inst. 57:995.
Kidokoro, Y., 1975, Spontaneous calcium action potentials in a
    clonal pituitary cell line and their relationship to pro-
    lactin secretion, Nature 58:741.
Leuschen, M. P., Tobin, R., and Moriarty, M., 1978, Enriched
    populations of pituitary thyrotrophs in monolayer culture,
    Endocrinology 102:509.
Matthews, E. K., and Sakamoto, Y., 1975, Electrical character-
    istics of pancreatic islet cells, J. Physiol. 246:421.
Meissmer, H. P., and Schmelz, H., 1974, Membrane potential of
    beta-cells in pancreatic islets, Pflügers Arch. 351:195.
Milligan, J. V., and Kraicer, J., 1974, Physical characteristics
    of the Ca^{2+} compartments associated with in vitro ACTH
    release, Endocrinology 94:435.
Moriarty, C. M., 1977, Involvement of intracellular calcium in
    hormone secretion from rat pituitary cells, Mol. Cell.
    Endocrinol. 6:349.
Ostlund, R. E., Leung, J. T., Hajek, S. V., Winokur, T.,
    and Melman, M., 1978, Acute stimulated hormone release
    from cultured GH3 pituitary cells, Endocrinology
    103:1245.
Ozawa, S., and Kimura, N., 1979, Membrane potential changes
    caused by thyrotropin-releasing hormone in the clonal
    GH3 cell and their relationship to secretion of pituitary
    hormone, Proc. Natl. Acad. Sci. USA 76:6017.
Pearse, A. G. E., and Takor, T., 1976, Neuroendocrine embryology
    and the APUD concept, Clin. Endocrinol. 5:2299.
Rotsztejn, W. H., Benoist, L., Besson, J., Beraud, G., Bluet-
    Pajot, M. T., Kordon, C., Rosselin, G., and Duval, J.,
    1980, Effect of vasoactive intestinal peptide (VIP) on the
    release of adenohypophyseal hormones from purified cells
    obtained by unit gravity sedimentation. Inhibition by

dexamethasone of VIP-induced prolactin release, Neuroendocrinology 31:282.

Ruberg, M., Rotsztejn, W. H., Arancibia, S., Besson, J., and
Enjalbert, A., 1978, Stimulation of prolactin release by
vasoactive intestinal polypeptide (VIP), Eur. J. Pharmacol.
51:319.

Sand, O., Haug, E., and Gautvik, K. M., 1980, Effects of thyroliberin and 4-amino-pyridine on action potentials and
prolactin release and synthesis in rat pituitary cells in
culture, Acta. Physiol. Scan. 108:247.

Taraskevich, P. S., and Douglas, W. W., 1977, Action potentials
occur in cells of normal anterior pituitary gland and are
stimulated by the hypophysiotropic peptide thyrotropin-
releasing hormone, Proc. Natl. Acad. Sci. USA 74:4064.

Taraskevich, P. S., and Douglas, W. W., 1978, Catecholamines of
supposed inhibitory hypophysiotropic function suppress
action potentials in prolactin cells, Nature 276:832.

Taraskevich, P. S., and Douglas, W. W., 1980, Electrical
behavior in a line of anterior pituitary cells (GH cells)
and the influence of the hypothalamic peptide thyrotropin-
releasing factor, Neuroscience 5:421.

Tashjian, A. H., Bancroft, F. C., and Levine, L., 1970, Production of both prolactin and growth hormone by clonal strains
of rat pituitary tumor cells, J. Cell. Biol. 47:61.

Tixier-Vidal, A., and Gourdji, D., 1981, Mechanism of action of
synthetic hypothalamic peptides on anterior pituitary
cells, Physiol. Reviews 61:974.

Tixier-Vidal, A., Gourdji, D., Pradelles, P., Morgat, J. L.,
Fromageot, P., and Kerdeluhex, B., 1975, A cell culture
approach to the study of TRH receptors, in: "Hypothalamic
Hormones", M. Motta, P. Grosignani, and L. Martini, eds.,
pp. 89-107, Academic Press, London.

Trifaro, J. M., 1977, Common mechanism of hormone secretion,
Ann. Rev. Pharmacol. Toxicol., 17:27.

York, D. H., Baker, F., and Kraicer, J., 1973, Electrical
changes induced in rat adenohypophysial cells, in vivo,
with hypothalamic extract, Neuroendocrinology 11:212.

Zyzek, E., Dufy-Barbe, L., Dufy, B., and Vincent, J. D., 1981,
Short-term effect of estrogen on release of prolactin by
pituitary cells in culture, Biochem. Biophys. Res. Commun.
102:1151.

Regulation of Insulin Responsiveness

HORMONAL REGULATION OF ADENYLYL CYCLASE ACTIVITY

Howard J. Kirchick[a], Juan Codina[a], John D.
Hildebrandt[a], Ravi Iyengar[a], Francisco J. Rojas[a],
Joel Abramowitz[b], Mary Hunzicker-Dunn[c], and
Lutz Birnbaumer[a]

[a]Department of Cell Biology, Baylor College of
Medicine, Houston, TX 77030
[b]Iowa State University, Department of Zoology,
Ames, IO
[c]Northwestern University School of Medicine,
Department of Biochemistry, Chicago, IL 60611

1. Introduction

Peptide and protein hormones such as glucagon and gonadotropins and neurotransmitters such as chatecholamines exert
their action on target cells by binding to their respective
receptors (R). These interactions lead to stimulation of
cAMP formation by the adenylyl cyclase systems in these
cells. In what follows we shall review and present key
experimental evidences on functional aspects of cAMP formation by adenylyl cyclases as seen both in the absence and
presence of hormonal influence. We shall present current
knowledge on the molecular composition and structure of
hormone sensitive adenylyl cyclases. Taking structural as
well as functional aspects into account we shall discuss
current thoughts on how both hormonal stimulation and the
ensuing desensitization to hormonal stimulation come about.
Finally we shall present some speculations as to other forms
of regulation, especially attenuation of cAMP formation
and raise some of the most pertinent questions in signal
transduction research.

2.   Kinetic and Molecular Aspects of Adenylyl Cyclase
      Regulation in the Absence of Hormone

The active substrate for adenylyl cyclase is MgATP
(Sutherland and Rall, 1962; Birnbaumer et al., 1969). It is
converted to cAMP and MgPP$_i$ by the system's catalyst $\underline{C}$. The
activity of $\underline{C}$, however, is dependent on being associated with
the active form (or conformation) of the system's regulatory
component $\underline{N}$ (Pfeuffer, 1977; Ross and Gilman, 1977; Northup
et al., 1980). $\underline{N}$ is a Mg-binding (Iyengar, 1981; Iyengar and
Birnbaumer, 1981), GTP-binding (Iyengar, 1981; Pfeuffer,
1977; Stenweis et al., 1980) and presumably GTP-degrading
(Cassel and Selinger, 1976, 1977) protein that interacts with
both $\underline{C}$ (Rodbell et al., 1971a; Ross et al., 1978; Strittmatter
and $\underline{N}$eer, 1980) and $\underline{HR}$ complex (Rodbell et al., 1971a;
Sternwis and Gilman, 1979). The active form of $\underline{N}$ is dependent
on it being under the influence of both Mg and GTP or GTP
analog (Iyengar and Birnbaumer, 1981; Iyengar, 1981). In the
absence of hormone, it is thought that GTP to GDP conversion
at the GTP binding site of $\underline{N}$, a reaction that appears to be
inhibited upon ADP-ribosylation by cholera toxin (Cassel and
Selinger, 1977; Cassel and Pfeuffer, 1978; Gill and Meren,
1978) leads to relaxation of its active conformation (Strittmatter and Neer, 1980) and very likely, to dissociation of $\underline{C}$
from $\underline{N}$ (Pfeuffer, 1979; Limbrid et al., 1980). Alternatively,
simple dissociation of GTP from $\underline{N}$ leads to its relaxation
(Birnbaumer et al., 1980; Abramowitz et al., 1980). Since
free $\underline{C}$ is inactive in forming cAMP from MgATP (Ross et al.,
1978), dissociation of GTP and/or GTPase activity of $\underline{N}$ leads
to inactivation of the system. Inhibition of this putative
GTPase activity or simple modification of the GTP binding
site by cholera toxin (Birnbaumer et al., 1980; Abramowitz et
al., 1980) leads to stimulation of GTP-mediated activation of
cAMP formation. The K_m of the adenylyl cyclase for GTP is in
the uM range, well below the cellular concentration of GTP
(Iyengar and Birnbaumer, 1979; Iyengar et al., 1980a).
Hence, the GTP binding site of $\underline{N}$ is always saturated and
physiologic regulation of the system by modification of the
affinity for GTP is not likely. In contrast, the Mg binding
site of $\underline{N}$ is not saturated under physiologic conditions. Its
apparent K_m for Mg, in the absence of hormonal influence, is
about 5-10^m mM (Iyengar, 1981; Iyengar and Birnbaumer, 1981),
well above the intracellular concentration of free Mg which
is about 0.5 mM. Assuming that $\underline{N}$ is indeed a GTPase, it is
thought that the combination of this GTPase activity and the
low apparent affinity of $\underline{N}$ for Mg, determines that the resting

equilibrium between $\underline{N}$ and $\underline{C}$ is towards the inactive and dissociated side, such that basal activities of the system, as seen in the absence of hormonal influence, are in the order of 1-2% of maximum in intact cells and 10-30% of maximum in isolated membranes, where higher Mg concentrations are used for its determination.

2.1. Composition of N

As shown in liver (Northup et al., 1980; Sternweis et al., 1982), turkey erythrocytes (Hanski et al., 1982) and human erythrocytes (see below), $\underline{N}$ is a heterodimeric protein formed of two types of subunit. One type, which will be called $\underline{n_\alpha}$, is ADP-ribosylated by cholera toxin, has M_r values that vary between 42,000 and 52,000, has the binding site for GTP (Pfeuffer, 1977) and appears to be the subunit that binds to the $\underline{C}$ component of the system (Strittmatter and Neer, 1980). The other subunit, here called $\underline{n_\beta}$ has an M_r value of 35,000 and is not ADP-ribosylated by cholera toxin. Kinetic arguments (Iyengar and Birnbaumer, 1982) suggest that it may be the subunit that both binds Mg ion and interacts with $\underline{HR}$ complex (see below). A schematic view of an adenylyl cyclase system is shown in Fig. 1. The heterodimeric composition of the human erythrocyte $\underline{N}$ is illustrated in Fig. 2.

2.2. Mechanism of N Activation

As assessed in model systems (Ross et al., 1978; Iyengar, 1981; Sternweis et al., 1982) inactive $\underline{N}$, free of $\underline{C}$ and formed of both $\underline{n_\alpha}$ and $\underline{n_\beta}$ subunits, can be "activated" by pretreatment with Mg and either NaF (a universal adenylyl cyclase stimulator) or the non-hydrolyzable GTP analogs (GMP-P(NH)P and GTPγS. As a consequence, when this pre-activated $\underline{N}$ is combined with $\underline{C}$ after dilution of GTP analog or NaF to ineffective concentrations, a rapid reconstitution takes place with resulting activities being those that would have been obtained if $\underline{C}$ and $\underline{N}$ had been mixed and assayed in the presence of Mg and either guanine nucleotide or NaF, even though the latter two are no longer present. Figure 3 illustrates both the requirement and the effect of Mg concentration in the pre-activation of $\underline{N}$ by GMP-P(NH)P. It can be seen that Mg is not only required for the preactivation, but also that it influences in a concentration dependent manner the rate at which "activation" occurs in the presence of the

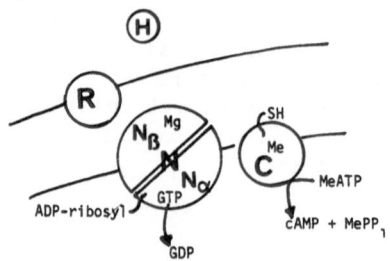

Figure 1. Subunit structure and components that form hormone
stimulable adenylyl cyclases. H: hormone; R: receptor; N:
nucleotide and Mg binding regulatory component; C: catalytic
unit; n_α: ADP-ribosylatable and GTP-binding subunit of N;
n_β.: 35,000 subunit of N assumed to be responsible for
binding of Mg. N is depicted as a GTPase. C is depicted as
having both an allosteric regulatory site for divalent metal
(Me) which may either be Mg or Mn (Somkuti et al., 1982)
and a critical -SH group essential for interaction with N.
The reaction catalyzed by C is shown with MeATP being either
MgATP or MnATP.

(saturating) concentration of GMP-P(NH)P used. As mentioned
above the Mg concentration necessary for this process of
preactivation of N is in the range of 5 to 10 mM for 50%
effect (Iyengar, 1981).

The necessity of Mg for obtaining a guanine nucleotide
effect and its action to accelerate the rate of activation by
saturating concentrations of guanine neucleotide appears to
be relevant to the mechanism of regulation of adenylyl cyclase
in intact membranes. This is illustrated in Figs. 4 and 5
where it is shown that preincubation of liver membranes with
GMP-P(NH)P results in pre-activation of this adenylyl cyclase
system only if carried out in the presence of Mg ion and that
increasing concentrations of Mg ion lead to a concentration
dependent increase in the rate of activation of adenylyl
cyclase by both GMP-P(NH)P and GTP. This is shown here for
liver membrane adenylyl cyclase. The same phenomenon is
observed also in membranes from other systems such as corpus
luteum (Abramowitz and Birnbaumer, 1982) and S49 lymphoma
cells (Iyengar and Birnbaumer, 1981).

It has been shown that the molecular dimension of N
decreases during preactivation from its native value of
approximately 80,000 daltons to a mere 50,000 daltons

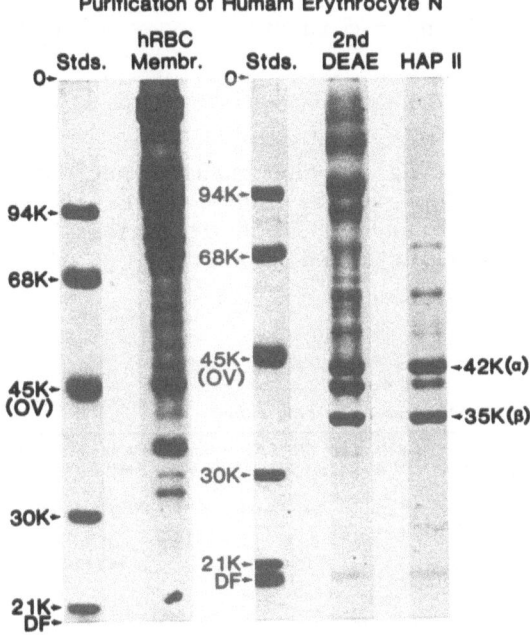

Purification of Humam Erythrocyte N

Figure 2. SDS-Page analysis of human erythrocyte membrane proteins (hRBC membranes: lane 2), of a partially purified $\underline{N}$ compenent (DEAE II fraction: lane 4) and of the fully purified $\underline{N}$ protein obtained after chromatography of the material of lane 4 over hydrpxyapatite (HAP II: lane 5). Lanes 1 and 3: Molecular weight standards.

(Sternweis et al., 1982; Hanski et al., 1982). These data strongly suggest that $\underline{N}$ activation is associated with a subunit dissociation reaction of the type:

$$\underline{N}_{\alpha\beta} \xrightarrow{\quad G, \ Mg \quad} \underline{n}_{\alpha}^{*G} + \underline{n}_{\beta}^{(Mg)} \qquad [1]$$

where $\underline{n}_{\alpha}^{*G}$ represents the activated form of the ADP-ribosylated subunit of $\underline{N}$ with guanine nucleotide bound to it, and $\underline{n}_{\beta}^{(Mg)}$ represents the non-ADP-ribosylated subunit assumed to have Mg bound to it. It is currently believed that $\underline{C}$ activation by guanine nucleotide and Mg results from the reaction:

$$\underset{n}{\overset{*G}{\underset{-\alpha}{}}} + c \text{ inactive} \longrightarrow \underset{n}{\overset{*G}{\underset{-\alpha}{}}} C \text{ active}$$

with $\underset{n}{\overset{*\,G}{\underset{-\alpha}{}}}C$ accumulating if the guanine nucleotide is a non-hydrolyzable analog (e.g., GMP-P(NH)P or GTPγS). This activation sequence and possible mechanisms for inactivation of the system are illustrated in Fig. 6.

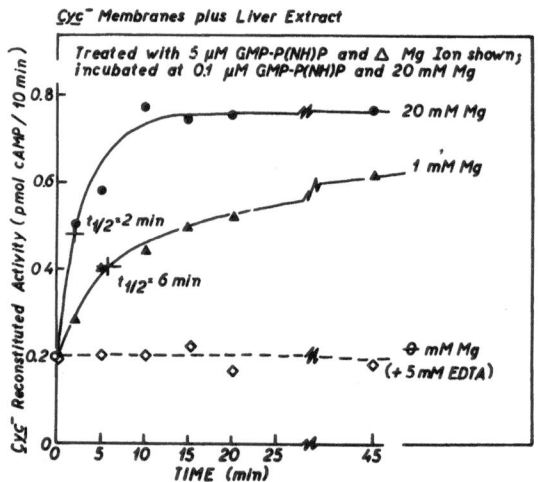

Figure 3. Mg and guanine nucleotide mediated "activation" of solubilized N component. Liver membranes were extracted with cholate, the extracts heated to inactivate endogenous C activity and incubated in the presence of either 1.0 mM Mg ion (in excess of chelators) or 25 mM Mg, for the indicated times. The samples were then diluted and analyzed for N activity in a cyc- reconstitution assay at final concentrations of 0.1 uM GMP-P(NH)P and 25 mN MgCl$_2$. Note that only when Mg was present did the preincubation lead to preactivation of N and that the rate of preactivation is dependent on the concentration of Mg ion in the medium (for details see Iyengar, 1981).

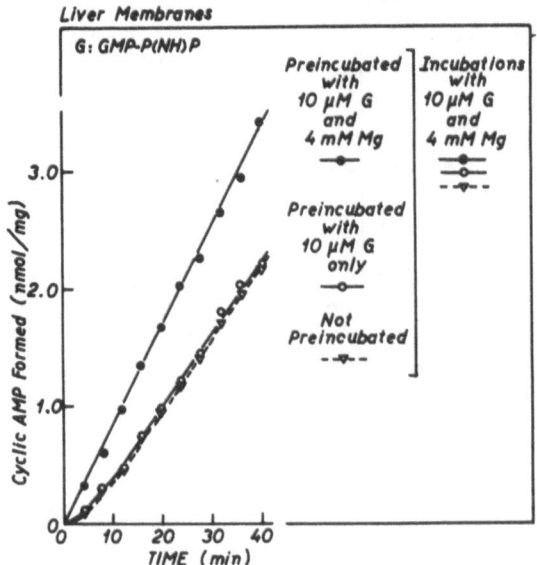

Figure 4. Requirement of Mg for GMP-(NH)P mediated activation in liver membrane adenylyl cyclase. Liver membranes were pre-incubated with saturating guanine nucleotide in the absence and presence of $MgCl_2$ and then assayed for adenylyl cyclase activity as a function of time. Note that only the pretreatment with both nucleotide and Mg leads to activation (for details see Iyengar and Birnbaumer, 1981).

3.   Regulation of Adenylyl Cyclase in the Presence of Hormone

HR complexes interact with N to stimulate the adenylyl cyclase system (Iyengar and Birnbaumer, 1982). It has been shown that they do so by lowering the apparent K_m of N for Mg to values in the range of 5 uM (Iyengar and Birnbaumer, 1982), well below the cellular concentration of Mg, and, at the same time, by facilitating in some tissues the exchange of inhibitory GDP for stimulatory GTP (Cassel and Selinger, 1978; Dufau et al., 1980). Figure 7 illustrates the effect of hormonal stimulation of liver membrane N and its action to lower the requirement for Mg in the guanine nucleotide dependent activation of the system. As exemplified above for

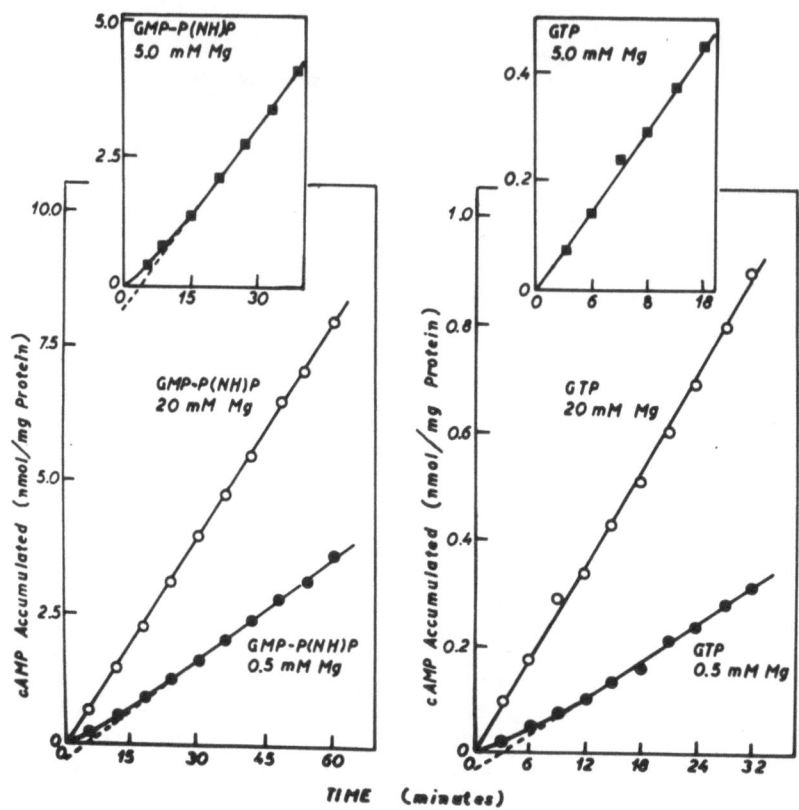

Figure 5.   Mg mediated modulation of the rate of activation of adenylyl cyclase by guanine nucleotide in intact membranes. Liver membranes were incubated with either 10 uM GMP-P(NH)P or GTP in the presence of 0.5, 5 and 25 mN Mg ion in excess of chelators.   Adenylyl cyclase was determined as a function of incubation time.   Note that not only extent, but also and importantly rate of activation is affected by Mg ion.

the effect of Mg ion on guanine nucleotide-mediated activation of $\underline{N}$ in the absence of hormone, the observed effect of hormone to reduce the Mg requirement for the guanine nucleotide-mediated increase in chloate extracted $\underline{cyc}$- reconstituting

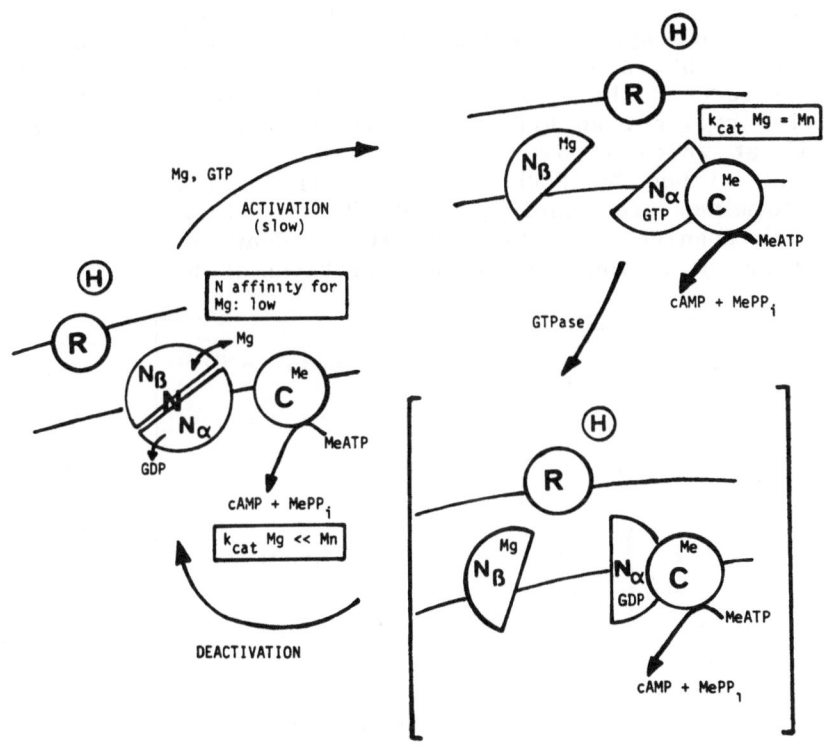

Figure 6. Schematic representation of the GTP and Mg-dependent activation cycle of adenylyl cyclase as it is believed to apply in the absence of hormonal stimulation. $\underline{N}$ is assumed to be a GTPase and two possible routes are represented for the deactivation of the activated and dissociated $\underline{N}$ protein: (1) the active $\underline{n}^{*GTP}$ subunit is an active GTPase leading to formation of the intermediary $\underline{n}_\alpha^{*GTP}$ $\underline{C}$ complex which then deactivates by sequential release of GDP, dissociation of $\underline{n}_\alpha$ from $\underline{C}$ and recombination with $\underline{n}\beta$ and concomitant release of Mg; (2) the active $\underline{n}_\alpha^{*GTP}$ is not active as a GTPase and becomes active with $\underline{n}_\alpha^{*G}\underline{C}$ accumulating if the guanine nucleotide is a non-hydrolyzable analog (e.g., GMP-P(NH)P or GTPγS). This activation sequence and possible mechanisms for inactivation of the system are illustrated in Fig. 6.

activity, appears to be relevant to the mode by which hormones act on intact systems in membranes. This is illustrated by two experiments shown in Fig. 8 and 9. Figure 8 shows that hormone reduces the apparent K_m for Mg in the activation of adenylyl cyclase, an effect that is independent of the level of ATP at which it is tested, and Fig. 9 shows the effect first described by Rodbell's group (Rodbell et al., 1974) that hormones are "anti-hysteretic", i.e. increase the rate at which guanine nucleotides activate adenylyl cyclase, thus mimicking the action of high concentrations of Mg.

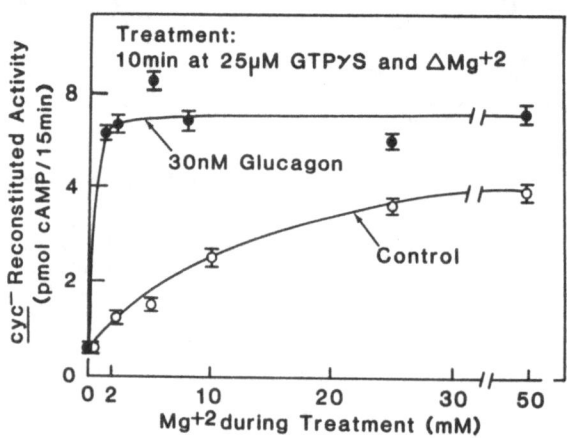

Figure 7. Effect of hormone (receptor) on Mg requirement for guanine nucleotide dependent activation of $\underline{N}$. Liver membranes were treated with N-ethyl maleimide to inactivate $\underline{C}$ and un-couple it from $\underline{N}$. The "$\underline{C}$" membranes thus obtained were incubated in the presence and absence of glucagon with saturating GTPγS and the varying concentrations of Mg ion depicted on the figure. $\underline{N}$ activity was assayed after washing the membranes, resuspending in 1% cholate, mixing with $\underline{cyc}$- membranes and determining reconsitution of cyc- adenylyl cyclase activity. It can be seen that $\underline{N}$ activity being extracted from such membrane incubated in the absence of Mg ion is relatively low but can be increased upon inclusion of divalent cation during incubation with GTPγS. Further, the concentration of Mg required for half-maximal effectiveness is lowered dramatically by hormone (30 nM glucagon) from a value of about 10 mM to concentrations well below 1.0 mM. In other experiments 50% effects were obtained with as little as 10 uM Mg ion, indicating that hormone receptors should be considered as "Mg switches".

Taken together the results shown in Fig. 3 and 7 demonstrate that the guanine nucleotide activation of adenylyl cyclase is due to activation of $\underline{N}$ component, that this activation is not only dependent on, but also regulated by Mg and that hormonal stimulation is due to the receptor-dependent modulation of the regulation of the system by Mg. How the basal system is restored after hormonal stimulation is not yet well understood. But it is likely that relaxation is the result of a combination of $\underline{H}$ dissociating from $\underline{R}$, Mg dissociating from $\underline{N}$, GTP dissociating from $\underline{N}$ (either as such or after conversion to GDP), and $\underline{N}$ dissociating from both $\underline{C}$ and $\underline{R}$. In terms of the two-subunit structure of $\underline{N}$ presented above, the most likely sequence of events leading to hormonal stimulation of adenylyl cyclase is that $\underline{HR}$ complex, by interacting with the $\underline{n}\beta$ subunit of $\underline{N}$, increases its affinity for Mg from being below ambient to being above ambient, with resulting facilitated dissociation of $\underline{n}_\alpha$. This subunit in turn either associates with GTP and activates $\underline{C}$ or exchanges GDP for GTP and then activates $\underline{C}$ according to the reaction:

$$HR + \underline{N}_{\alpha\beta} \xrightarrow{\text{G, Mg}} HR\underline{n}^{*}_{\beta}(Mg) + \overset{*G}{\underline{n}_\alpha} \qquad [3]$$

where $\overset{*G}{\underline{n}_\alpha}$ interacts with inactive $\underline{C}$ as described above in reaction [2].

Several laboratories are currently investigating with pure $\underline{N}$ whether this sequence of events, suggested by kinetic (Iyengar, 1981; Iyengar and Birnbaumer, 1982) and structural (Sternweis et al., 1982; Hanski et al., 1982) analyses and illustrated in Fig. 10 is indeed correct.

4.   Desensitization

Continued occupancy of $\underline{R}$ by $\underline{H}$ due either to continued presence of $\underline{H}$ or to persistence of slowly dissociating $\underline{RH}$ complex does not result in continued activation of the adenylyl cyclase system. Rather, as shown in response to gonadotropin stimulation of gonadal cells (Lamprecht et al., 1973; Marsh et al., 1973; Hsueh et al., 1976; Hunzicker-Dunn and Birnbaumer, 1976a,b, and c; Hunzicker-Dunn et al., 1979b), a two step process sets in whereby first the $\underline{HR}$ complex becomes altered and uncouples from adenylyl cyclase

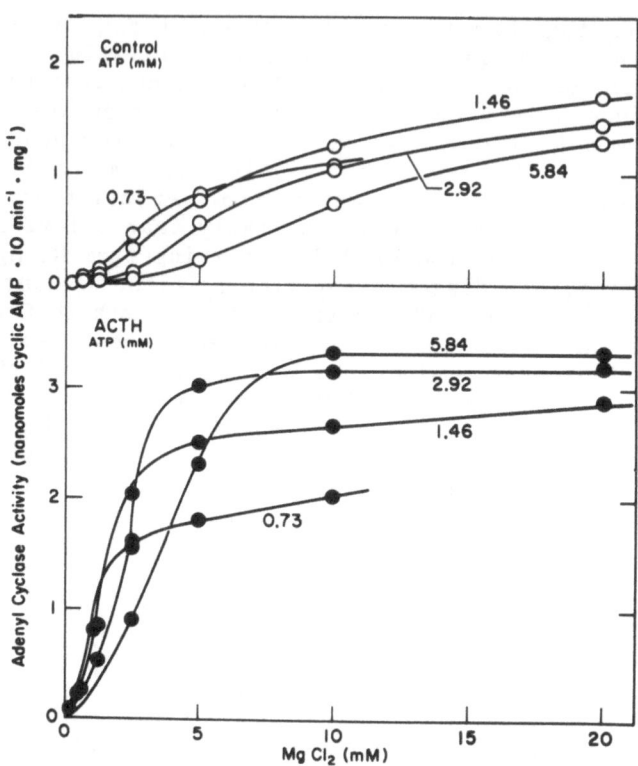

Figure 8. Effect of ACTH to reduce the apparent K_m for $MgCl_2$ in activation of fat cell adenylyl cyclase. Adenylyl cyclase activity was tested at concentrations of ATP indicated next to each of the curves, in the presence of varying concentrations of $MgCl_2$. Adapted from Birnbaumer et al. (1969).

and then the R (alone or in combination with H) is removed from the cell surface. The first step is called hormone-specific or homologous desensitization and the second is called "down regulation". These steps may occur temporally well separated from each other, as demonstrated in response to catecholamines in human astrocytoma cells (Su et al., 1980) and S49 lymphoma cells (Iyengar et al., 1981), and also seen in gonads in response to gonadotropins (Katikineni et al., 1980). They may occur almost simultaneously as well,

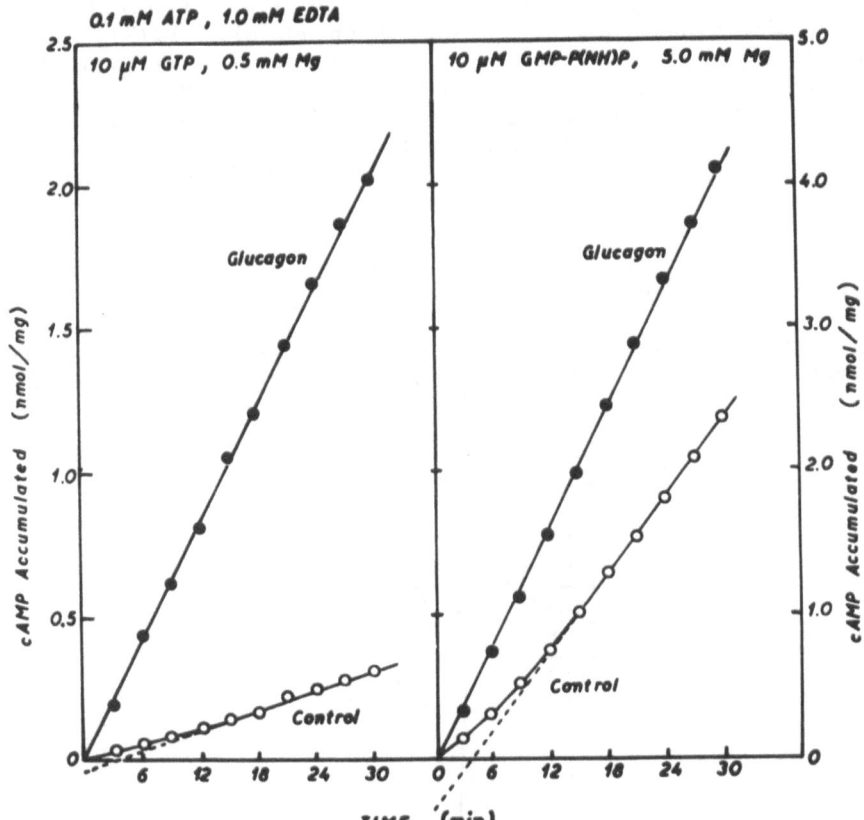

Figure 9. Effect of hormonal stimulation on rate of activation of liver adenylyl cyclase by guanine nucleotides. Adenylyl cyclase activity was determined as a function of time with either GTP or GMP-P(NH)P as the stimulating nucleotide. Glucagon was added as shown. Compare to results on Fig. 5 and note that glucagon acts to allow the system to behave at low Mg as if high Mg had been added.

rendering their separate observation difficult or impossible. In some cell systems, the first step is reversible with $t_{1/2}$ values in the order of 10-15 min (Su et al., 1980). Such reversals require ready dissociation of $\underline{H}$ from $\underline{R}$, such as happens if $\underline{H}$ is a catecholamine. Gonadotropins dissociate much more slowly (Abramowitz et al., 1982; Conti et al., 1976; Katikineni et al., 1980; Koch et al., 1973). Hence gonadotropin desensitizations are essentially irreversible, provided they are triggered by saturating H (Hunzicker-Dunn et al., 1979b; Katikineni et al., 1980). If not all R's are occupied, desensitization is partial and upon early clearance of H, reversal to the original sensitive state occurs (Harwood et al., 1978).

4.1. Homologous Desensitization

This type of desensitization can be obtained in isolated membranes (Bockaert et al., 1976; Iyengar et al., 1980b) and

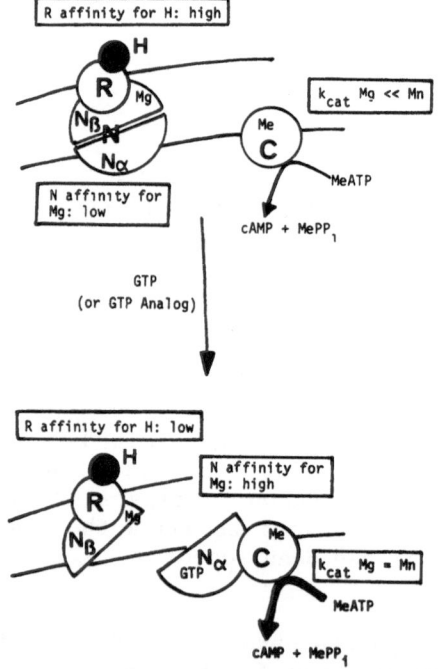

Figure 10. Schematic representation of the most likely mode by which hormone receptors stimulate GTP-dependent activation of adenylyl cyclase. Although R is shown to interact only with nβ, its simultaneous interaction with n_α has by no means been excluded.

is independent of cAMP. It requires HR complex formation, activation of HR complex by GTP and presence of Mg and ATP (Iyengar et al., 1980b). It does not occur in the absence of ATP or upon substituting AMP-P(NH)P for ATP (Bockaret et al., 1976; Iyengar et al., 1980b). This is illustrated in Fig. 11 and 12. A cell-free membrane-bound desensitization process dependent on LH and GTP, but apparently not on ATP, has been reported in membranes from ovaries of E_2 and PSMG-treated rats (Ezra and Salomon, 1980, 1981). Its relation to the above described ATP dependent phenomenon, which is also observed in membranes from cultured cells (Anderson and

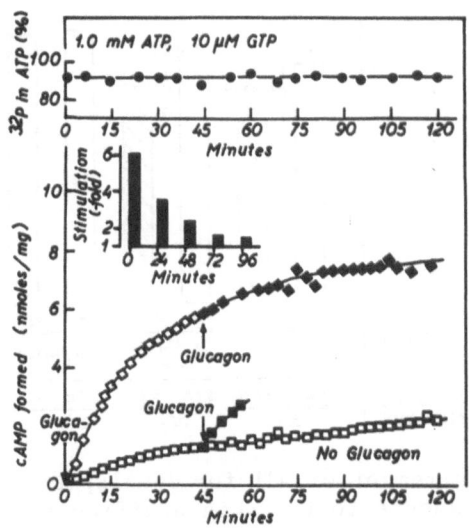

Figure 11. Glucagon induced desensitization of liver adenylyl cyclase. Liver membranes were incubated under adenylyl cyclase assay conditions with 1.5 mM ATP, 5.0 mM $MgCl_2$ and 10 uM GTP in the absence (open symbols) and the presence of a saturating concentration of glucagon (closed symbols); cAMP formation was then determined as a function of time. Note that the rate of accumulation of cAMP decreased in the presence but not in the absence of glucagon. As shown by the hormonal effect obtained upon post-addition of glucagon to a system incubated without it, the loss of accumulation rate obtained in its presence (insert) was not due to nonspecific inactivation of this system. (For further details see Iyengar et al., 1980b).

Jaworski, 1979), is not clear. As seen in S49 cells and illustrated in Fig. 13 and 14, homologous desentization does not appear to be due to modification of N and has been proposed, but not yet been unequivocally proven, to be due to phosphorylation of H-occupied R by a membrane-bound enzyme (Iyengar et al., 1981b). This phosphorylation would render HR complex incapable of continued coupling (Bockaert et al., 1976; Iyengar et al., 1980b). In support of this contention, a phosphorprotein phosphatase-containing membrane extract was found to reverse in a Mn-dependent manner LH-, GTP-, ATP- and Mg-induced desensitization of LH-sensitive adenylyl cyclase of pig Graafian follicles (Hunzicker-Dunn et al., 1979a) but

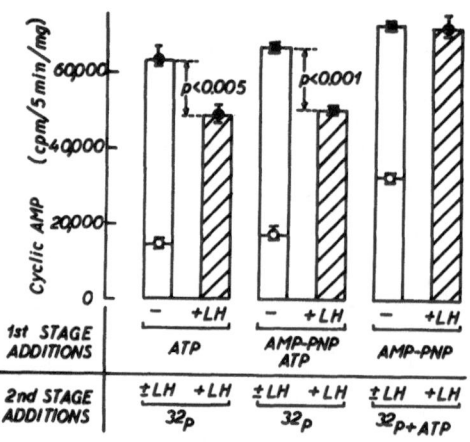

Figure 12. Requirement of ATP for development of desensitized state in the response to LH. Pig Graffian follicle membranes were incubated in the presence and absence of LH with or without the indicated additions of ATP and/or AMP-P(NH)P. After 25 min of incubation in the presence of adenylyl cyclase assay reagents containing 5 mM $MgCl_2$ and guanine nucleotides, the responsiveness of the system was studied by pulsing it with [alpha-^{32}P]ATP of high specific activity to monitor cAMP forming capacity. Note that in the presence of ATP an LH-dependent loss of LH response developed. This loss of response was not interfered with by AMP-P(NH)P, a substrate for adenylyl cyclase but not for protein kinases, but was not apparent if ATP was replaced by AMP-P(NH)P. (For further details see Bockaert et al., 1976).

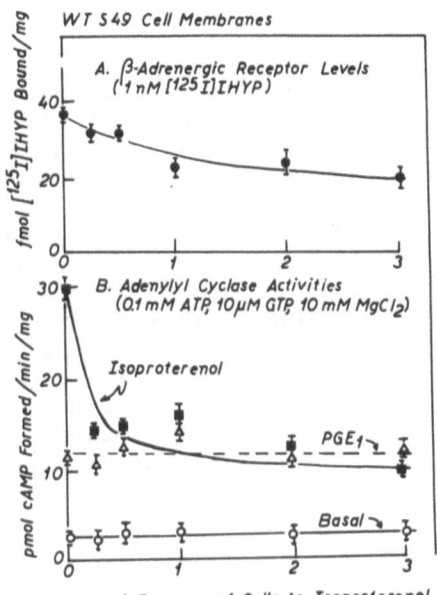

Figure 13. Homologous nature of desensitization obtained in S49 cells upon exposure to isoproterenol. S49 cells were incubated for the indicated times with $10^{-5}M$ isoproterenol, harvested, lysed and membranes prepared for the determination of <u>beta</u>-receptors via ^{125}I-HYP binding (top panel) and isoproterenol and prostaglandin stimulated adenylyl cyclase activities (bottom panel). Note that treatment with isoproterenol leads to a selective loss of isoproterenol-stimulated activity <u>without</u> change in basal or prostaglandin stimulated activities, and that, at least initially, this occurs without concurrent loss of <u>beta</u>-receptor sites. This type of desensitization is termed homologous (from Iyengar et al., 1981b).

was ineffective in reversing a glucagon, GTP-, ATP- and Mg-induced desensitization in liver membranes (Iyengar, Hunzicker-Dunn, and Birnbaumer, unpublished). A model for the possible mechanism of homologous desensitization involving receptor phosphorylation is schematized in Fig. 15.

4.2. Heterologous Desensitization

This is the phenomenon by which stimulation of the cell by one hormone leads to a variable loss of responsiveness to all hormones that affect the adenylyl cyclase of that cell (Su et al., 1976). This process leads subsequently to loss not only of the R whose occupancy triggered it, but also of all other R's whose responses are lost. Such a heterologous process is responsible for final loss of FSH responsiveness in mature Graafian follicles upon hCG treatment (Jonassen and Richards, 1980). Heterologous desensitization is less well understood than homologous desensitization, and its mechanism of action has just begun to be explored. A preliminary study suggests that modification of N and/or R's that couple to N may be involved (Kirchick and Birnbaumer, 1982). This is illustrated in Fig. 16 where hCG-induced changes were shown

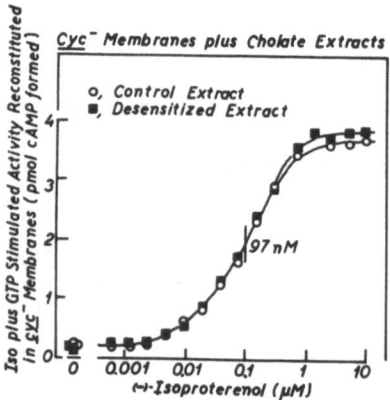

Figure 14. Lack of impairment of N component activity upon homologous desensitization. N component was extracted from control and 30 min desensitized S49 cell membranes and assayed for its capacity to reconstitute hormone (isoproterenol)-stimulable cyc- adenylyl cyclase activity. Note that N activity of desensitized membranes is both quantitatively (total activity reconstituted) and qualitatively (position of the response curve to isoproterinol of the reconstituted system) indistinguishable from N activity of control membranes.

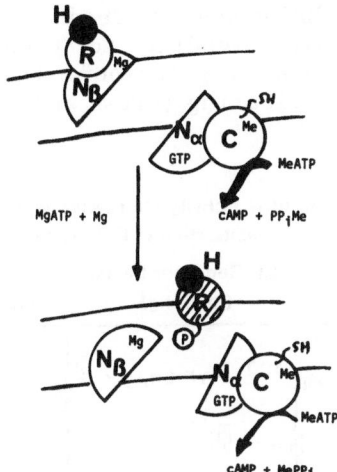

Figure 15. Proposed model for homologous (hormone-specific) desensitization of adenylyl cyclases. The model is based on the findings that this type of desensitization does not affect N component activity and that when obtained in isolated membranes it depends on receptor activation (requiring GTP and hormone), presence of high levels of ATP and Mg and is reversed at least in one system by treatment with phosphatase-containing fractions.

to include not only loss of availability of gonadatropin receptors and of LH responsiveness, but also a partial loss of catecholamine responsiveness of adenylyl cyclase activity which was concomitant with a partial loss in the levels of N activity. As shown recently by Hunzicker-Dunn and Birnbaumer (1981) and illustrated in Fig. 17, heterologous effects of this kind may be the result of negative feedback regulation of adenylyl cyclase responsiveness by cAMP. Thus, cAMP or, as illustrated on the figure, its analogue db-cAMP, can induce loss of LH responsiveness in rabbit Graffian follicles. Similarly, cAMP appears to be responsible for loss of catecholamine action in astrocytoma cells (Nickols and Brooker, 1979). It can therefore be envisioned that hetero-logous desensitization and subsequent loss of receptors is

the result of a cAMP-dependent feedback physphorylation at
N of the HRN complex leading to uncoupled HR complexes
susceptible to "down regulation" (Rao et al., 1977;
Conn et al., 1978) or clearing (Brown and Goldstein, 1976)

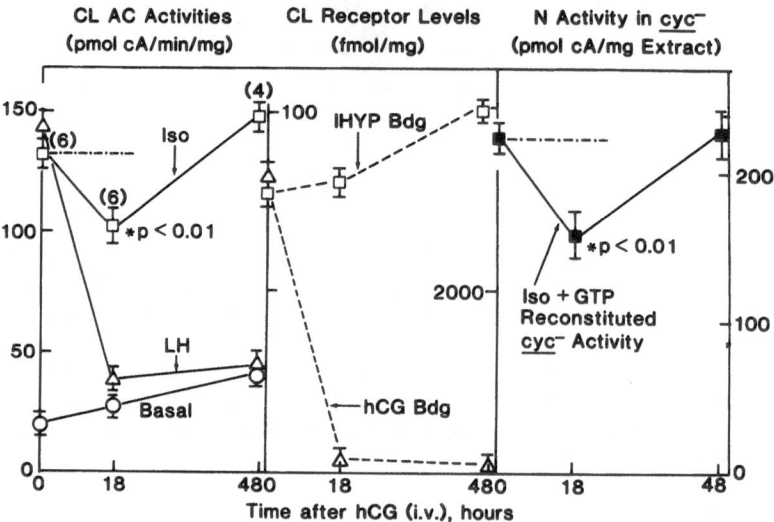

Figure 16. Association of impairment of N component activity
with heterologous effects of hCG on rat corpus luteum receptors and adenylyl cyclase. Immature rats were superovulated
by PMS priming and hCG administration 56 hours afterwards.
Seven days later (days 0 of graph) they received a luteolytic
dose of hCG (for details see Hunzicker-Dunn et al., 1979b)
and were killed at the indicated times. Their ovaries (90+%
luteal tissue) were excised, homogenized, and membranes
prepared for the determination of available LH receptor sites
(^{125}I-hCG binding), catecholamine beta-receptors (^{125}I-HYP
binding), basal, LH and catecholamine (isoproterenol) stimulated adenylyl cyclase activities, and N activity as assessed
by reconstitution of either NaF-stimulable or isoproterenol-
stimulable activity in cyc- S49 cell membranes. Adenylyl
cyclase assays (panel A), receptor assays (panel B) and
N activity assays by reconstitution of cyc- S49 cell
adenylyl cyclase were performed as described by Hunzicker-
Dunn et al. (1979b), Abramowitz et al. (1982) and Iyengar
et al. (1981a), respectively.

from the membrane and to altered (phosphorylated) $\underline{N}$ units incapable of mediating coupling of any new $\underline{HR}$ complex that may form. Figure 18 presents a tentative model for heterologous desensitization based on this hypothesis.

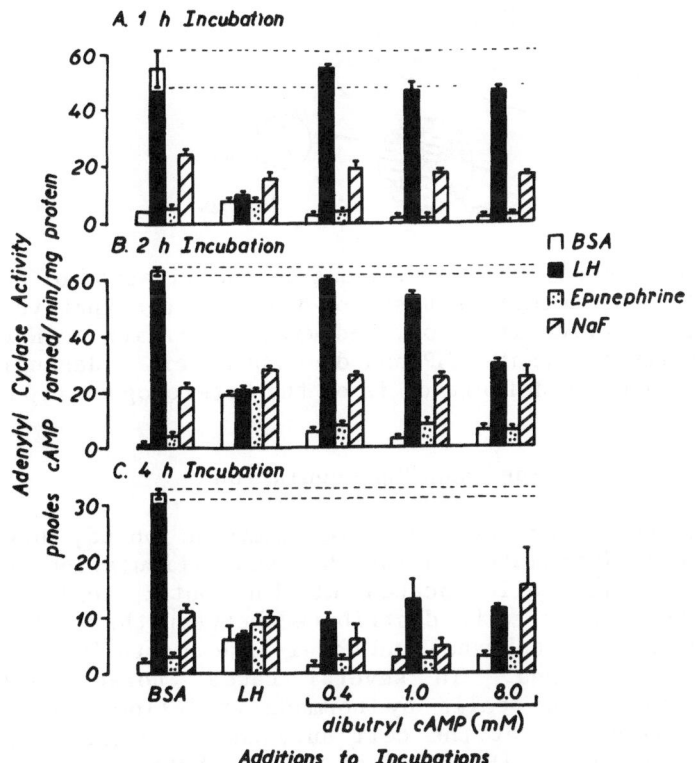

Figure 17. cAMP-induced desensitization of LH responsive adenylyl cyclase. Grafian follicles were dissected from rabbit ovaries and incubated in glucose-containing Krebs-Ringer bicarbonate buffer under an atmosphere of 95% O_2-5% CO_2 at 37°C for the indicated times in the absence and presence of LH or db-cAMP as shown. Note that incubation with the dibutyryl derivative of cAMP caused loss of LH responsiveness suggesting strongly the existence of an inhibitory feed-back loop that operates to insure development of loss of hormonal stimulability after massive stimulation of adenylyl cyclase. In contrast to cAMP, AMP was without effect (not shown). (For further details see Hunzicker-Dunn and Birnbaumer, 1981.)

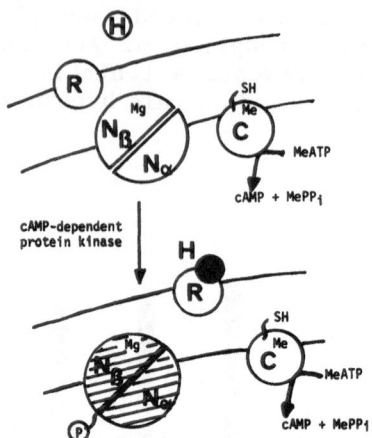

Figure 18. Model for heterologous desensitization of adenylyl
cyclases. This model is based on the findings that this type
of desensitization is associated with alteration in N̲ component activity and that cAMP and db-cAMP elicit a desensitizing
response which by definition is of the heterologous type.

4.3. "Down-Regulation" and "Up-Regulation"

Receptors for hormones are membrane bound, but in a
resting cell immediately before hormonal stimulation they are
not necessarily all located at the outer cell surface.
Rather they appear to be distributed between the cell surface
membrane (plasma membrane) and Golgi-like smooth intracellular
membrane structures. In several cases, notably with LH,
stimulation of the cells by hormone is followed by a rapid
transient increase at the cell surface of receptors for the
stimulating hormone (Hsueh et al., 1977; Suter et al., 1980).
This phenomenon has been termed "up-regulation" and preceeds
that of "down-regulation." The mechanisms involved in
"up-regulation," i.e., in recruitment of new receptors to the
cell surface, are unknown but are surely dependent on cytoskeletal elements. The mechanism by wich desensitized receptors (with or without H̲ bound to them) are cleared is also
largely unknown. It is likely that prior to internalization,
desensitized receptors are collected at or near coated pits
and that their internalization path is similar to that
followed by LDL (for review see Brown and Goldstein, 1976).

In this case the receptors end in lysosomes where they are proteolytically degraded. Evidence for "patching" and internalization of hCG associated with macromolecular elements supposed to be receptors, followed by accumulation in lysosomes, has been presented in granulosa cells (Amsterdam et al., 1974). It is conceivable that internalized receptors may be slowly recycled to the intracellular pool of receptors awaiting restimulation. This could account for some of the slow reacquisitions of hormonal sensitivity seen after LH or hCG treatment of ovarian and testicular tissues in vivo (Harwood et al., 1978).

5. Final Comments

On the basis of studies on preactivation of N by Mg and guanine nucleotides influenced or not by hormone receptors (Iyengar et al., 1981; Iyengar and Birnbaumer, 1982; Sternweis et al., 1982), it seems that a rather good explanation exists for the mode of action of stimulatory hormone receptors (Fig. 6 and 10). However, many questions relating to hormonal regulation of adenylyl cyclase still exist. These four stand out.

5.1. Meaning of N-Mediated Regulation of Receptor Affinities

Although the effect of guanine nucleotides on adenylyl cyclases was discovered on the basis of their effects on hormone or agonist binding to the receptors (Rodbell et al., 1971a), there is still no clear explanation as to the mechanistic meaning of the nucleotide regulation of receptor-hormone interaction. Thus, catecholamine receptors are regulated not only by guanine nucleotides (which cause a decrease in receptor affinity for agonist), but also by Mg ion (Bird and Maguire, 1978; Williams et al., 1978). In fact, as illustrated in Fig 19, a Mg-induced increase in receptor affinity for catecholamines is a prerequisite for observing a guanine nucleotide-induced decrease in affinity. As is also illustrated in Fig. 19, the effect of Mg and hence guanine nucleotides is dependent on presence of a functionally fully active N component, being absent in both the cyc- and the UNC variants of S49 cells. This is the situation depicted in the model of Fig. 8 where the changes in agonist (hormone) binding affinities upon guanine nucleotide addition to a Mg-dominated system are shown. Glucagon receptors, on the other hand, show

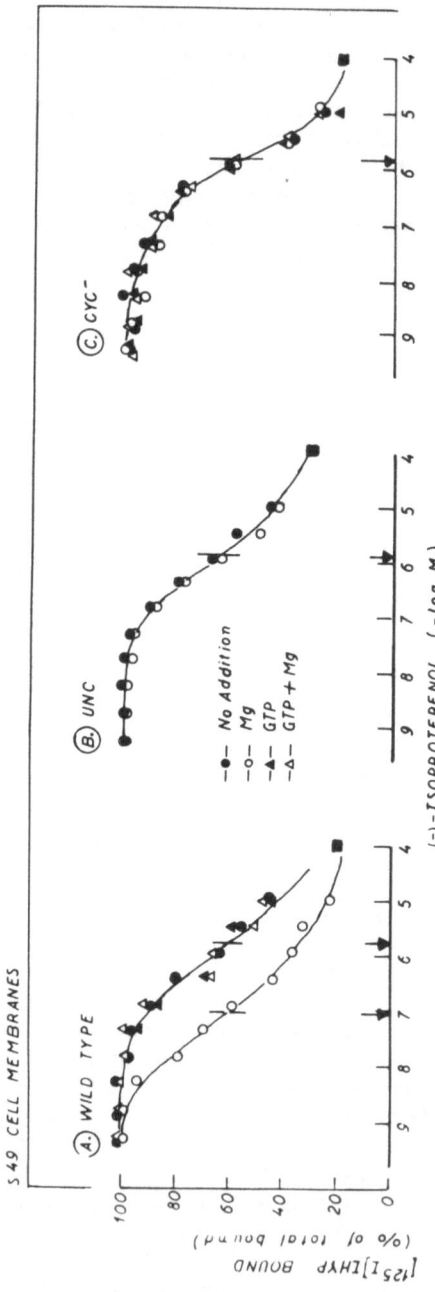

Figure 19. Mg dependence of guanine nucleotide effects on agonist (catecholamine) binding to beta-adrenergic receptors of S49 lymphoma cells and absence of these effects in catecholamine unresponsive, receptor-replete and N̲ component-defective UNC and cyc⁻ variants of these cells. Assays for specific binding of ¹²⁵I-HYP and displacement by increasing concentrations of isoproterenol were performed as described by Iyengar et al. (1980a). When present MgCl₂ was 5 mM and GTP was 100 uM.

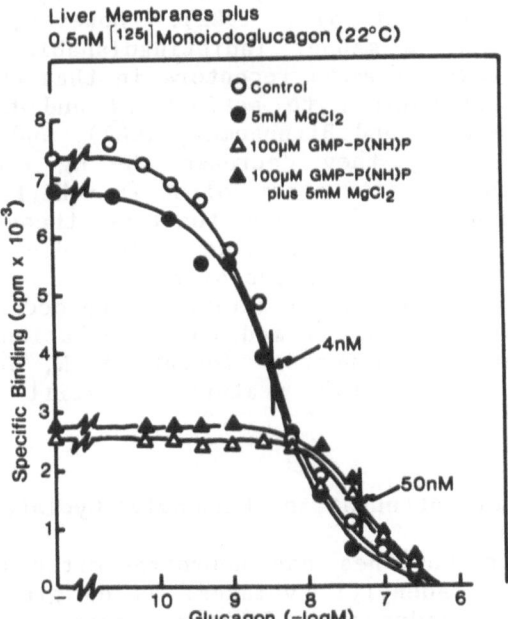

Figure 20.   Guanine nucleotides, but not Mg, affect binding of glucagon to liver membrane glucagon receptor.   [^{125}I-Tyr^{10}] Monoiodoglucagon used as receptor probe was synthesized, purified and characterized as described in Birnbaumer et al. (1983).   Specific binding was assayed as described in Birnbaumer and Swartz (1982).

no regulation by Mg ion (Fig. 20) and the presence of Mg is not a prerequisite for observing the induction of a low-affinity state of the receptor by guanine nucleotides. Yet, in the absence of Mg, there is no activation of $\underline{N}$ protein, even though the $\underline{N}$ protein-induced receptor affinity change does occur. With respect to gonadotropin in receptors, the situation is different still. Thus, as illustrated for hCG binding in Fig. 21, these receptors show regulation of their hormone-binding function by Mg ion, but not by guanine nucleotides (Abramowitz et al., 1982). However, gonadotropin receptors act in a manner indistinguishable from that of glucagon and catecholamine receptors in that they require Mg and guanine nucleotides to activate $\underline{N}$ and hence adenylyl cyclase (Abramowitz and Birnbaumer, 1982), and in that, like glucagon receptors, they decrease the Mg requirement for guanine nucleotide activation of $\underline{N}$ (Kirchick, Iyengar and Birnbaumer, unpublished). Taken together, these data indicate that possibly neither the guanine nucleotide-induced nor the Mg-induced shifts in affinities of receptors for hormones are mechanistically required for activation to occur. Yet, it is relatively certain that $\underline{N}$-mediated regulation of receptor binding reflects an important feature of $\underline{N}$, or $\underline{R}$, or of $\underline{RN}$ interactions. What this feature is still needs to $\underline{be}$ discovered.

5.2. Mechanism of Attenuation of Adenylyl Cyclases by Hormones

There are hormones and neurotransmitters that rather than activating adenylyl cyclases, as do glucagon, gonado-tropins and beta-adrenergic ligands, cause a partial (up to 50-60%) inhibition, e.i., cause attenuation of adenylyl cyclase activity. The mechanism by which this attenuation comes about is a center of current research in several laboratories. Among the hormones or hormonal effects that cause attenuation are $alpha_2$-adrenoceptor effects on platelets (Aktories and Jakobs, 1981), muscarinic receptor effects on heart (Jakobs et al., 1979), angiotensin II effects on liver (Jard et al., 1981), opioid receptor effects on neuroblastoma cells (Sharma et al., 1977; Blume et al., 1979), and prosta-glandin effects on adipose tissue (Aktories et al., 1979). Like stimulatory effects, inhibitory effects on adenylyl cyclase are dependent on presence of guanine nucleotides and Mg ion. As with stimulatory effects, attenuation is the result of a potentiation of an intrinsic, in this case negative, effect of GTP. Higher concentrations of GTP are required for inhibition that for stimulation of adenylyl cyclase, giving rise to "bell-shaped" dose-response curves (Londos et al., 1978, Cooper et al., 1979). On kinetic grounds, it has been proposed that positive and negative regulation by nucleotides (and hormonal regulation of these effects) are mediated by separate $\underline{N}$ proteins: $\underline{N}_s$ and $\underline{N}_i$, respectively (for review, see Cooper, 1982). More direct evidence for existence of functionally independent $\underline{N}_s$ and $\underline{N}_i$ units was recently provided by the finding that inhibitory regulation of adenylyl cyclase is blocked by toxin from <u>Bordetella</u> <u>pertussis</u>, the so-called islet-activating protein,

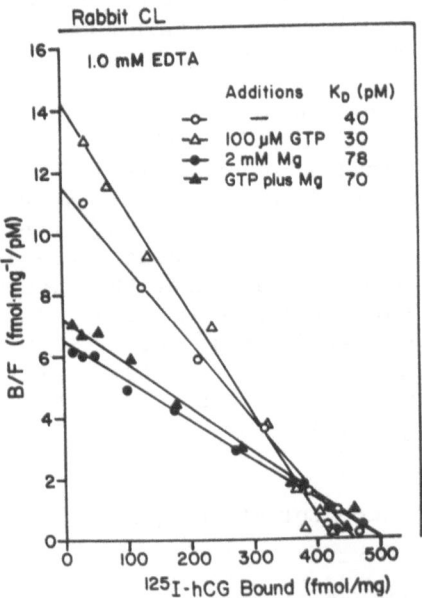

Figure 21. Mg, but not guanine nucleotides, affects LH receptor binding. Luteal membranes were incubated with increasing concentrations of biologically active ^{125}I-hCG and specifically bound ^{125}I-hCG was represented as a function of free ^{125}I-hCG in the incubations according to Scatchard. Labeling of hCG and determination of binding are described in Abramowitz et al. (1982). Note that the result obtained here is essentially opposite to that obtained when Mg and guanine nucleotide effects were tested for in glucagon receptor assays (Fig. 20).

or IAP (Hazeki and Ui, 1981; Katada and Ui, 1981; Cronin et al., 1982). Furthermore, this toxin, like cholera toxin, is an ADP-ribosylating enzyme which ADP-ribosylates a peptide of $M_r \cong 40,000$ distinct from the 42-45,000 and 50-52,000 n_α subunits of $\underline{N}$ that are ADP-ribosylated by cholera toxin (Katada and Ui, 1982a and b). Research is currently underway to purify $\underline{N}_i$ (containing the ca. 40,000 dalton pertussis toxin substrate) and to determine whether this protein resembles $\underline{N}_s$ in its $\alpha\beta$-type heterodimeric composition and if so, whether the β-type subunit of $\underline{N}_i$ is related to the β-type subunit of $\underline{N}_s$. The possibility exists that $\underline{N}_i$ and $\underline{N}_s$ are functions embedded in an $\underline{N}$ protein of $\alpha_s \alpha_i \beta$ composition with $\underline{n}\alpha_i$ being the pertussis toxin substrate responsible for mediation of attenuating effects of nucleotides (enhanced by receptors that mediate attentuating effects onto adenylyl cyclase), $\underline{n}\alpha_s$ being the cholera toxin substrate(s) responsible for mediation of stimulatory regulation of adenylyl cyclases and the $\underline{n}\beta$ subunit being responsible for interaction with receptors and both α_s and α_i subunits of $\underline{N}$. Chemical isolation of $\underline{N}_i$ and comparison to $\underline{N}_s$ will yield answers to some of these questions. In this context it is of interest to note that cyc- S49 cell membranes that are void of the $\underline{n}\alpha_s$ type subunit of $\underline{N}$ (Ferguson et al., 1982) contain an adenylyl cyclase activity that is readily measurable after stimulation by the diterpene forskolin and that this activity is inhibitable by guanine nucleotides (Fig. 22). This suggests that cyc- S49 membranes while void of $\underline{N}_s$-type N-protein, are constitutive for the $\underline{N}_i$-type N protein. This cell line will therefore aid further in the elucidation of regulatory features of adenylyl cyclases.

5.3. Comparison of Receptor Affinity Regulation by $\underline{N}_i$ to that by $\underline{N}_s$

As are stimulatory receptors, attenuating receptors are also regulated by guanine nucleotides and Mg ion in terms of their affinity for agonist (Hoffman et al., 1980; Wei and Sulakhe, 1980). These regulatory effects, however, are in no way different for attenuating receptors from those seen for stimulatory receptors. Thus, when present, Mg causes an increase in binding affinities and guanine nucleotides decrease binding affinities. This raises further questions as to the meaning of $\underline{N}$-mediated regulation of receptor-agonist interactions. It becomes clear, therefore, that if opposing effects are to be elicited and Mg and guanine nucleotide regulation of receptor affinity for hormone do not differ, the message that lies in regulation of receptor affinities has up until now eluded us.

5.4 $\underline{N}$ Proteins as a Family of Signal Transducing Proteins: $\underline{N}_s$, $\underline{N}_i$, $\underline{N}_x$, and $\underline{N}_{h\mu}$

As mentioned above, two types of $\underline{N}$ components or proteins have been defined that couple to adenylyl cyclase: $\underline{N}_s$ and $\underline{N}_i$. They share the properties of having ADP-ribosylatable subunits, of binding GTP or its analogs, of transducing the receptor occupancy signal into altered cAMP formation and of regulating in an as yet not well understood manner receptor binding. These are not the only guanine nucleotide regulatory proteins involved in signal transduction, however. As illustrated in Fig. 23, Goodhardt et al. (1982), have recently described guanine nucleotide regulation of the liver

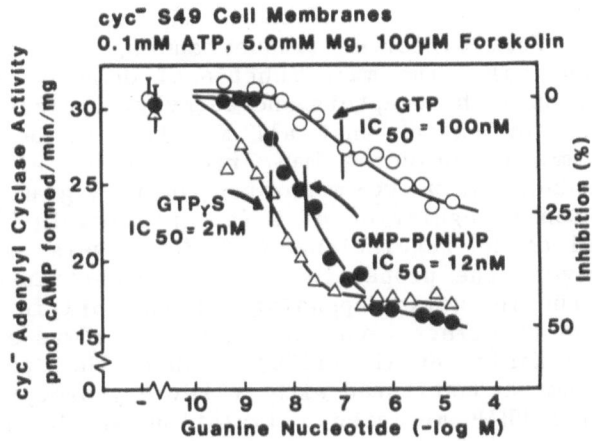

Figure 22. Inhibition of cyc- S49 cell adenylyl cyclase by nucleotides. The assays were carried out using MgATP as substrate with forskolin present throughout. Inhibition by guanine nucleotides is equally effective on a percent basis in the absence of forskolin (not shown). (For further details see Hildebrandt et al., 1982.)

alpha-adrenergic receptor. This receptor affects intracellular Ca fluxes and distributions, phosphatidyl inositol breakdown and leads to phosphorylase b kinase activation without
affecting cAMP. Similarly Yamada et al. (1980) have shown
guanine nucleotide regulation of $alpha_1$-adrenergic receptors
in heart. The term N_x may be used to describe the guanine
nucleotide regulatory component involved in mediating $alpha_1$-
adrenergic receptors. In liver, effects of N_x are under
control of glucocorticoids and disappear upon adrenalectomy
(Fig. 23). Still another guanine nucleotide binding regulatory component involved in signal transduction has been
purified from rod outer segments of retinas. This component
mediates the photoreceptor-dependent activation of cGMP-
specific phosphodiesterase in this tissue. Here, as is the
case with adenylyl cyclase, the transduction process is GTP
and Mg dependent. This protein, which we shall call $N_{h\mu}$ was
christened transducin by Stryer et al. (1982). $N_{h\mu}$, like N_s
and N_i may be a GTPase. Comparison of the structural data
known for $N_{h\mu}$ to that of N_s is complex for $N_{h\mu}$ appears to be
composed of at leat two proteins. One of them, however, is
also a heterodimer of $\alpha\beta$ composition. Interestingly, the β
subunit of $N_{h\mu}$ is of $Mr \cong 35000$.

In addition to the existence of various types of N
proteins, N_s from different tissues and species are similar
but not identical. The main functional domains responsible
for interaction with receptors and adenylyl cyclase have been
preserved to the extent that all N_s studied, be they from
birds or mammals including man, reconstitute all forms of
signal transduction in cyc- membranes, be they guanine nucleotide or hormonal regulation of C (exemplified in Fig. 14) or
guanine nucleotide regulation of R (Sternweis and Gilman,
1979). However, the properties of the reconstituted systems
differ in subtle ways depending on the origin of the N
proteins used to effect reconstitution. This was exemplified
by a study of Kaslow et al. (1979) in which the cyc- adenylyl
cyclase system reconstituted with turkey erythrocyte N showed
lags in GMP-P(NH)P mediated stimulation which were longer
than those observed when reconstitutions had been obtained
with wild type S49 cell N. This is precisely the main kinetic
difference between turkey erythrocyte adenylyl clase and S49
(and other mammalian) adenylyl cyclases. Property differences
of this kind may relate to differing proportions of isoforms
of n_α subunits of N_s. Thus, as seen upon ADP-ribosylation of
membranes with cholera toxin, turkey erythrocytes have single
Mr 42,000 n_α peptide, S49 cells have an Mr 42,000 peptide

(predominating) and an Mr 51-52,000 doublet, liver membranes have an Mr 42,000 (also reported as Mr 45,000) predominating peptide and an Mr 52,000 minor peptide, and transformed lung fibroblasts contain only an Mr 52,000 n_α peptide and lack the Mr 42,000 peptide that predominates in almost all other cells. Although the characteristics of the turkey erythrocyte adenylyl cyclase might therefore be ascribed at least in part to a lack of a 50-52,000 dalton ADP-ribosylatable isoform of $n_{-\alpha}$ subunit of N_{-s}, this argument vanishes upon examination of human erythrocyte n_α which in membranes exists only in a 42,000 dalton ADP-ribosylated form yet reconstitutes in <u>cyc</u>- a system that has very short lags as compared to what is observed with turkey erythrocyte <u>N</u>.

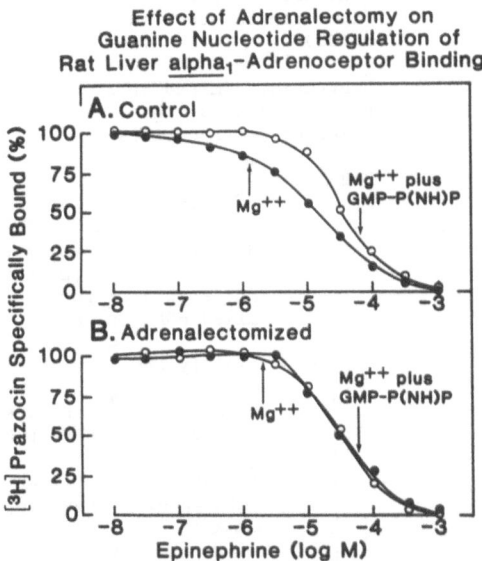

Figure 23. Guanine nucleotide effect on agonist (epinephrine) binding to liver membrane <u>alpha</u>₁-adrenergic receptor and abolishment upon adrenalectomy. Liver membranes from control (top panel) and adrenalectomized rats (bottom panel) were incubated with 1 nM [³H]prazocin and the indicated concentrations of agonist in buffer containing 10 mM MgCl₂. After incubation the samples were filtered through Whatman GF/C filters, washed and analyzed for bound [³H]prazosin by liquid scintillation counting. (For further details see Goodhardt et al., 1982).

Table I.

Strategy for the Determination of the Primary Sequence Structure

N proteins via Molecular Cloning

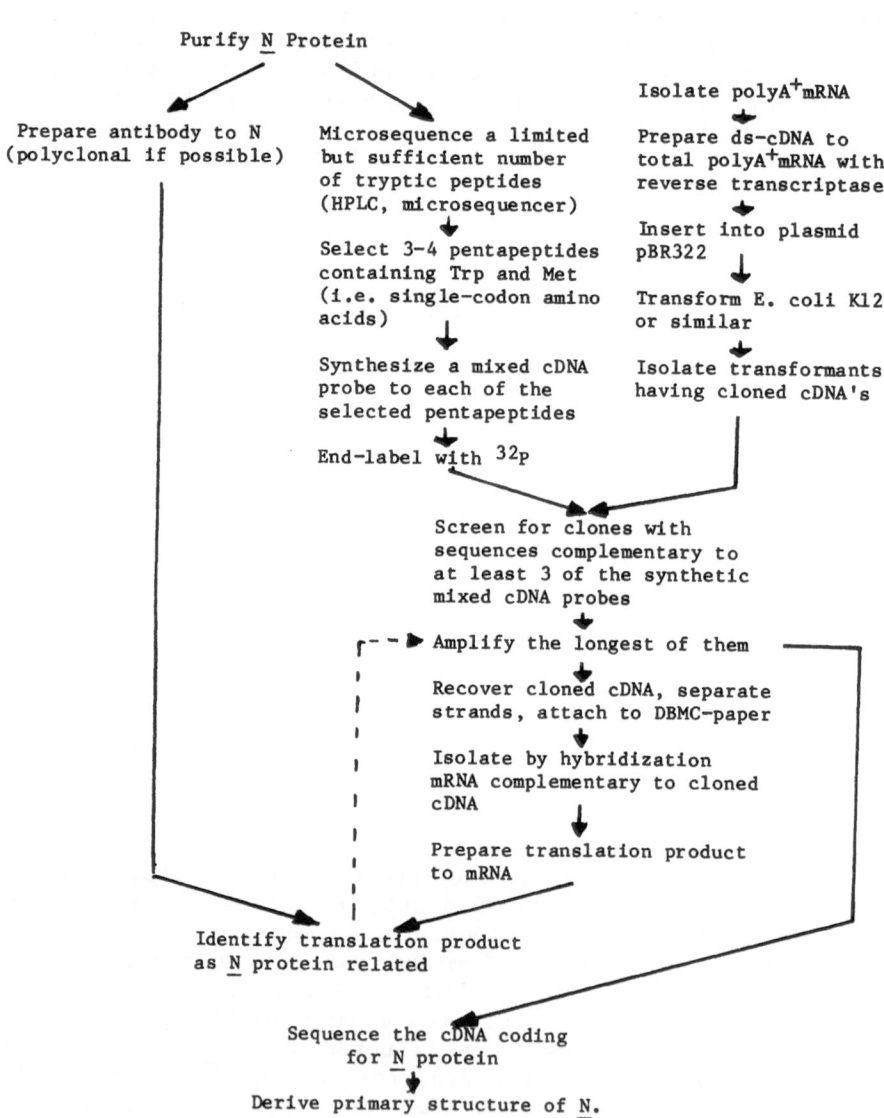

Purify N Protein

Prepare antibody to N
(polyclonal if possible)

Microsequence a limited
but sufficient number
of tryptic peptides
(HPLC, microsequencer)

Select 3-4 pentapeptides
containing Trp and Met
(i.e. single-codon amino
acids)

Synthesize a mixed cDNA
probe to each of the
selected pentapeptides

End-label with ^{32}P

Isolate polyA^{+}mRNA

Prepare ds-cDNA to
total polyA^{+}mRNA with
reverse transcriptase

Insert into plasmid
pBR322

Transform E. coli K12
or similar

Isolate transformants
having cloned cDNA's

Screen for clones with
sequences complementary to
at least 3 of the synthetic
mixed cDNA probes

Amplify the longest of them

Recover cloned cDNA, separate
strands, attach to DBMC-paper

Isolate by hybridization
mRNA complementary to cloned
cDNA

Prepare translation product
to mRNA

Identify translation product
as N protein related

Sequence the cDNA coding
for N protein

Derive primary structure of N.

In conclusion, N_s seems to be polymorphic and appears to belong to a family of signal tranducing proteins. An investigation into structural aspects of N proteins to elucidate the basis for their similar and differential properties seems to be called for. However, because of the extreme scarcity of these proteins standard protein sequencing techniques can not be used to obtain this information. One approach that we are currently following is outlined in Table I. It involves molecular cloning of total messenger RNA, identification of the desired clones with a 14 to 15 nucleotide long synthetic cDNA -- made on the basis of partial amino acid sequencing of the protein -- and sequencing of the cDNA coding for the protein to deduce the total amino acid sequence and structural organization of the protein. By carrying out this approach for each subunit of N_s first and then for subunits for other N proteins (N_i, N_x and N_{hu}) it can be expected that a unique insight into common and differential features of these signal tranducing proteins will be obtained which due to the natural scarcity of these proteins (1/50,000th of cell protein), could not be obtained otherwise.

Some "minor" questions remain as well: Are N proteins GTPases? What is the stoichiometry between N, R and C? Does physical dissociation of R from N, and N from C, and n_α from n_β actually occur, or are changes in degree of subunit and component interaction all that happens under the various regulatory conditions thus far defined? These and all of the questions raised earlier will surely find answers in the near future. And, other new ones are going to emerge.

ACKNOWLEDGMENT. This work was supported in part by NIH research grants HD-09581 and AM-19318 to LB, CA-29808 to RI, HD-16594 to JA and HD-11356 to MHD; NIH center grants HD-07495 and AM-27685; and by Postdoctoral Fellowship HD-05823 to HJK, New Investigator Research Award AM-26905 to RI and Research Career Development Award HD-00292 to MHD. JC is a trainee of Diabetes Training Grant AM-07348 to Dr. J. B. Field.

REFERENCES

Abramowitz, J., and Birnbaumer, L., 1982, Properties of the hormonally responsive rabbit luteal adenylyl cyclase: effects of guanine nucleotides and magnesium ion on stimulation by gonadotropin and catecholamines, Endocrinology 110:773.

Abramowitz, J., Iyengar, R., and Birnbaumer, L., 1980, On the
    mode of action of catecholamines on the turkey erythrocyte
    adenylyl cyclase: Evaluation of basic activity states
    after removal of endogenous GDP and interpretation of
    nucleotide regulation and hormone activation in terms of a
    two state model, J. Biol. Chem. 255:8259.
Abramowitz, J., Iyengar, R., and Birnbaumer, L., 1982, Guanine
    nucleotide and magnesium ion regulation of the interaction
    of gonadotropic and β-adrenergic receptors with their
    hormones: a comparative study using a single membrane
    system, Endocrinology 110:336.
Aktories, K., and Jakobs, K. H., 1981, Epinephrine inhibits
    adenylate cyclase and stimulates a GTPase in human platelet
    membranes via α-adrenoceptors, FEBS Letters 130:235.
Aktories, K., Schultz, G., and Jakobs, K. H., 1979, Inhibition
    of hamster fat cell adenylate cyclase by prostaglandin E_1
    and epinephrine: requirement for GTP and sodium ions,
    FEBS Letters 107:100.
Amsterdam, A., Nimrod, A., Lamprecht, S. A., Bernstein, Y., and
    Lindner, H. R., 1974, Internalization and degradation of
    receptor-bound hCG in granulosa cell cultures, Am. J.
    Physiol. 236:E129.
Anderson, W. B., and Jaworski, C. J., 1979, Isoproteronol
    induced desensitization of adenylyl cyclase responsiveness
    in a cell-free system, J. Biol. Chem. 254:4596.
Bird, S. J., and Maguire, M. E., 1978, The agonist-specific
    effect of magnesium action of magnesium action of GTP and
    magnesium in adenylate cyclase activation, J. Biol. Chem.
    253:8826.
Birnbaumer, L., Pohl, S. L., and Rodbell, M., 1969, Adenyl
    cyclase in fat cells. I. Properties and effects of adreno-
    corticotropin and fluoride, J. Biol. Chem. 244:3468.
Birnbaumer, L., Swartz, T. L., Abramowitz, J., Mintz, P. W., and
    Iyengar, R., 1980, Transient and steady state kenetics of
    the interaction of nucleotides with the adenylyl cyclase
    system from rat liver plasma membranes: Interpretation in
    terms of a simple two-state model, J. Biol. Chem. 255:3542.
Birnbaumer, L., Swartz, T. L., Rojas, F. J., and Garber, A. J.,
    1983, Synthesis, purification by HPLC and characterization
    of monoiodoglucagon labeled with carrier-free ^{125}I: use as
    a glucagon receptor probe, J. Receptor Res. (in press).
Blume, A. J., Lichtstein, D., and Boone, G., 1979, Coupling of
    opiate receptors to adenylate cyclase: Requirement for
    Na^+ and GTP, Proc. Natl. Acad. Sci. USA 76:5626.
Blockaert, J., Hunzicker-Dunn, M., and Birnbaumer, L., 1976,
    Hormone-stimulated desensitization of hormone-dependent
    adenylyl cyclase, J. Biol. Chem. 251:2653.

Brown, M. S., and Goldstein, J. L., 1976, Receptor mediated
    control of cholesterol metabolism, Science 191:150.
Cassel, D., and Pfeuffer, T., 1978, Mechanism of cholera toxin
    action: covalent modification of the guanyl nucleotide-
    binding protein of the adenylate cyclase system, Proc.
    Natl. Acad. Sci. USA 75:2669.
Cassel, D., and Selinger, Z., 1976, Catecholamine-stimulated
    GTPase activity in turkey erythrocyte membranes, Biochim.
    Biophys. Acta 452:538.
Cassel, D., and Selinger, Z., 1977, Mechanism of adenylate
    cyclase activation by cholera toxin: inhibition of GTP
    hydrolysis at the regulatory site, Proc. Natl. Acad. Sci.
    USA 74:3307.
Cassel, D., and Selinger, Z., 1978, Mechanism of adenylate
    cyclase activation through the beta-adrenergic receptor.
    Catecholamine-induced displacement of bound GDP by GTP.
    Proc. Natl. Acad. Sci. USA 75:4155.
Conn, P. M., Conti, M., Harwood, J. P., Dufau, M. L., and Catt,
    K. J., 1978, Internalization of gonadotropin receptor
    complex in ovarian luteal cells, Nature 274:598.
Conti, M., Harwood, J. P., Hsueh, A. J. W., Dufau, M. L., and
    Catt, K. J., 1978, Internalization of gonadotropin receptor
    and desensitization of adenylate cyclase in the ovary, J.
    Biol. Chem. 251:7729.
Cooper, D. M. F., 1982, Biomodal regulation of adenylate
    cyclase, FEBS Letters 138:157.
Cooper, D. M. F., Schlegel, W., Lin, M. C., and Rodbell, M.,
    1979, The fat cell adenylate cyclase system; characteriza-
    tion and manipulation of its bimodal regulation by GTP, J.
    Biol. Chem. 254:8927.
Cronin, M. J., Myers, G. A., Dabney, L. G., and Hewlett, E. L.,
    1982, Pertussis toxin uncouples dopamine receptor-mediated
    inhibition of prolactin release. 64th Annual Meeting of
    the Endocrine Society, Abstract, No. 857, p. 294.
Dufau, M. L., Baukal, A. J., and Catt, K. J., 1980, Hormone-
    induced guanyl nucleotide binding and activation of aden-
    ylate cyclase in the Leydig cell, Proc. Natl. Acad. Sci.
    USA 77:5837.
Ezra, E., and Salomon, Y., 1980, Mechanism of desensitization
    of adenylate cyclase by lutropin. GTP-dependent uncoupling
    of the receptor, J. Biol. Chem. 255:65.
Ezra, E., and Salomon, Y., 1981, Mechanism of adenylate cyclase
    by lutropin. Impaired introduction of GTP into the regula-
    tory site, J. Biol. Chem. 256:5377.
Ferguson, K. M., Northup, J. K., and Gilman, A. G., 1982, Goat
    antibodies to the regulatory component of adenylate
    cyclase, Fed. Proc. 41:1407 (Abstract No. 6642).

Fung, B. K.-K., Hurley, J. B., and Stryer, L., 1981, Flow of information in the light-triggered cyclic nucleotide cascade of vision, Proc. Natl. Acad. Sci. 78:152.

Gill, P. M., and Meren, R., 1978, ADP-ribosylation of membrane proteins catalyzed by cholera toxin. Basis of the activation of adenylate cyclase, Proc. Natl. Acad. Sci. USA 75:3050.

Goodhardt, M., Ferry, N., Geynet, P., and Hanoune, J., 1982, Hepatic alpha$_1$-adrenergic receptors show agonist-specific regulation by guanine nucleotides: Loss of nucleotide effect after adrenalectomy, J. Biol. Chem., 257:11577.

Hanski, E., Sternweis, P. C., Northrup, J. K., Domerick, A. W., and Gilman, A. G., 1981, The regulatory component of adenylate cyclase, J. Biol. Chem. 256:12911.

Harwood, J. P., Conti, M., Conn, P. M., Dufau, M. L., and Catt, K. J., 1978, Receptor regulation and target cell responses: studies in the ovarian luteal cell, Mol. Cell. Endocrinol. 11:121.

Hazeki, O., and Ui, M., 1980, Modification by islet-activating protein of receptor-mediated regulation of cyclic AMP accumulation in isolated rat heart cells, J. Biol. Chem. 256:2856.

Hildebrandt, J., Hanoune, J., and Birnbaumer, L., 1982, Guanine nucleotide inhibition of cyc⁻ S49 mouse lymphoma cell membrane adenylyl cyclase, J. Biol. Chem., 257:14723.

Hoffman, B., Mullikin-Kilpatrick, D., and Lefkowitz, R. J., 1980, Heterogeneity of radioligand binding to α-adrenergic receptors; analysis of guanine nucleotide regulation of agonist binding in relation to receptor subtypes, J. Biol. Chem. 255:4645.

Hsueh, A. J. W., Dufau, M. L., and Catt, K. J., 1976, Regulation of luteinzing hormone receptors in testicular interstitial cells by gonadotropin, Biochem. Biophys. Res. Commun. 72:1145.

Hsueh, A. J. W., Dufau, M. L., and Catt, K. J., 1977, Gonadotropin-induced regulation of luteinizing hormone receptors and desensitization of testicular 3'5'-cyclic AMP and testosterone responses, Proc. Natl. Acad. Sci. USA 74:592.

Hunzicker-Dunn, M., and Birnbaumer, L., 1976a, Adenylyl cyclase in ovarian tissues. II. Regulation of responsiveness to LH, FSH, and PGE$_1$ in the rabbit, Endocrinology 99:185.

Hunzicker-Dunn, M., and Birnbaumer, L., 1976b, Adenylyl cyclase activities in ovarian tissues. III. Regulation of responsiveness to LH, FSH and PGE$_1$ in prepubertal, cycling, pregnant and pseudopregnant rats, Endocrinology 99:198.

Hunzicker-Dunn, M., and Birnbaumer, L., 1976c, Adenylyl cyclase activities in ovarian tissues. IV. Gonadotropin-induced desensitization of the luteal adenylyl cyclase throughout pregnancy and pseudopregnancy in the rabbit and the rat, Endocrinology 99:211.

Hunzicker-Dunn, M., and Birnbaumer, L., 1981, Studies on the mechanism of LH-induced desensitization of the rabbit follicular adenylyl cyclase system in vitro, Endocrilology 109:345.

Hunzicker-Dunn, M., Derda, D., Jungmann, R. A., and Birnbaumer, L., 1979a, Resensitization of the desensitized follicular adenylyl cyclase system to LH, Endocrinology 104:1785.

Hunzicker-Dunn, M., Day, S. L., Abramowitz, J., and Birnbaumer, L., 1979b, Ovarian responses of pregnant mare serum gonadotropin- and human chorionic gonadotropin-primed rats: desensitizing, luteolytic and ovulatory effects of a single dose of human chorionic gonadotropin, Endocrinology 105:442.

Iyengar, R., 1981, Hysteretic activation of adenylyl cyclases. II. Mg ion regulation of the activation of the regulatory component as seen in reconstitution assays, J. Biol. Chem. 256:11042.

Iyengar, R., and Birnbaumer, L., 1979, GDP promotes coupling and activation of cyclizing activity in the glucagon-sensitive adenylate cyclase system of rat liver plasma membranes. Evidence for two levels of regulation in adenylyl cyclase, Proc. Natl. Acad. Sci. USA 76:3189.

Iyengar, R., and Birnbaumer, L., 1981, Hysteretic activation of adenylyl cyclases. I. Effects of Mg ion on the rate of activation by guanine nucleotides and fluoride, J. Biol. Chem. 256:11036.

Iyengar, R., and Birnbaumer, L., 1982, Hormone receptor modulates the regulatory component of adenylyl cyclase by reducing its requirement for Mg and enhancing its extent of activation, Proc. Natl. Acad. Sci. USA (in press).

Iyengar, R., Abramowitz, J., Bordelon-Riser, M. E., Blume, A. J., and Birnbaumer, L., 1980a, Regulation of hormone-receptor coupling to adenylyl cyclase: effects of GTP and GDP, J. Biol. Chem. 255:10312.

Iyengar, R., Mintz, P. W., Swartz, T. L., and Birnbaumer, L., 1980b, Divalent cation-induced desensitization of glucagon stimulable adenylyl cyclase in rat liver plasma membranes: GTP-dependent stimulation by glucagon, J. Biol. Chem. 255:11875.

Iyengar, R., Bhat, M. K., Riser, M. E., and Birnbaumer, L.,
    1981, Receptor-specific desensitization of the S49 cell
    adenylyl cyclase: unaltered behavior of the regulatory
    component, J. Biol. Chem. 256:4810.
Jakobs, K. H., Actories, K., and Schultz, G., 1979, GTP-depend-
    ent inhibition of cardiac adenylate cyclase by muscarinic
    cholinergic agonists, Naunyn-Achmiedeberg's Arch.
    Pharmacol. 310:113.
Jard, S., Cantau, B., and Jakobs, K. R., 1981, Angiotensin II
    and α-adrenergic agonists inhibit rat liver adenylate
    cyclase, J. Biol. Chem. 256:2603.
Jonassen, J. A., and Richards, J. S., 1980, Granulosa cell
    desensitization: effects of gonadotropins in antral and
    preantral follicles, Endocrinology 106:1786.
Kaslow, H. R., Farfel, Z., Johnson, G. L., and Bourne, H. R.,
    1979, Adenylate cyclase assembled in vitro: cholera toxin
    substrates determines different patterns of regulation by
    isoproterenol and guanosine 5'-triphosphate, Mol.
    Pharmacol. 15:472.
Katada, T., and Ui, M., 1981, Islet-activating protein; a modi-
    fier of receptor-mediated regulation of rat islet adenylate
    cyclase, J. Biol. Chem. 256:8310.
Katada, T., and Ui, M., 1982a, ADP ribosylation of the specific
    membrane protein of C6 cells by islet-activating protein
    associated with modification of adenylate cyclase activity,
    J. Biol. Chem. 257:7210.
Katada, T., and Ui, M., 1982b, Direct modification of the
    membrane adenylate cyclase system by islet-activating
    protein due to ADP-ribosylation of a membrane protein,
    Proc. Natl. Acad. Sci. USA 79:3129.
Katikineni, M., Davies, T. F., Huhtaniemi, I. T., and Catt, K.
    J., 1980, Luteinizing hormone-receptor interaction in the
    testis: progressive decrease in reversibility of the
    hormone-receptor complex, Endocrinology 107:1980.
Kirchick, H. J., and Birnbaumer, L., 1982, hCG-induced desensi-
    tization of luteal catecholamine-responsive adenylyl
    cyclase is a result of alterations in the nucleotide
    binding regulatory (N)-component, Biol. Reprod. 26
    (Suppl. # 1), 41A (Abstract #10).
Koch, Y., Zor, U., Pomerantz, S. H., Chobsieng, P., and LIndner,
    H. R., 1973, Intrinsic stimulatory action of follicle
    stimulating hormone on ovarian adenylate cyclase, J
    Endocrinol. 58:677.
Lamprecht, S. A., Zor, U., Tsafriri, A., and Lindner, H. R.,
    1973, Action of prostaglandin E_2 and of luteinizing hormone
    on ovarian adenylate cyclase, protein kinase and ornithine

decarboxylase activity during postnatal development and
maturity in the rat, J. Endocrinol. 57:217.

Limbird, L. E., Gill, D. M., and Lefkowitz, R. J., 1980,
Agonist-promoted coupling of the B-adrenergic receptor with
the guanine nucleotide protein of the adenylate cyclase
system, Proc. Natl. Acad. Sci. 77:775.

Londos, C., Cooper, D. M. F., Schlegel, W., and Rodbell, M.,
1978, Adenosine analogs inhibit adipocyte adenylate
cyclase by a GTP-dependent process: basis for actions
of adenosine and methylxanthines on cyclic AMP production and lipolysis, Proc. Natl. Acad. Sci.
USA 75:5362.

Marsh, J. M., Mills, T. M., and LeMaire, W. J., 1972, Cyclic AMP
synthesis in the rabbit Graafian follicle and the effect of
luteinizing hormone, Biochim. Biophys. Acta 273:197.

Nickols, G. A., and Brooker, G., 1979, Induction of refractoriness to isoproterenol by prior treatment of C6-2B rat
astrocytoma cells with cholera toxin, J. Cyclic Nucleo.
Res. 5:435.

Northup, J. K., Sternweis, P. C., Smigel, M. D., Schleifer,
L. S., Ross, E. M., and Gilman, A. G., 1980, Purification
of the regulatory component of adenylate cyclase, Proc.
Natl. Acad. Sci. USA 77:6515.

Pfeuffer, T., 1977, GTP-binding proteins in membranes and the
control of adenylate cyclase activity, J. Biol. Chem.
252:7224.

Pfeuffer, T., 1979, Guanine nucleotide-controlled interactions
between components of adenylate cyclase, FEBS Letters
101:85.

Rao, M. C., Richards, J. S., Midgley, A. R. Jr., and Reichert,
L. E., 1977, Regulation of gonadotropin receptors by LH in
granulosa cells, Endocrinology 101:512.

Rodbell, M., Krans, H. M. J., Pohl, S. L., and Birnbaumer, L.,
1971a, The glucagon-sensitive adenyl cyclase system in
plasma membranes of rat liver. IV. Effects of guanyl
nucleotides on binding of ^{125}I-glucagon, J. Biol. Chem.
246:1872.

Rodbell, M., Birnbaumer, L., Pohl, S. L., and Krans, H. M. J.,
1971b, The glucagon-sensitive adenyl cyclase system in
plasma membranes of rat liver. V. An obligatory role of
guanylnucleotides in glucagon action, J. Biol. Chem.
246:1877.

Rodbell, M., Lin, M. C., and Salomon, Y., 1974, Evidence
for interdependent action of glucagon and nucleotides
on the hepatic adenylate cyclase system, J. Biol.
Chem. 249:59.

Ross, E. M., and Gilman, A. G., 1977, Resolution of some components of adenylate cyclase necessary for catalytic activity,
J. Biol. Chem. 252:6966.

Ross, E. M., Howlett, A. C., Fergusson, K. M., and Gilman, A.
G., 1978, Reconstitution of hormone-sensitive adenylate
cyclase activity with resolved components of the enzyme,
J. Biol. Chem. 253:6401.

Sharma, S. K., Klee, W. A., and Nirenberg, M., 1977, Opiate-
dependent modulation of adenylate cyclase, Proc. Natl.
Acad. Sci. USA 74:3365.

Somkuti, S. G., Hildebrandt, J. D., Herberg, J. T., and Iyengar,
R., 1982, Divalent cation regulation of adenylyl cyclase;
an allosteroic site on the catalytic component, J. Biol.
Chem. 257:6387.

Sternweis, P. C., and Gilman, A. G., 1979, Reconstitution of
chatecholamine-sensitive adenylate cyclase. Reconstitution
of the uncoupled variant of S49 lymphoma cell, J. Biol.
Chem. 254:3333.

Sternweis, P. C., Northup, J. K., Smigel, M. D., and Gilman, A.
G., 1981, The regulatory component of adenylate cyclase.
Purification and properties, J. Biol. Chem. 256:11517.

Strittmatter, S., and Neer, E. J., 1980, Properties of the
separated catalytic and regulatory units of brain adenylate
cyclase, Proc. Natl. Acad. Sci. USA 77:6344.

Su, Y. F., Cubeddu, X. L., and Perkins, J. P., 1976, Regulation
of adenosine 3',5'-monophosphate content in human astrocytoma cells: desensitization to catecholamines and prostaglandins, J. Cycle. Nucleo. Res. 2L257,

Su, Y. P., Harden, T. K., and Perkins, J. P., 1980, Catechola-
mine-specific desensitization of adenylate cyclase:
evidence for multistep process, J. Biol. Chem. 255:7410.

Suter, D. E., Fletcher, P. W., Sluss, P. M., Reichert, L. E.
Jr., and Niswender, G. D., 1980, Alterations in the number
of ovine luteal receptors for LH and progesterone secretion
induced by homologous hormone, Biol. Repro. 22:205.

Sutherland, E. W., and Rall, T. W., 1962, Adenyl cyclase. I.
Distribution, preparation and properties, J. Biol. Chem.
237:1220.

Yamada, S., Yamamura, H., and Roeske, W. R., 1980, The regulation of cardiac $alpha_1$-adrenergic receptors by guanine
nucleotides and muscarinic cholinergic agonists, Eur. J.
Pharm. 63:239.

Wei, J. W., and Sulakhe, P. V., 1980, Requirement for sulfhydryl
groups in the differential effects of magnesium ion and GTP
on agonist binding of muscarinic cholinergic receptor sites

in rat atrial membrane fraction, Naunym-Schmeideberg's Arch
Pharma. 314:51.
Williams, L. T., Mullikin, D., and Lefkowitz, R. J., 1978,
    Magnesium dependence of agonist binding to adenylate
    cyclase-coupled hormone receptors, J. Biol. Chem. 253:2984.
Birnbaumer, L., and Swartz, T., 1982, Membrane receptors:
    criteria and selected methods of study, in: "Laboratory
    Methods Manual for Hormone action and Molecular Endocrin-
    ology", W. T. Schrader and B. W. O'Malley, eds., Chapter 3,
    Houston Biological Associates.

DISCUSSION

NAOR: I. It seems that the effect of the hormone on increased affinity of Mg^{2+} to the regulatory subunit can only
partly explain the hormone activity, since even in the presence of saturating concentration of Mg^{2+}, there was further
increase in enzyme activity in the presence of the hormone.
2. In the case of homologous desensitization, is the coupling
of the receptor to the regulatory subunit affected?

BIRNBAUMER: In response to your first question; you are
right in that the change in affinity of regulatory component
for Mg is not the sole effect of HR complex. There is a
second effect (for details, see Iyengar and Birnbaumer, 1982)
which consists in a displacement of the equilibrium reaction
between inactive $(N_{\alpha\beta})$ and active (n_α^G) forms of the component
from being at about 50/50 towards formation of more n_α^G. This
is probably due to simultaneous formation of complex $HR \cdot n_\beta(Mg)$
as we explain in the main body of our article. With respect
to your second question, this is precisely the type of effect
we feel the receptor modification has on receptor behavior:
a decrease of the capacity of receptor to interact with the
regulatory subunit.

ROMMERTS: Have interactions between hormone receptor complexes and the regulatory subunit been investigated?

BIRNBAUMER: Very little. Sternweis and Gilman (1980)
demonstrated that reconstitution of cyc- S49 lymphoma cells
with N-containing cholate extracts leads to reappearance
of Mg and G nucleotide mediated regulation of agonist
(isoproterenol) binding to beta-receptors. Schramm and
collaborators showed that turkey solubilized N is activated by

solubilized turkey erythrocyte beta-receptor when combined in a phospholipid vesicle. These are functional measures of RN interactions obtained upon reconstitution. However, physical interactions between R and N have not been reported on as yet and have not as yet been studied by us.

RITZEN: In homologous desensitization, you indicated that the hormone binding to the receptor may be decreased in affinity. Can you discuss this against the recent report by Haour from Lyon, who found (by immunocytochemical methods) thet hCG binding to Leydig cells may be tightened, not even extractable by acid treatment?

BIRNBAUMER: When I referred to the decrease in receptor affinity for agonist in association with homologous (or also heterologous) desensitization, I referred specifically to catcholamine receptors. These are the receptors that (as we discuss in the main body of the above article) show both Mg and GTP shifts in binding. As mentioned too, hCG does not show GTP effects and Mg^{2+} addition, rather than increasing affinity, decreases the affinity of hCG for receptors. Assuming that with hCG receptors, as is the case for catechol-amine receptor regulation, the Mg effect is N-mediated, then one may predict desensitization to lead to a (modest) increase of hCG binding affinity. This, coupled to the inherent high affinity and low reversibility of hCG binding to receptor, could account for Dr. F. Haour's recent findings.

MEANS: Is the purified N component phosphorylated by cAMP-dependent protein kinase? If so, can this be added to cyc-membranes in order to demonstrate hormone-dependent dephosphorylation? Such would be a required corollary of your heterologous desensitization model.

BIRNBAUMER: You are right in that this is a way to test the hypothesis that heterologous desensitization involves phos-phorylation of N. We are currently setting up the conditions to do these experiments and should soon know the answer.

LABRIE: Which other data are available on the characteristics of N_s and N_i, especially those ivolved with their interaction with the receptor and C, similarity or dissimilarity of binding components?

BIRNBAUMER: Since we wrote up the manuscript, we succeeded in purifying N_i, i.e., a protein that has an ADP-ribosylatable subunit (substrate for B. pertussis toxin) of M_r = 39,000 and a non-ADP-ribosylatable subunit of M_r = 35,000. This work was carried out in collaboration with Drs. Sekura and Manclark. We determined further that the 35,000 subunits of N_s and N_i are identical by peptide mapping but their 42,000 and 39,000 ADP-ribosyltable subunits differ not only among themselves but also from the 35,000 subunits. Nothing is as yet published on the possible mode of interaction of the 39,000 α_i subunit of N_i with C. This will require a reconstitution assay for N_i which, at least to our laboratory, is not yet available. As assessed by measurement of ADP-ribosylation of the 39,000 α_i subunit of N_i this protein resembles N_s in that treatment with nucleotide and Mg^{2+} causes the ca. M_r = 80,000 molecule to "dissociate" to a form of M_r = 40,000.

ROMMERTS: Different mechanisms of desensitization have been described. In most of the studies high concentrations of hormones or ions have been employed. I wonder which mechanisms operate when physiological concentrations are used.

BIRNBAUMER: In general desensitization reactions become noticeable only after massive stimulation by high concentrations of hormones and neurotransmitters. Although one can speculate that low ("tonic") levels of hormones and neurotransmitters cause or induce low degrees of desensitization, experimental evidence for such an ongoing process is scant.

NAOR: Most of the data regarding regulation of adenylate cyclase activity came from studies on the coupling of the regulatory subunit (N) to the catalytic subunit (C), what about regulation at the level of the receptor (R)-N coupling and whether the N protein is exposed to the outside of the cell?

BIRNBAUMER: At this time we do not know whether the N protein is exposed towards the outside of the cell. However, as shown by Perkins' group, desensitization reactions are associated with loss of N regulation of R binding to H, and therefore it is most likely that the homologous desensitization reaction involves principally RN uncoupling due to R alteration.

NICHOLSON: Is there any experimental evidence for a steroid-induced desensitization of adenylyl cyclase activity and if so what mechanisms are involved?

BIRNBAUMER: Dr. Howard Kirchick has recently determined (see Abstracts of the 1982 Meeting of the Endocrine Society), that E_2 treatment of rabbits leads to an about 60% loss of LH-stimulable adenylyl cyclase. These changes were associated with a ca. 70% decrease in LH (hCG) receptors, no change in beta-adrenergic receptors and an 20-25% decrease in N_s activity. The mechanisms by which these changes came about are not known at the moment. Their existence, however, indicates that hormonal responses at the adenylyl cyclase level can be under steroid hormone control and that this control is complex and multifaceted.

RAO: Is there a difference in the desensitizing ability of LH and hCG? Do the gonadotropin surges that occur in reproductive cycles cause desensitization?

BIRNBAUMER: In answer to the second part of your question: Yes. We showed some time ago that at the time of ovulation follicles are partially or totally desensitized (see Hunzicker-Dunn and Birnbaumer, 1976a,b,c).

With regards to the first part of your question, we also showed that not only hCG but also LH causes desensitization when injected in large amounts into animals. However, larger doses of LH than of hCG are needed. This is probably due to a combination of LH having a shorter circulating half-life and LH binding in a more reversible manner to receptors.

Regulation of Insulin Responsiveness

RECEPTOR DEFECTS IN GENETIC FORMS OF EXTREME

INSULIN RESISTANCE

Simeon I. Taylor

Diabetes Branch
National Institute of Arthritis, Diabetes, Digestive
    and Kidney Diseases
National Institutes of Health
Bethesda, MD 20205 USA

1. Introduction

The responsiveness of target cells to insulin is carefully regulated under many physiological conditions (Grunberger
et al., 1983; Olefsky, 1981). Thus, two mechanisms work in
concert to regulate the biological effect of insulin upon
target cells: (1) changes in circulating levels of insulin
in plasma; and (2) alterations in the sensitivity of the
target cell to insulin. Abnormalities in the regulation of
insulin sensitivity contribute importantly to the pathophysiology of many disease states: e.g., obesity, type II diabetes
(non-insulin-dependent diabetes mellitus), acromegaly, and
Cushing's syndrome.

In the intact organism, there are many steps involved in
coordinating the synthesis, secretion, and delivery of insulin
to the target cells where insulin ultimately acts. Defects
in many of these steps have been described (Table I). This
chapter will focus primarily on those conditions where insulin
resistance results from an intrinsic defect in the target
cell, despite delivery of a normal amount of insulin in
bioactive form. When the insulin molecule arrives at a
target cell, the first step in insulin action is binding to
the insulin receptor which is located in the plasma membrane.
This binding step is the best understood among the early
steps in insulin action. Consequently, most of what is known
about the mechanisms of regulation of insulin sensitivity

derives from studies of the insulin receptor. Very little is
known with regard to the importance of post-receptor steps in
the regulation of insulin sensitivity.

Table I. Differential Diagnosis of Extreme Insulin
Resistance and Hyperinsulinemia

Cause	Reference
Anti-insulin antibodies	Kahn & Rosenthal (1979)
Subcutaneous degradation of exogenous insulin	Friedenberg et al. (1981)
Defects in insulin biosynthesis	
a. Familial hyperpro- insulinemia	Gabbay et al. (1979) Robbins et al. (1981)
b. Biologically inactive insulin molecule	Given et al. (1980) Haneda et al. (1982)
Syndromes of extreme insulin resistance associated with acanthosis nigricans	
a. Autoantibodies to the insulin receptor	Flier et al. (1976) Kahn et al. (1976)
b. Primary (? genetic) target cell resistance to insulin	(See Table II)

2.   Classification of Genetic Syndromes of Extreme
Insulin Resistance

Among the many clinical syndromes associated with extreme
insulin resistance, several syndromes are usually presumed to
be genetic in etiology (Table II). This presumption is based
almost exclusively on circumstantial evidence:

(1) Parental consaguinity has occasionally been documented (Barnes et al., 1974).

(2) In some syndromes, multiple cases have been identified within the same kindred (Rosenberg et al., 1980; Barnes et al., 1974; Huseman et al., 1978; Scarlett et al., 1982; West et al., 1975).

(3) Biochemical evidence of insulin resistance may be preserved in patients' cells cultivated in vitro (Kobayashi et al., 1978; Schilling et al., 1980; Taylor et al., 1981, 1982a; Podskalny and Kahn, 1982a,b).

These "genetic" syndromes, although rare, are of special interest because they provide an unparalleled opportunity to define the biochemical mechanisms of insulin resistance in human disease. The severity of the insulin resistance in these rare syndromes contrasts markedly with the milder insulin resistance associated with common syndromes such as type II diabetes. Thus, the molecular defects in these rare syndromes of extreme insulin resistance are more severe and, as a result, easier to detect. Moreover, if one assumes that the syndromes result from point mutations in a single gene, this should facilitate the identification of the primary lesion(s) causing insulin resistance.

A priori, one might have predicted that each distinct clinical syndrome would have been associated with a different defect, and that each biochemical defect would cause a specific syndrome. However, this does not seem to be the case. Curiously, in any given clinical syndrome (e.g., leprechaunism), multiple different biochemical mechanisms for insulin resistance have been identified in individual patients (Taylor et al., 1981, 1982a; D'Ercole et al., 1979; Schilling et al., 1980). Moreover, any particular biochemical mechanism causing insulin resistance (e.g., a decrease in the number of insulin receptors) may give rise to several clinical syndromes (Taylor et al., 1982a). On the other hand, this confusing situation may arise in part from the fact that we have not completely defined the genetic defect in any case. For example, two patients with different clinical syndromes may both have a decrease in the number of insulin receptors per cell. However, it is possible that the decrease in receptor number might result from different molecular defects in the two syndromes.

Table II. Primary (? genetic) Target Cell Resistance

Cause	Reference
Lipoatrophic diabetes	Wachslicht-Rodbard et al. (1981) Rossini and Cahill (1979)
Type A extreme insulin resistance	Kahn et al. (1976) Barnes et al. (1974) Flier et al. (1980) Scarlett et al. (1982) Bar et al. (1980)
Leprechaunism	Donohue and Uchida (1954) Rosenberg et al. (1980) D'Ercole et al. (1979) Kobayashi et al. (1978) Schilling et al. (1979) Taylor et al. (1981, 1982a,b) Podskalny and Kahn (1982a,b) Knight et al. (1981)
Rabson-Mendenhall Syndrome	Rabson and Mendenhall (1956) West, Lloyd, and Turner (1975) West and Leonard (1980) Perez Corral et al. (1980) Taylor et al. (1983)

3.   Mechanisms Causing Extreme Insulin Resistance

3.1. Decreased Number of Insulin Receptors

The most straightforward mechanism for insulin resistance is a decrease in the number of insulin receptors on the
surface of each cell. If insulin binding to the cell is
impaired, the cell's ability to respond to insulin is
decreased. This mechanism was first recognized in patients
with the syndrome of type A extreme insulin resistance (Kahn
et al., 1976; Bar et al., 1980). The initial demonstration
of a decrease in the number of insulin receptors depended on

the use of circulating monocytes which were studied immediately after they were obtained from the patients. Of course,
in this setting, it was impossible to be certain whether the
decrease in insulin binding was the result or the cause of
the insulin resistance. This uncertainty arises from the
fact that insulin resistance - regardless of mechanism - may
be associated with a compensatory rise in the level of plasma
insulin. Hyperinsulinemia, in turn, would be expected to
give rise to a decrease in the number of insulin receptors by
a process known as down-regulation (Gavin et al., 1974).
Using cultured lymphocytes from the patients, we demonstrated
that this decrease in receptor number was an intrinsic
property of the patients' cells - not the consequence of
down-regulation induced by hyperinsulinemia. After transformation with Epstein-Barr virus, the patients' lymphocytes may
be grown indefinitely in vitro under defined conditions free
from the influence of the patients' internal milieu. These
cultured lymphocytes retained the same binding defect which
was expressed in the patients' fresh cells (Fig. 1). With
cultured cells from four patients with various syndromes of
extreme insulin resistance (i.e., leprechaunism, type A
extreme insulin resistance and the Rabson-Mendenhall
syndrome), the number of insulin receptors per cell was
decreased by approximately 80-90% below the lower limit of
normal (Taylor et al., 1982a). Moreover, the residual insulin
receptors on these patients' cells appeared to be qualitatively normal as judged by their specificity for insulin
analogs (Fig. 2) and their ability to be recognized by anti-
receptor antibody (Fig. 3).

In theory, many possible defects might give rise to a
decrease in the number of insulin receptors in the plasma
membrane. For example, there might be a decrease in the rate
of synthesis and insertion of receptors into the membrane
because of a block at the level of any of a number of steps:
(1) transcription of RNA; (2) post-translational processing
of the receptor (e.g., glycosylation); or (3) insertion of the
finished receptor into the plasma membrane. Alternatively,
there might be an increase in the rate of degradation of
the receptor either because of an intrinsic instability
of the altered receptor or because of a defect in the
pathways of receptor recycling. In beginning to address these
questions, we have studied the structure of the insulin receptors in cultured lymphocytes from these patients. The normal
insulin receptor consists of two major subunits which are

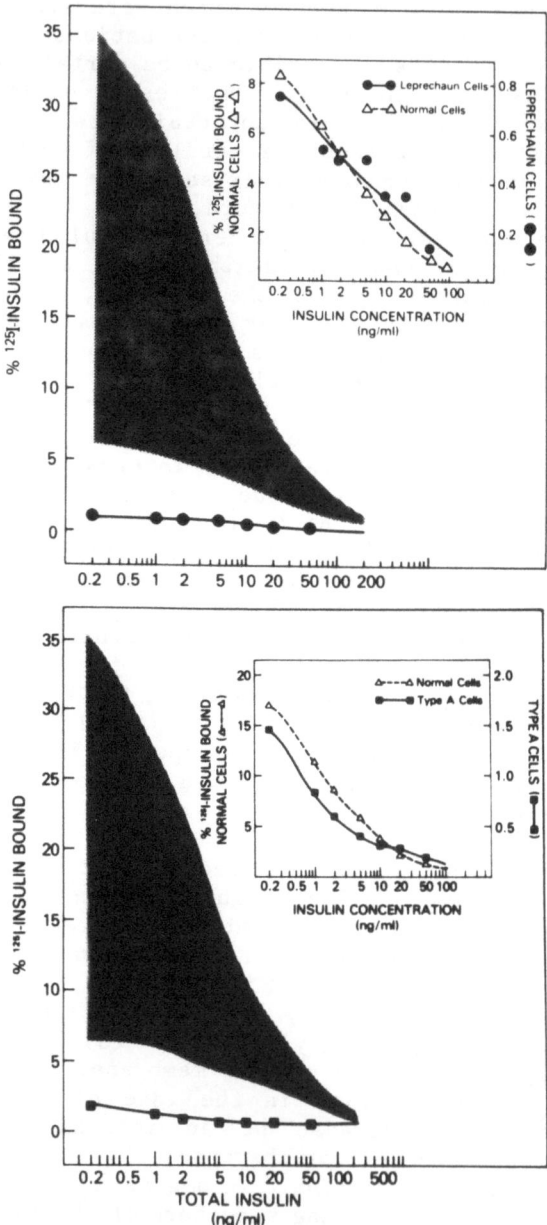

Figure 1. ^{125}I-insulin binding to cultured lymphocytes from patients with a reduced number of insulin receptors. The binding of ^{125}I-insulin (0.1 ng/ml) is plotted as a function of the concentration of unlabelled insulin for cells from

glycoproteins with apparent molecular weights of approximately 135,000 and 95,000 (Pilch and Czech, 1979; Jacobs et al., 1979; Van Obberghen et al., 1980). When cultured cells are iodinated usng $Na^{125}I$ and lactoperoxidase, it is possible to identify the subunits of the insulin receptor using SDS-poly-acrylamide gel electrophoresis to analyze immunoprecipitates of cell extracts (Kasuga et al., 1981a). According to this method as well as other labelling techniques, the subunit structure of the insulin receptor appears to be normal in cultured lymphocytes from these insulin resistant patients (Fig. 4).

What is the quantitative significance of this decrease in the number of insulin receptors? According to a model assuming spare receptors (Kono and Barham, 1971; Roth and Grunfeld, 1981), small decreases in the number of insulin receptors would be expected to shift the dose-response curve for insulin to the right without affecting the maximal response to insulin. However, when the number of receptors per cell is decreased below a critical number, the maximal biological response may be decreased as well. This question has been addressed in detail in one patient studied by Scarlett and collaborators (1982). In their patient, the number of receptors appeared to be so markedly reduced that it was not possible to obtain a normal maximal biological effect even in the presence of a huge excess of insulin. Moreover, because there were no longer any spare receptors, the dose-response curve was shifted rightward. These observations were made using two techniques: in vivo euglycemic clamp studies and in vitro studies of adipocyte hexose transport. While we have not carried out similar studies in our own patients, this patient closely resembled our patients in the magnitude of the binding defect. Thus, it seems likely that our four patients also have a drastic reduction in receptor number to the point that there are no longer

---

Figure 1 (continued). a 6 week old girl with leprechaunism (left hand panel) and a 20 year old woman with type A extreme insulin resistance (right hand panel). The shaded areas represent the total range of binding we have observed with 15 control subjects. Specific binding of ^{125}I-insulin is plotted on an expanded scale in the insets. Reproduced from Taylor et al. (1982a).

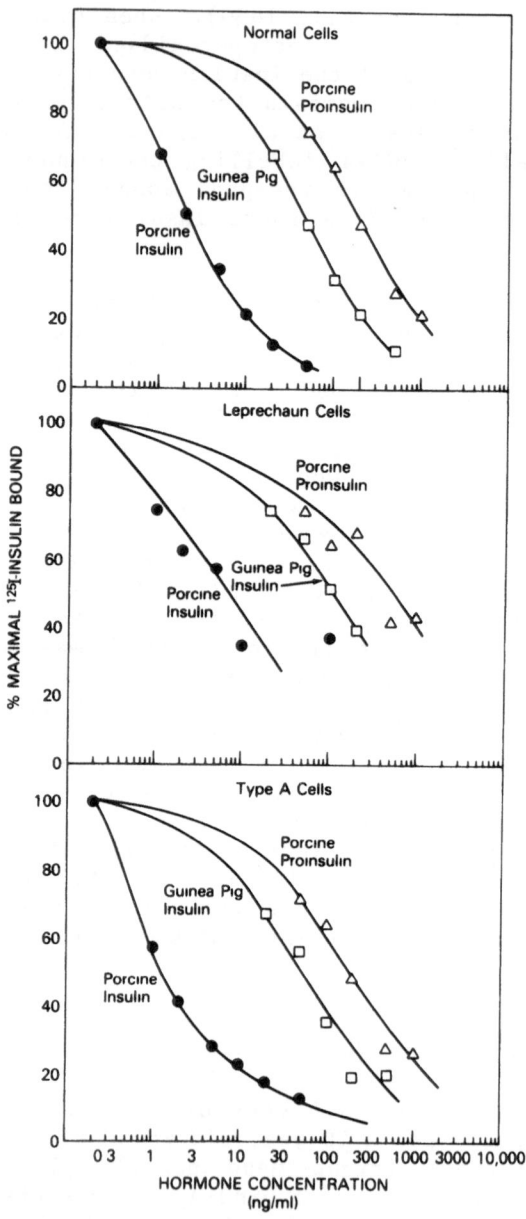

"spare receptors", and that this receptor defect is the explanation of their clinical insulin resistance.

3.2 Qualitative Abnormalities in the Insulin Receptor

Insulin receptors have at least two functions: (1) to bind insulin, and (2) to couple insulin binding to insulin action. Insulin resistance may result from defects compromising either of these functions. However, at present, limitations in our understanding of insulin receptor function prevent us from studying the receptor's coupling function directly. Consequently, defects in the insulin receptor reveal themselves only if they affect the binding function of the receptor. We have characterized one such qualitative receptor defect in detail (Taylor et al., 1981, 1982b; Taylor and Leventhal, 1982). Earlier studies with this patient (leprechaun/Ark-1) had suggested that the binding properties of the receptors were normal (Kobayashi et al. 1978). However this initial impression was based on limited studies carried out at low temperature and unphysiological pH. When a broader range of conditions was considered, it became clear that the binding properties of this patient's receptors were strikingly abnormal. Normal insulin receptors are exquisitely sensitive to changes in temperature and pH (Waelbrock et al., 1979; Waelbrock, 1982). Thus, the apparent affinity of the normal receptor to bind insulin falls by approximately 75% as the temperature is increased from 12° to 37°. In contrast, there is only a 20% fall in the affinity of receptors from leprechaun/Ark-1 (Fig. 5). Similarly, ^{125}I-insulin binding to receptors from leprechaun/Ark-1 had markedly reduced sensitivity to changes in pH (Fig. 6). This qualitative abnormality in ^{125}I-insulin binding was observed not only with intact cells, but with solubilized and partially purified receptors as well (Fig. 6). These observations led to a surprising conclusion: that the receptor from leprechaun/-Ark-1 actually bound an abnormally large amount of insulin

←——

Figure 2. Analog specificity of insulin receptors on cultured lymphocytes from insulin resistant patients. The binding of ^{125}I-insulin (0.1 ng/ml) is plotted as a function of the concentration of unlabelled porcine insulin, guinea pig insulin, or porcine proinsulin. The patients are the same as in Fig. 1. Data are expressed as a percentage of the specific binding of ^{125}I-insulin (0.1 ng/ml) observed in the absence of unlabelled insulin. Reproduced from Taylor et al. (1982a).

under physiological conditions of pH and temperature (i.e., pH 7.4 at 37°C). Because it is hard to attribute insulin resistance to increased insulin binding per se, it seems likely that the binding abnormalities noted in receptors from leprechaun/Ark-1 are a biochemical marker for a structural abnormality in the insulin receptor. Presumably, the major pathophysiological significance of this structural defect is to compromise the receptor's ability to couple insulin binding to insulin action.

We have had limited success in directly demonstrating the presumed structural defect in the insulin receptor of leprechaun/Ark-1. The apparent size of the detergent-solubilized receptor as judged by gel filtration chromatography appears normal (Taylor et al., 1982b). In addition, the subunit structure of the receptor appears normal (Fig. 7).

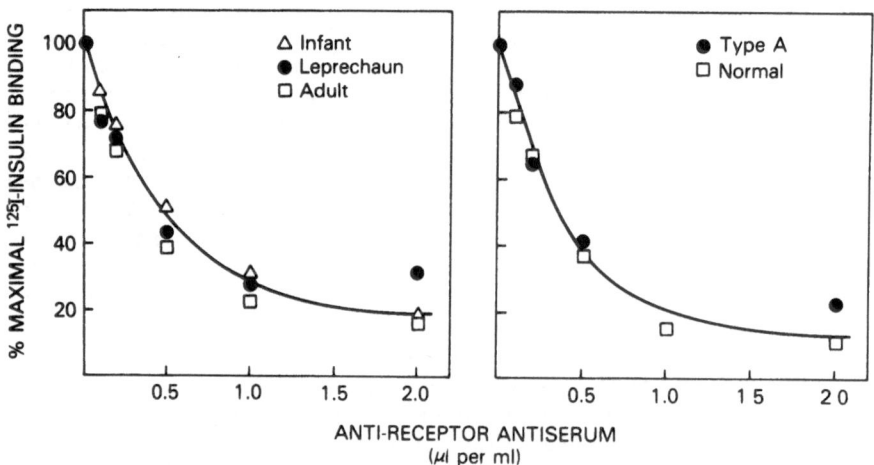

Figure 3. Inhibition of ^{125}I-insulin binding by anti-receptor antiserum. Cultured lymphocytes were incubated for 90 min at 20°C with varying concentrations of antiserum from a patient (B-2) with autoantibodies to the insulin receptor. After the cells were washed to remove the unbound antiserum, binding of ^{125}I-insulin was determined. Data are plotted as a percentage of the specific binding observed with cells which were preincubated in the absence of anti-receptor antiserum. The patients are the same as in Fig. 1. Reproduced from Taylor et al. (1982a).

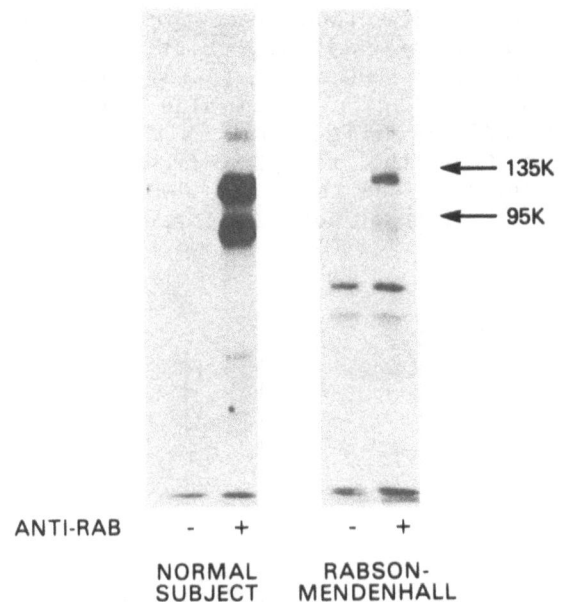

Figure 4.   Subunit structure of insulin receptors on cultured
lymphocytes.   Insulin receptors on the surface of cultured
cells were iodinated using a lactoperoxidase method (Kasuga
et al., 1981a).   After solubilization using Triton X-100,
labelled receptors were immunoprecipitated with either anti-
receptor antiserum (lanes 2 and 4) or control human serum
(lanes 1 and 3).   The immunoprecipitates were analyzed by
NaDodSO$_4$ polyacrylamide gel electrophoresis carried out under
reducing conditions.   The radioautograms of these gels are
shown here.   The two major subunits of the receptor are
depicted by the arrows at apparent molecular weights of
135,000 (135K) and 95,000 (95K).   Two cell lines are used:
one derived from a normal adult (lanes 1 and 2) and another
derived from an insulin-resistant patient with the Rabson-
Mendenhall syndrome (Perez-Corral et al. 1980) who manifested
a decreased number of insulin receptors (lanes 3 and 4).
These are previously unpublished studies carried out in
collaboration with Dr. Jose A. Hedo.

Of course, these methods would not detect a subtle structural
abnormality such as a point mutation or a minor change in the
post-translational processing (e.g., glycosylation).   Using
one antiserum (B-2) directed against the insulin receptor, we

could not distinguish between receptors on normal cells vs. cells from leprechaun/Ark-1 (Taylor et al., 1981). However, another anti-receptor antibody (B-10) appeared to have a three-fold increased affinity to bind solubilized receptors from leprechaun/Ark-1 (Fig. 8). This observation supports the inference that the receptor from leprechaun/Ark-1 is structurally abnormal and that this abnormality is recognized by antibody B-10, although not by antibody B-2.

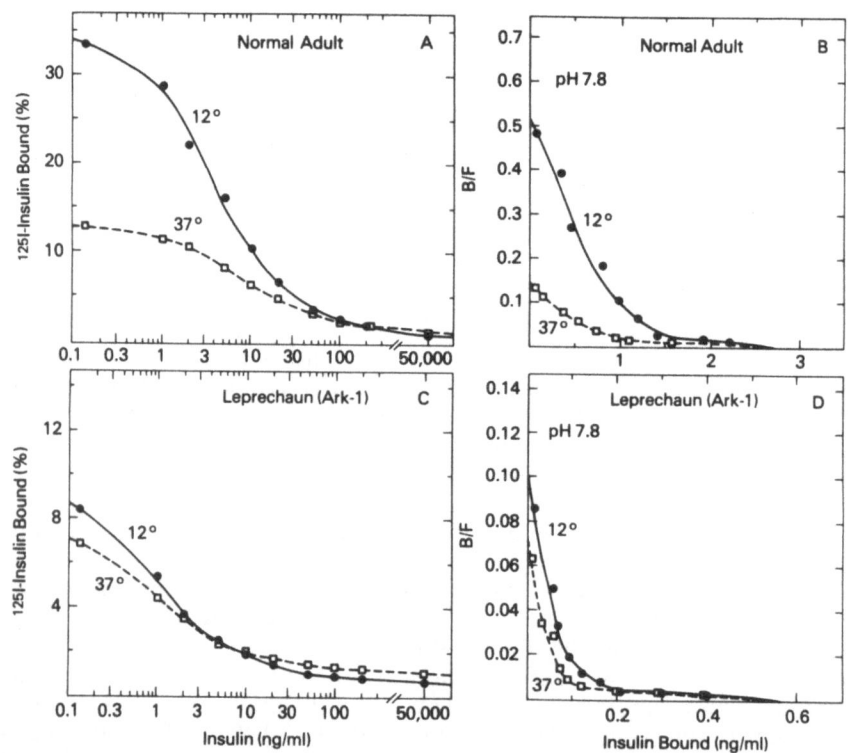

Figure 5. Steady-state insulin binding at 12° and 37°. ^{125}I-insulin binding studies were carried out at either 12° or 37° using cultured lymphocytes from a normal adult (panels A and B) or leprechaun/Ark-1 (panels C and D). Data are presented either as binding-competition experiments (panels A and C) or Scatchard plots (panels B and D). Reproduced from Taylor et al., 1981.

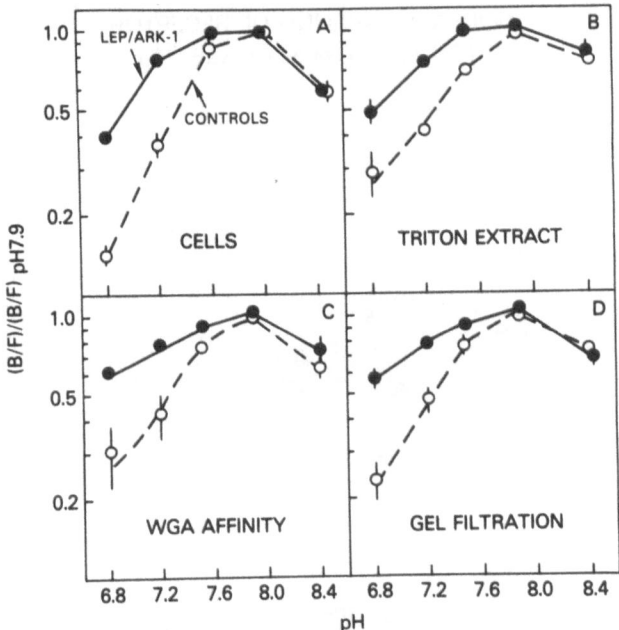

Figure 6. Effect of pH on ^{125}I-insulin binding. Binding of ^{125}I-insulin (0.2 ng/ml) was studied as a function of pH with receptors from lymphocytes of leprechaun/Ark-1 (closed circles) and control subjects (open circles). Specific binding of ^{125}I-insulin to intact cells (15°) is presented in panel A (Taylor et al., 1981). Specific binding of ^{125}I-insulin to solubilized receptors (4°C) is presented in panels B-D: panel B, crude Triton X-100 extracts of plasma membrane; panel C, insulin receptors partially purified by chromatography over wheat germ agglutinin-agarose; panel D, insulin receptors partially purified by gel filtration chromatography. For each point, the magnitude of SEM is represented by a vertical bar. (Error bars are omitted where the magnitude of the SEM is smaller than the radius of the circular symbol.) Reproduced from Taylor, et al., 1982b.

Unfortunately, we do not understand the mechanism by which insulin binding is coupled to insulin action. However, we have hypothesized that the mechanism may possibly resemble the coupling mechanism for hormones which activate adenylate

SURFACE LABELING OF RECEPTOR
(Galactose Oxidase + NaB ^{3}H$_4$)

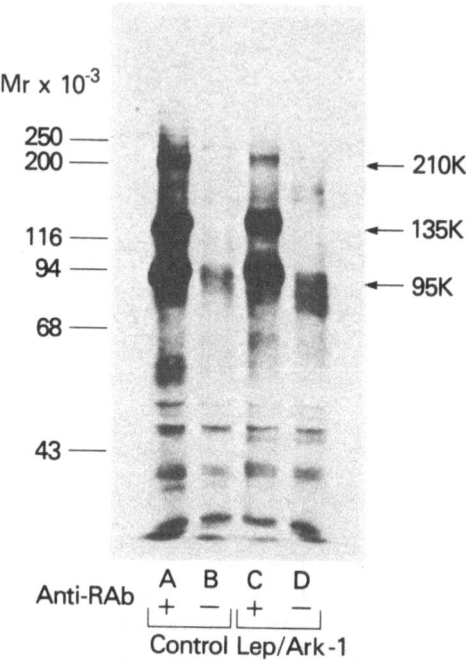

Figure 7. Subunit structure of insulin receptors from leprechaun/Ark-1. After treatment of intact cells with neuraminidase and galactose oxidase, insulin receptors on the surface of cultured lymphocytes were labelled in the carbohydrate moiety with ^{3}H by reduction with NaB^{3}H$_4$ (Hedo et al., 1981). After this labelling procedure, receptors were solubilized with Triton X-100 and immunoprecipitated with either anti-receptor antiserum (anti-R Ab) or normal human serum. The receptor subunits are indicated in this fluorograph of the gel with arrows as "210K", "135K", and "95K" according to the nomenclature of Kasuga et al. (1981). Note that digestion with neuraminidase as employed in this experiment alters the mobility of the subunits so that the apparent molecular weights appear smaller than suggested by the above numbers. Reproduced from Taylor et al., 1982b.

cyclase (Fig. 9). In that case, coupling results from an interaction between the guanine nucleotide binding subunit

(G/F subunit) and the hormone receptor. Not only does the guanine nucleotide binding subunit effect coupling of binding to bioactivity; in addition, the interaction between the receptor and the guanine nucleotide subunit serves to regulate the affinity of the receptor for hormone. Certain mutations affecting the guanine nucleotide binding subunit may give rise to hormone resistance as well as abnormalities in the affinity of receptor for hormone (Johnson et al., 1980).

Previous studies (Hedo et al., 1980) had suggested that purification of solubilized insulin receptors using lectin-affinity columns led to an increase in the receptor's binding

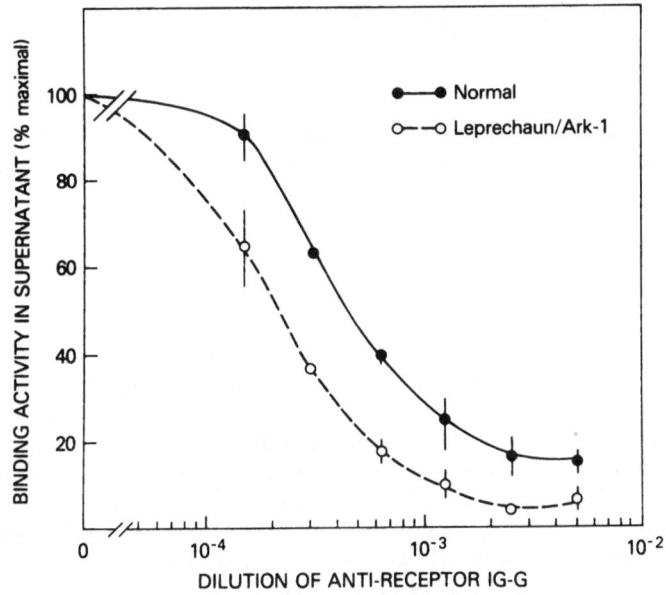

Figure 8. Immunodepletion of solubilized insulin receptors from leprechaun/Ark-1. Solublized insulin receptors were incubated with varying concentrations of anti-receptor IgG (B-10) for 24 hr at 4°. After precipitation of immune complexes using protein A (Pansorbin, Calbiochem), the supernatants were analyzed for specific binding of ^{125}I-insulin (0.1 ng/ml). The percentage of the initial ^{125}I-insulin binding activity remaining in the supernatant is plotted as a function of the concentration of anti-receptor IgG added during the immunodepletion step. The concentration of antireceptor IgG prior to dilution was 11 mg/ml.

ANALOGY OF INSULIN RECEPTOR WITH RECEPTORS LINKED
TO ADENYLATE CYCLASE

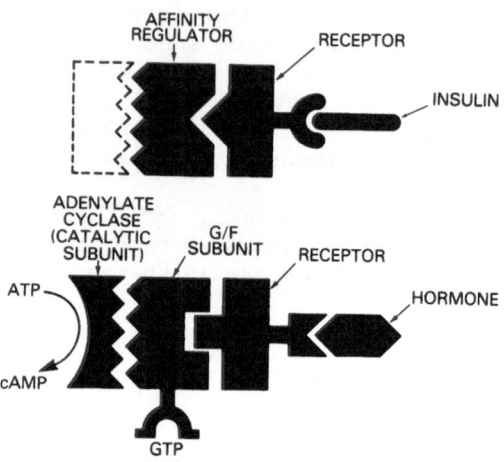

Figure 9. Speculative model for coupling of insulin binding to insulin action based on analogy to mechanism of hormonal regulation of adenylate cyclase.

affinity. This change in binding affinity was attributed to removal of the influence of a hypothetical receptor-associated component (i.e., an "affinity regulator"). We wondered whether a mutation which prevented the interaction between the receptor and the affinity regulator might explain the abnormally high binding affinity observed with receptors from leprechaun/Ark-1. Unlike the increase in affinity which was observed upon lectin-affinity purification of solubilized receptors from normal cells, the affinity of insulin receptors from leprechaun/Ark-1 was unaffected by purification over wheat germ agglutinin-agarose (Fig. 10). It is tempting to speculate that the affinity regulator may play a role similar to the guanine nucleotide binding subunit - i.e., to couple hormone binding to hormone action. According to this view, we can detect the defect in the interaction between the receptor and the "affinity regulator" because of the increased binding affinity. However, the pathophysiological significance of the defect is that the "affinity regulator" is impaired in its function to couple insulin binding to insulin action.

3.3. Receptors with Decreased Affinity for Insulin

In principle, insulin resistance might result from a decrease in the affinity of insulin receptors to bind insulin. This has been reported in some studies using cultured human fibroblasts (Kahn and Podskalny, 1980; Podskalny and Kahn, 1982a). However, some confusion has arisen from the observation that the binding affinity of insulin receptors has seemed to be normal in studies using fresh monocytes or cultured lymphocytes from the same patients (Bar et al., 1980; Taylor et al., 1982a, 1983). While the explanation of these apparently contradictory observations is not completely certain, it seems most likely that the confusion arises from the presence of receptors for insulin-like growth factors (IGF) on cultured fibroblasts (Rechler et al., 1977). With cultured human fibroblasts, insulin binds not only to insulin receptors, but to type I receptors for insulin-like growth factors (Massague et al., 1982). With fibroblasts from normal subjects, the observed ^{125}I-insulin binding represents the summation of binding to these two types of receptors (Fig. 11). Based on published data, it has been estimated that approximately 30% of the binding of tracer concentrations of ^{125}I-insulin may involve IGF-receptors with cultured fibroblasts from normal subjects (Taylor et al., 1982a). As shown in Fig. 12, in fibroblasts from normal subjects, the summation of binding to these two receptor types more closely resembles binding to the insulin receptor. However, if the number of insulin receptors were markedly reduced (as suggested by studies with monocytes and lymphocytes) without a change in the number of IGF receptors, then the binding would more closely resemble binding to the IGF-receptor (Fig. 12). Many of the observations of Podskalny and Kahn can be explained by the conclusion that most of the binding involves the IGF receptor with cultured fibroblasts from these insulin resistant patients: (1) the apparently reduced binding affinity of insulin; (2) the increase in the potency of an insulin-like growth factor (i.e., multiplication stimulating activity) to compete for ^{125}I-insulin binding; and (3) the decreased ability of antibody to the insulin receptor to inhibit ^{125}I-insulin binding. In addition, while Podskalny and Kahn (1982a) cite affinity cross-linking studies with ^{125}I-insulin to support the view that the binding they are studying involves insulin receptors, it is now known that the apparent molecular weights of the subunits of the IGF (type I) receptor are virtually identical to those of the insulin receptor (Kasuga et al., 1981b; Massague et al., 1982).

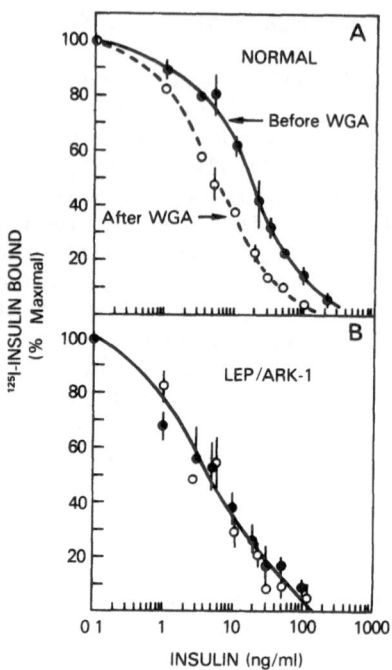

Figure 10. Effect of lectin-affinity purification of receptors on binding competition curves. Solubilized insulin receptors from lymphocytes of leprechaun/Ark-1 (panel B) and normal subjects (panel A) were purified by affinity chromatography over wheat germ agglutinin-agarose. ^{125}I-insulin binding was studied before (closed circles) or after (open circles) lectin-affinity purification. Data are presented as means ± SEM of six separate experiments. Specific binding was normalized by dividing by the maximal specific binding of ^{125}I-insulin (0.2 ng/ml) observed in the absence of unlabeled insulin. The magnitude of the SEM is represented by a vertical error bar except as noted in the legend to Fig. 6. Reproduced from Taylor et al., 1982b.

In summary, while a decrease in the binding affinity of the insulin receptor might cause insulin resistance, such a defect has not been convincingly demonstrated.

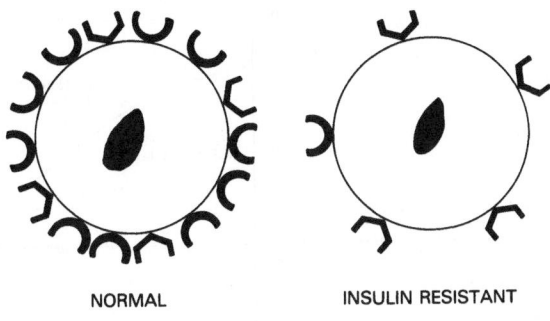

INSULIN RECEPTOR

IGF RECEPTOR

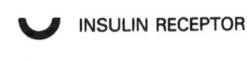

Figure 11. Schematic diagram of cell surface receptors
on cultured human fibroblasts. Cells from normal subjects ("normal") are depicted as having ten occupied
insulin receptors and four occupied receptors for insulin-
like growth factors ("IGF"). In the cells from insulin-
resistant subjects, it is assumed that there is a 90%
reduction in the number of insulin receptors in analogy
to the observations with cultured lymphocytes from the
same patients.

3.4. Normal Insulin Binding

Many, possibly most, of the patients with extreme insulin
resistance exhibit completely normal insulin binding (Bar et
al., 1978; Wachslicht-Rodbard et al., 1981). It seems likely
that the insulin receptors from these patients may be normal.
Presumably, the defect causing insulin resistance affects a
post-binding event in the mechanism of insulin action.
Because of our limited understanding of the molecular mechanism of insulin action, it has not been possible to identify
the precise defects in this group of patients.

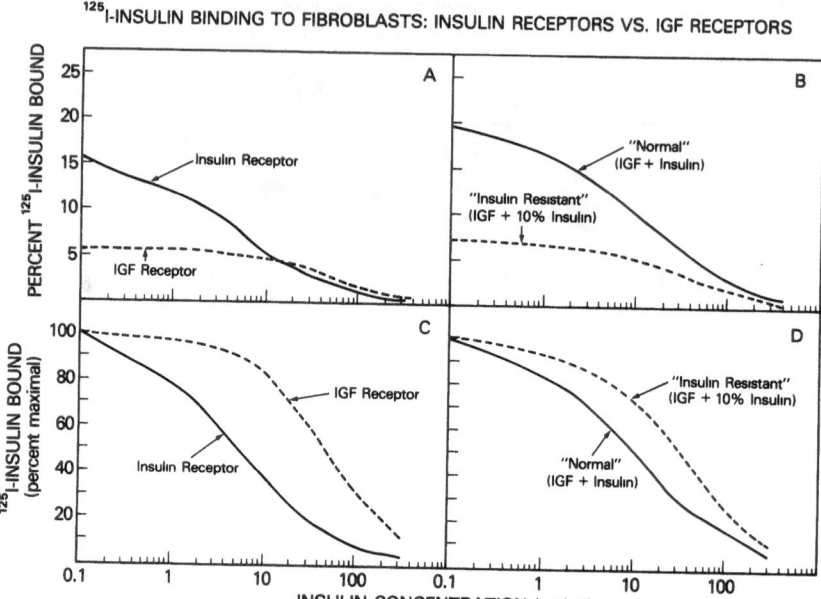

Figure 12. Theoretical calculation of ^{125}I-insulin binding
to cells with receptors for both insulin and insulin-like
growth factors. Binding-competition curves for binding of
^{125}I-insulin to receptors for insulin and insulin-like growth
factors (IGF) are presented in panels A and C. The curves
for binding to an insulin receptor derive from actual data
obtained using cultured human lymphocytes, a cell type which
seems not to possess a detectable number of IGF receptors
(Taylor et al., 1982a). The curves for ^{125}I-insulin binding
to IGF receptors were calculated making the following assumptions: (1) that the Scatchard plot for binding to the IGF
receptor is linear; (2) that a concentration of insulin of
approximately 50 ng/ml displaces 50% of the binding of
^{125}I-labelled tracer to the IGF receptor; (3) that 30%
of the binding of ^{125}I-insulin (0.1 ng/ml) to normal skin
fibroblasts involves IGF receptors while 70% involves
insulin receptors. As discussed elsewhere (Taylor et al.,
1982a), these assumptions are probably a realistic approximation of the situation in cultured human fibroblasts. In
panels B and D, the curves denoted as "normal" are derived
from Scatchard plots by assuming that the binding to the two
types of receptors is independent and additive. The curves
denoted as "Insulin Resistant" are derived under the same

4. Conclusions

The syndromes of extreme insulin resistance have given us insight into some of the pathophysiologic mechanisms which may play a role in regulating target cell sensitivity to insulin. Remarkably, even in such a rare syndrome as lepre-chaunism, the few patients who have been studied have exhibited a multiplicity of biochemical defects despite the similarity of their phenotypic features. It seems likely that a similar diversity of molecular mechanisms may be involved in such common syndromes as obesity and type II diabetes.

ACKNOWLEDGMENTS. I would like to thank Ms. Laurie Tuchman for her excellent help in preparing this manuscript. In addition, I am grateful to Ms. Lisa Underhill for her assistance in carrying out much of the work described herein. Drs. José A. Hedo, Masato Kasuga, Jonathan Whittaker, C. Ronald Kahn, Philip Gorden, and Jesse Roth have provided much helpful discussion and advice. Finally, I thank the American Diabetes Association for their support (Roger Staubach Feasibility Grant Award).

REFERENCES

Bar, R. S., Muggeo, M., Kahn, C. R., Gorden, P., and Roth, J., 1980, Characterization of insulin receptors in patients with the syndrome of insulin resistance and acanthosis nigricans, Diabetologia 18:209.
Bar, R. S., Muggeo, M., Roth, J., Kahn, C. R., Havrankova, J., and Imperato-McGinley, J., 1978, Insulin resistance, acanthosis nigricans, and normal insulin receptors in a young woman: Evidence for a post-receptor defect, J. Clin. Endocrinol. Metab. 47:620.

Figure 12 (continued) assumptions except that the number of insulin receptors is assumed to be reduced by 90% as compared to the cells from normals without any change in the number of IGF receptors. This is also a realistic assumption for fibro-blasts from the patients studied by Podskalny and Kahn (1982a) based on studies of fresh monocytes and cultured lymphocytes obtained from the same patients.

Barnes, N. D., Polumbo, P. J., Hayles, A. B., and Folgar, H.,
    1974, Insulin resistance, skin changes, and virilization:
    A recessively inherited syndrome possibly due to pineal
    gland dysfunction, Diabetologia 10:285.
D'Ercole, A. J., Underwood, L. E., Groelke, J., and Plet, A.,
    1979, Leprechaunism: Studies of the relationship among
    hyperinsulinism, insulin resistance, and growth retarda-
    tion, J. Clin. Endocrinol. Metab. 48:495.
Donohue, W. L., and Uchida, I., 1954, Leprechaunism. A euphuism
    for a rare familial disorder, J. Pediatrics 45:505.
Flier, J. S., Kahn, C. R., Jarrett, D. B., and Roth, J., 1976,
    Characterization of antibodies to the insulin receptor: A
    cause of insulin-resistant diabetes in man, J. Clin.
    Invest. 58:1442.
Flier, J. S., Young, J. B., and Landsberg, L., 1980, Familial
    insulin resistance with acanthosis nigricans, acral hyper-
    trophy, and muscle cramps, N. Eng. J. Med. 303:970.
Friedenberg, G. R., White, N., Cataland, S., O'Dorisio, T. M.,
    Sotos, J. F., and Santiago, J. V., 1981, Diabetes respon-
    sive to intravenous but not subcutaneous insulin: Effect-
    iveness of aprotinin, N. Eng. J. Med. 305:363.
Gabbay, K. H., Bergenstal, R. M., Wolff, J., Mako, M. E., and
    Rubenstein, A. H., 1979, Familial hyperproinsulinemia:
    Partial characterization of circulating proinsulin-like
    material, Proc. Natl. Acad. Sci. USA 76:2881
Gavin, J. R., III, Roth, J., Neville, D. M. Jr., De Meyts, P.,
    and Buell, D. N., 1974, Insulin-dependent regulation of
    insulin receptor concentrations: A direct demonstration
    in cell culture, Proc. Natl. Acad. Sci. USA 71:84.
Given, B. D., Mako, M. E., Tager, H., Baldwin, D., Markese, J.,
    Rubenstein, A. H., Olefsky, J., Kobayashi, M., Kolterman,
    O., and Poucher, R., 1980, Diabetes due to secretion of an
    abnormal insulin, N. Eng. J. Med. 302:129.
Grunberger, G., Taylor, S. I., Dons, R. F., and Gorden, P.,
    1983, Insulin receptor in normal and disease states, Clin.
    Endocrinol. Metab. (in press).
Haneda, M., Bergenstal, R., Freidenberg, G., Wishner, W., Blix,
    P., Provow, S., Polonsky, K., and Rubenstein, A., 1982,
    Familial diabetes associated with a possible structural
    defect in circulating insulin, Diabetes 31 (suppl. 2):4A
    (abstract #13).
Hedo, J. A., Harrison, L. C., and Roth, J., 1981, Binding of
    insulin receptors to lectins: Evidence for common carbo-
    hydrate determinants on several membrane receptors,
    Biochemistry 20:3385.

and II and their relationship to the insulin receptor,
   J. Biol. Chem. 257:5038.
Olefsky, J. M., 1981, Insulin resistance and insulin action:
   An in vitro and in vivo perspective, Diabetes 30:148.
Perez-Corral, F., de la Vina, S., Carbo, M., Barrio, R.,
   Yturriaga, R., Perez-Meceda, B., Alonso, M., and Serrano-
   Rios, M., 1980, Rabson syndrome: Model of insulin resist-
   ance due to decreased number and affinity of insulin
   receptors in erythrocytes, Diabetologia 19:306 (abstract).
Pilch, P. F., and Czech, M., 1979, Interaction of cross-linking
   agents with the insulin effector system of isolated fat
   cells, J. Biol. Chem. 254:3375.
Podskalny, J. M., and Kahn, C. R., 1982a, Cell culture studies
   on patients with extreme insulin resistance. I. Receptor
   defects on cultured fibroblasts, J. Clin. Endo. Metab.
   54:261.
Podskalny, J. M., and Kahn, C. R., 1982b, Cell culture studies
   on patients with extreme insulin resistance. II. Abnormal
   biological responses in cultured fibroblasts, J. Clin.
   Endocrinol. Metab. 54:269.
Rabson, S. M., and Mendenhall, E. N., 1956, Familial hypertrophy
   of pineal body, hyperplasia of adrenal cortex and diabetes
   mellitus, Amer. J. Clin. Path. 26:283.
Rechler, M. M., Nissley, S. P., Podskalny, J. M., Moses, A. C.,
   and Fryklund, L., 1977, Identification of a receptor for
   somatomedin-like polypeptides in human fibroblasts, J.
   Clin. Endocrinol. Metab. 44:820.
Robbins, D. C., Blix, P. M., Rubenstein, A. H., Kanazawa, Y.,
   Kosaka, K., and Tager, H. S., 1981, A human proinsulin
   variant at arginine 65, Nature 291:679.
Rosenberg, A. M., Haworth, J. C., Degroot, G. W., Trevenen,
   C. L., and Rechler, M. M., 1980, A case of leprechaunism
   with severe hyperinsulinemia, Am. J. Dis. Child 134:170.
Roth, J., and Grunfeld, C., 1981, Endocrine systems: Mechanisms
   of disease, target cells, and receptors, in: "Textbook of
   Endocrinology", R. H. Williams, ed., p. 15, Philadelphia:
   W. B. Saunders, p. 1270.
Scarlett, J. A., Kolterman, O. G., Moore, P., Saekow, M., Insel,
   J., Griffin, J., Mako, M., Rubenstein, A. H., Olefsky, J.
   M., 1982, Insulin resistance and diabetes due to a genetic
   defect in insulin receptors, J. Clin. Endocrinol. Metab.
   55:123.
Schilling, E. E., Rechler, M. M., Grunfeld, C., and Rosenberg,
   A. M., 1979, Primary defect of insulin receptors in skin
   fibroblasts cultured from an infant with leprechaunism and
   insulin resistance, Proc. Natl. Acad. Sci. USA 76:5877.

Huseman, C., Johanson, A., Varma, M., and Blizzard, R. M., 1978,
    Congenital lipodystrophy: An endocrine study in three
    siblings. I. Disorders of carbohydrate metabolism, J.
    Pediatr. 93:221.
Jacobs, S., Hazum, E., Shechter, Y., and Cuatrecasas, P., 1979,
    Insulin receptor: Covalent labeling and identification of
    subunits, Proc. Natl. Acad. Sci. USA 76:4918.
Kahn, C. R., Flier, J. S., Bar, R. S., Archer, J. A., Gorden,
    P., Martin, M. M., and Roth, J., 1976, The syndromes
    of insulin resistance and acanthosis nigricans.
    Insulin-receptor disorders in man, N. Eng. J. Med.
    294:739.
Kahn, C. R., and Podskalny, J. R., 1980, Demonstration of a
    primary (? genetic) defect in insulin receptors in fibro-
    blasts from a patient with the syndrome of insulin resist-
    ance and acanthosis nigricans type A, J. Clin. Endocrinol.
    Metab. 50:1139.
Kahn, C. R., and Rosenthal, A. S., 1979, Immunologic reactions
    to insulin: Insulin allergy, insulin resistance, and the
    autoimmune insulin syndrome, Diabetes Care 2:283.
Kasuga, M., Kahn, C. R., Hedo, J. A., Van Obberghen, E., Yamada,
    K. M., 1981a, Insulin-induced receptor loss in cultured
    human lymphocytes is due to accelerated receptor degrada-
    tion, Proc. Natl. Acad. Sci. USA 78:6917.
Kasuga, M., Van Obberghen, E., Nissley, S. P., and Rechler,
    M. M., 1981b, Demonstration of two subtypes of insulin-like
    growth factor receptors by affinity cross-linking, J. Biol.
    Chem. 256:5308.
Knight, A. B., Rechler, M. M., Romanus, J. A., Van Obberghen-
    Schilling, E. E., and Nissley, S. P., 1981, Stimulation
    of glucose incorporation and amino acid transport by
    insulin and an insulin-like growth factor in fibroblasts
    with defective insulin receptors cultured from a patient
    with leprechaunism, Proc. Natl. Acad. Sci. USA 78:2554.
Kobayashi, M., Olefsky, J. M., Elders, J., Mako, M. E., Given,
    B. D., Schedewie, H. K., Fiser, R. H., Hintz, R. L.,
    Horner, J. A., Rubenstein, A. H., 1978, Insulin resistance
    due to a defect distal to the insulin receptor: Demon-
    stration in a patient with leprechaunism, Proc. Natl.
    Acad. Sci. USA 75:3469.
Kono, T., and Barham, F. W., 1971, The relationship between the
    insulin-binding capacity of fat cells and the cellular
    respone to insulin, J. Biol. Chem. 246:6210.
Massague, J., and Czech, M., 1982, The subunit structures of
    two distinct receptors for insulin-like growth factors I

Taylor, S. I., and Leventhal, S., 1982, Absence of positive
    cooperativity in insulin receptors from a patient with
    congenital extreme insulin resistance (leprechaunism),
    Diabetes 31:131A (abstract #501).
Taylor, S. I., Roth, J., Blizzard, R. M., and Elders, M. J.,
    1981, Qualitative abnormalities in insulin binding in a
    patient with extreme insulin resistance: Decreased sensi-
    tivity to alterations in temperature and pH, Proc. Natl.
    Acad. Sci. USA 78:7157.
Taylor, S. I., Samuels, B., Roth, J., Kasuga, M., Hedo, J. A.,
    Gorden, P., Brasel, D. E., Pokora, T., and Engel, R. R.,
    1982a, Decreased insulin binding in cultured lymphocytes
    from patients with extreme insulin resistance, J. Clin.
    Endocrinol. Metab. 54:919.
Taylor, S. I., Hedo, J. A., Underhill, L. H., Kasuga, M.,
    Elders, M. J., and Roth, J., 1982b, Extreme insulin resist-
    ance in association with abnormally high binding affinity
    of insulin receptors from a patient with leprechaunism:
    Evidence for a defect intrinsic to the receptor, J. Clin.
    Endocrinol. Metab. 55:1108.
Taylor, S. I., Underhill, L. H., Roth, J., Serrano,Rios, M.,
    and Blizzard, R. M., 1983, Decreased insulin binding to
    cultured cells from a patient with the Rabson-Mendenhall
    syndrome: Dichotomy between studies with cultured lympho-
    cytes and cultured fibroblasts, J. Clin. Endocrinol. Metab.
    (in press)
Van Obberghen, E., Kasuga, M., Le Cam, A., Hedo, J. A., Itin, A.,
    and Harrison, L. C., 1981, Biosynthetic labeling of insulin
    receptors: Studies of subunits in cultured human IM-9
    lymphocytes, Proc. Natl. Acad. Sci. USA 78:1052.
Wachslicht-Rodbard, H., Muggeo, M., Kahn, C. R., Saviolakis,
    G. A., Harrison, L. C., and Flier, J. A., 1981, Hetero-
    geneity of the insulin-receptor interaction in lipostrophic
    diabetes, J. Clin. Endocrinol. Metab. 52:416.
Waelbroeck, M., 1982, The pH dependence of insulin binding, J.
    Biol. Chem. 257:8284.
Waelbroeck, M., Van Obberghen, E., and De Meyts, P., 1979,
    Thermodynamics of the interaction of insulin with its
    receptor, J. Biol. Chem. 254:7736.
West, R. J., and Leonard, J. V., 1980, Familial insulin resist-
    ance with pineal hyperplasia: Metabolic studies and effect
    of hypophysectomy, Arch. Dis. Child 55:619.
West, R. J., Lloyd, J. K., and Turner, W. M. L., 1975, Familial
    insulin-resistant diabetes, multiple somatic anomalies,
    and pineal hyperplasia, Archs. Dis. Child 50:703.

DISCUSSION

HALL: 1. Can you be sure that transformation of lymphocytes does not alter coupling and other details of function of normal receptor? 2. What criteria do you use for determining number of receptors? If the number of receptors is decreased, it can be difficult to measure affinity accurately. 3. Have you tested the patients' cells by fluorescent microscopy?

TAYLOR: 1. As discussed in detail elsewhere (Taylor et al., 1982a), we do not believe this is a problem although we have worried about it a great deal. While we have studied a large number of cell lines (derived from both normal subjects as well as patients with a variety of diseases), we have found only five patients with abnormal binding. All of these patients displayed a clinical syndrome of extreme insulin resistance. Moreover, in every case where it has been possible to obtain circulating monocytes for study, studies with fresh cells have confirmed the data with EB-virus transformed cells. Of course, it will be necessary to keep an open mind as we get the opportunity to study additional patients.

2. Estimation of receptor number is complicated by the curvilinearity of the Scatchard plot and the controversy with respect to the correct kinetic model to apply. Thus we have carried out studies using independent methods - e.g. binding of anti-receptor antibody (Taylor et al., 1982a) as well as direct labelling studies (Fig. 4 and 7) - to estimate the receptor number. All of these approaches have yielded similar conclusions.

3. No. We have not carried out studies with fluorescently labelled insulin.

HAZUM: Could it be that the insulin receptors from normal patients and abnormal patients differ with regard to the structure of the subunits and/or the sialic acid content?

TAYLOR: Most of our studies with SDS-polyacrylamide gel electrophoresis have been carried out under reducing conditions. However, in collaboration with Drs. Masato Kasuga and José A. Hedo, we have done preliminary experiments in the absence of reductant but have not noted any clear differences with respect to the oxidation state of insulin receptors from the patients.

We have direct data with respect to the sialic acid content of the receptor. When receptors are digested with neuraminidase to remove sialic acid, the migration of the receptor subunits is altered so as to suggest a decrease in the apparent molecular weight as judged by SDS-polyacrylamide gel electrophoresis. In leprechaun/Ark-1, this shift in apparent molecular weight occurs normally (Fig. 7). This suggests that there is not a gross difference in the sialic content. Of course, we cannot rule out a selective abnormality in a single sialic acid residue.

GOLDFINE: Do these patients have a phospholipid abnormality which in turn causes the altered binding?

TAYLOR: Possibly, but since the solubilized receptor has similar properties, most likely phospholipid abnormalities are not the major cause of the problem.

CHRISTOFFERSON: Is the insulin binding in any of your preparations, from patients or normal subjects, influenced by GTP or cholera toxin?

TAYLOR: In preliminary studies, we have not observed an effect of GTP on insulin binding. Although we have never studied the effects of cholera toxin, I agree the experiment would be interesting.

ROY: You presented some data showing that the anti-receptor antibody binds more tightly with the defective receptor. What about the biological response after the addition of the anti-receptor antibody - is it also higher in these cells?

TAYLOR: First, let me emphasize that this one particular antiserum (i.e., B-10) differed from other antisera (e.g., B-2) in being able to distinguish the normal insulin receptor from the receptor of leprechaun/Ark-1. Unfortunately, we cannot answer your main question because we have not identified biological effects of insulin upon these cultured lymphocyte cell lines. Ultimately, these studies might be carried out with another cell type (e.g., adipocytes). It is clearly of interest to know whether the mechanism of coupling binding to biological activity is the same for the insulin-like effects of insulin and the insulin-like effects of anti-receptor antibody.

SCHRADER: Are the leprechaun phenotype patients in fact diabetic?

TAYLOR: The patients clearly manifest glucose intolerance - i.e. marked hyperglycemia in response to a glucose load. Moreover, they are highly resistant to large quantities of exogenous insulin. However, their syndrome differs from diabetes in that they usually are not hyperglycemic in the fasting state. Rather, they exhibit fasting hypoglycemia. This hypoglycemia appears not to result from hyperinsulinemia. Instead, it appears that the patients are unable to mobilize fuel for gluconeogenesis during prolonged starvation.

THE ROLE OF PROTEIN PHOSPHORYLATION IN INSULIN ACTION

Robert S. Horn[a] and Otto Walaas[a,b]

[a]Institute of Medical Biochemistry
University of Oslo, Norway
[b]California Metabolic Research Foundation
La Jolla, California, USA

1. Introduction

It has been well established that insulin exerts numerous effects on the metabolism of carbohydrates, lipids and amino acids as well as on membrane transport processes and protein synthesis. However, in spite of extensive studies the mechanism of insulin action at the molecular level is an unsolved problem (Walaas and Horn, 1981). At the present time there is general agreement that the initial event in insulin action involves interaction of the hormone with specific receptors in the plasma membrane of target cells. The receptor has now been purified and has a molecular weight of 350,000. The protein consists of two α-subunits (M_r 135,000) and two β-subunits (M_r 95,000) associated by disulfide bridges (Czech et al., 1981). The coupling system between the insulin-receptor complex and intracellular effector systems has yet to be elucidated. For many years research in this field has been concerned with identification of a "second messenger" of insulin action. A series of small molecules including cyclic AMP, cyclic GMP, unknown nucleotides, Ca^{2+}, H_2O_2, etc. have been proposed as mediators of insulin action. Until now these investigations have failed to identify a specific insulin dependent coupling system.

Insulin, after interaction with its specific receptor, is rapidly internalized by an endocytotic process. The internalized complex undergoes processing and is partly degraded in lysosomes (Schlessinger, 1980). It has been proposed that degradation products of insulin might act as

161

mediators of insulin action. However, there is little support for this hypothesis since the metabolic effects of insulin are expressed even when degradation of insulin is inhibited by lysomotropic drugs.

The insulin sensitive sugar transport system in membranes is associated with cytochalasin B binding sites. The interesting discovery was made that this system was partly localized in the microsomal fraction isolated from adipocytes. Treatment with insulin leads to transfer of cytochasalin B binding sites (and presumably sugar transporters) from the endoplasmic reticulum to the plasma membranes (Cushman and Wardzala, 1980, Suzuki and Kono, 1980). It seems most likely that the insulin-mediated transfer of the sugar transport system is secondary to a coupling system triggered by binding of insulin at its receptor in the plasma membrane.

The mechanism of insulin action still remains mysterious. Some progress has, however, been obtained by recent investigations along two different lines. These will be briefly reviewed:

A. Investigations on the influence of insulin on phosphorylation of insulin-sensitive enzymes and membrane proteins and the relationship to insulin effects on protein kinases and phosphoprotein phosphatases.

B. Investigations concerned with identification of a "second messenger" in the plasma membrane triggered by interaction of insulin with its specific receptor.

2.   The Influence of Insulin on the Phosphorylation of
      Enzymes and Membrane Proteins

2.1. The Glycogen Synthase System

It has been established that the activity of glycogen synthase is controlled through complex regulation involving phosphorylation/dephosphorylation of the enzyme. Five distinct protein kinases and four phosphoprotein phosphatases have been identified as regulators of the system (Cohen, 1982). The M_r 85,000 monomer of glycogen synthase is phosphorylated at 7 different serine residues (Picton et al., 1982). All of these sites have been found to be phosphorylated in vivo. Each of the protein kinases phosphorylates specific sites on the enzyme. Cyclic AMP-dependent protein kinase and glycogen synthase kinase 3 which is independent of both cyclic AMP and Ca^{2+} are the most important enzymes (Cohen et al., 1982). The key dephosphorylating enzyme in muscle seems to be phosphoprotein phosphatase-1 which is under control of the heat stable proteins inhibitor-1 and inhibitor-2 (Cohen, 1982).

Activation of glycogen synthase by insulin is attributed to dephosphorylation of the enzyme. How can insulin exert control of the complex regulatory system which results in dephosphorylation of glycogen synthase? Obviously, this effect could be obtained either by inhibition of protein kinase activity or activation of protein phosphatase. Experiments on isolated diaphragm muscle have demonstrated that insulin decreases the activity of cyclic AMP-dependent protein kinase without any increase in the concentration of cyclic AMP (Shen et al., 1970; Walaas et al., 1973). Subsequent work has shown that inactivation of cyclic AMP-dependent protein kinase by insulin can be attributed to decreased sensitivity of the enzyme to cyclic AMP (Walkenbach et al., 1978; Walkenbach et al., 1980; Mor et al., 1981).

Cohen and co-workers (Parker et al., 1982) have shown that cyclic AMP-dependent protein kinase phosphorylates a near N-terminal end site (Site 2) and two near C-terminal sites on the enzyme while protein kinase 3 phosphorylates three different sites (3a, 3b, 3c). The activity of glycogen synthase in vivo is largely determined by the state of phosphorylation of sites 3a, 3b, 3c and to a minor degree of site 2 (Parker et al., 1982). It has been recently reported that activation of muscle glycogen synthase by insulin is largely explained by decreased phosphorylation of sites 3a, 3b, 3c. This suggests that glycogen synthase kinase 3 is controlled by insulin (Cohen, 1982). It has been unexpectedly observed that in skeletal muscle adrenalin, which is known to activate cyclic AMP-dependent protein kinase, also increases the phosphorylation of the synthase kinase 3 sites (Parker et al., 1982).

Other experiments indicate that phosphoprotein phosphatases are involved in insulin activation and dephosphorylation of glycogen synthase. The activity of protein phosphatase-1 is inhibited by inhibitor-1 (M_r 22,000) which is an effective inhibitor only after phosphorylation by cyclic AMP-dependent protein kinase (Cohen, 1980). Administration of insulin in

vivo leads to decreased phosphorylation of inhibitor-1
(Foulkes et al., 1980). This would be expected to lead to an
increased activity of protein phosphatase-1 with increased
dephosphorylation of glycogen synthase. Protein phosphatase-1
also exists in an inactive form which can be activated by
incubation with Mg^{2+}-ATP and a protein factor now identified
as glycogen synthase kinase 3 (Vandenheede et al., 1981). It
has been suggested (Cohen, 1980) that this system is
controlled by insulin but no experimental support for this
hypothesis has yet been obtained. The data indicate complex
interactions between protein kinases and protein phosphatases
which are regulated by insulin.

2.2. The Pyruvate Dehydrogenase Complex

The activity of mammalian pyruvate dehydrogenase complex
is controlled through phosphorylation/dephosphorylation by a
mitochondrial protein kinase and a Ca^{2+}-activated phosphoprotein phosphatase. The complex is activated by dephosphorylation of the catalytic α-subunit (M_r 42,000) (Hughes et
al., 1980; Seals et al., 1979a). It has been demonstrated
that 3 different serine residues of this subunit are subjected to phosphorylation (Sale and Randle, 1980). Inactivation of the enzyme is associated with rapid phosphorylation
of one specific site. Phosphorylation of the two additional
sites is a slower process which leads to a decreased rate of
reactivation of the enzyme by the phosphoprotein phosphatase.
It has been well established that insulin rapidly increases
the activity of pyruvate dehydrogenase. This effect has been
associated with decreased phosphorylation of the α-subunit.
Insulin treatment leads to a dephosphorylation of all three
serine residues (Hughes et al., 1980). The effect of insulin
on pyruvate dehydrogenase appears to involve activation of a
specific protein phosphatase rather than inhibition of the
protein kinase. The effect has been attributed to release of
intramitochondrial Ca^{2+}. Jarett and co-workers (Seals et
al., 1979b) demonstrated that insulin could stimulate pyruvate dehydrogenase in a subcellular system from adipocytes
consisting of mitochondria and plasma membranes. Insulin
had, however, no effect on mitochondria pyruvate dehydrogenase
in the absence of plasma membranes. Activation of the enzyme
by insulin was associated with decreased phosphorylation of
the α-subunit. The action of insulin was blocked by sodium
fluoride which is known to inhibit phosphoprotein phosphatase.

These observations suggest that insulin causes release of
material from the plasma membrane which acts as a "second
messenger" and stimulates pyruvate dehydrogenase through
activation of the protein phosphatase.

2.3. Acetyl-CoA Carboxylase

Acetyl-CoA carboxylase from liver and adipose tissue
is phosphorylated by cyclic AMP-dependent protein kinase
with parallel inhibition of enzyme activity. These
effects are reversed by treatment of the enzyme with
phosphoprotein phosphatases (Brownsey and Denton, 1979).
Incubation of fat cells with adrenaline and liver cells
with glucagon leads to phosphorylation of this enzyme at
several sites, probably at the same sites as those phosphorylated by cyclic AMP-dependent protein kinase. Adipocytes
respond to insulin with a rapid increase in the activity
of acetyl-CoA carboxylase. It was expected that the
effect of insulin would be mediated by dephosphorylation
of the enzyme. It was, therefore, surprising that Brownsey
and Denton (1982) demonstrated a consistant increase in
the overall phosphorylation of the 230,000 (M_r) subunit
of the enzyme after treatment of adipocytes with insulin.
Further studies revealed that exposure of fat cells
to insulin leads to a marked increase in the incorporation
of $[^{32}P]$-phosphate into a peptide which is different from
those most extensively phosphorylated during exposure of
fat cells to adrenaline. The enhanced phosphorylation of
a specific site on the enzyme initiated by insulin suggested
that insulin stimulated a specific protein kinase which
is distinct from cyclic AMP-dependent protein kinase.
This hypothesis was supported by experiments in which
purified acetyl-CoA carboxylase was incubated with plasma
membranes from fat cells. In this system it was demonstrated (Brownsey et al., 1981) a membrane-bound protein
kinase which was independent of cyclic AMP and which
phosphorylated acetyl-CoA carboxylase and led to increased
enzyme activity. The activation brought about by this
protein kinase was similar to that seen after exposure
of fat cells to insulin. The results indicate that the
increased phosphorylation of acetyl-CoA carboxylase promoted
by insulin is mediated through stimulation of a membrane-bound
cyclic AMP-independent protein kinase.

2.4. ACT-Citrate Lyase

Several investigators have documented that ATP-citrate lyase is a phosphoprotein. The enzyme contains 2 mol acid-labile "catalytic" phosphate/mol enzyme and, in addition, 2 mol acid-stable "structural" phosphate/mol enzyme. The acid-labile phosphate is incorporated into the enzyme during the first step in its reaction mechanism. Some years ago it was reported that exposure of adipocytes or hepatocytes to insulin rapidly led to increased [^{32}P]-phosphorylation of a protein with mol. wt. 123,000 (Benjamin and Singer, 1974; Avruch et al., 1976). Subsequently this protein has been purified and identified as ATP-citrate lyase (Alexander et al., 1979). Insulin increases [^{32}P]-phosphorylation of this enzyme in vivo in adipose and liver tissue (Alexander et al., 1982). Furthermore, it has been shown that glucagon and β-adrenergic agents also increase phosphorylation of this enzyme through stimulation of cyclic AMP-dependent protein kinase. Recently, a cyclic AMP-independent protein kinase which phosphorylated ATP-citrate lyase was purified from rat liver (Ramakrishna and Benjamin, 1981). The acid-stable sites phosphorylated by the lyase kinase include both phospho-serine and phosphothreonine. Only phosphoserine was found in ATP-citrate lyase when the enzyme was phosphorylated with the catalytic subunit of cyclic AMP-dependent protein kinase (Ramakrishna et al., 1981). Somewhat different results were obtained in studies on phosphorylation of ATP-citrate lyase in 3T3-Ll adipocytes (Swergold et al., 1982). The effect of insulin and glucagon on phosphorylation of the enzyme were not additive and for both hormones the phosphorylated residues occur on a single small peptide. In hepatocytes Avruch and co-workers have shown that insulin stimulates incorporation of phosphate into serine residues of ATP-citrate lyase (Alexander et al., 1982). The exact mechanism of the insulin effect on phosphorylation of this enzyme is not known. A reasonable hypothesis is that insulin increases the activity of a cyclic AMP-independent protein kinase. However, other possibilities such as decreased phosphatase activity or structural changes in ATP-citrate lyase itself with alter-ation in sensitivity to the action of protein kinase or phosphatase remain open. The physiological significance of the insulin-stimulated phosphorylation of the ATP-citrate lyase is unknown.

2.5. Ribosomal Protein S6

3T3-L1 fibroblast-like cells differentiate to adipocytes. During this process insulin receptors in plasma membrane increase dramatically and the cells become sensitive to insulin action. Insulin treatment of the differentiated cells greatly enhance the incorporation of $[^{32}P]$-phosphate into the ribosomal protein S6 (M_r 31,000) (Smith et al., 1979). This effect was retained in cell-free extracts prepared from insulin-treated cells (Smith et al., 1980). Addition of insulin to a cell-free particulate system derived from 3T3-L1 adipocytes containing high affinity insulin receptors and ribosomes stimulated incorporation of ^{32}P from $[^{32}P]$-γ-ATP into the ribosomal protein S6 (Rosen et al., 1981). This insulin effect is mediated by a cyclic AMP-independent pathway. These results imply that insulin causes stimulation of a specific protein kinase which phosphorylates the ribosomal protein. The functional consequence of the phosphorylation state of the protein is not known.

2.6. Plasma Membrane Proteins

The recent work reported by Kahn and co-workers demonstrated that the β-subunit (M_r 95,000) of the lymphocyte hepatocyte insulin receptor is phosphorylated in the presence of $[^{32}P]$-phosphate and insulin (Kasuga et al., 1982a). Phosphorylation of the receptor-subunit was insulin specific and the phosphorylation induced by insulin was found to occur exclusively at tyrosine residues. Similarly, epidermal growth factor has been shown to stimulate phosphorylation of tyrosine residues on its specific receptor (Ushiro and Cohen, 1980). Phosphorylation of the insulin receptor has also been demonstrated in a cell-free system (Kasuga et al., 1982b). The results are extremely interesting and may indicate an early event in insulin action.

During the last years several reports on the effect of insulin on protein phosphorylation in membranes have been presented (Table I). We have demonstrated that addition of insulin to sarcolemma membranes increased phosphorylation of a polypeptide with mol. wt. 15,000 (Walaas et al., 1977). This insulin effect was independent of cyclic AMP but was increased 3-4 fold by GTP and to a lesser extent by GMP-P(NH)P

Table I. Effect of Insulin on Phosphorylation of Plasma Membrane Proteins

Plasma membranes	Authors	Protein M_r	cAMP dependent	Insulin effect on phosphorylation
Skeletal muscle sarcolemma	Walaas et al., 1977	15,000	–	Increased
		95,000	–	Decreased
Adipocyte membranes	Seals et al., 1979a	120,000	–	Decreased
	Belsham et al., 1980	61,000	–	Increased
		22,000	–	Increased
	Chan and McDonald, 1982	110,000 (catalytic intermediate)	–	Decreased
Liver cell membranes	Tarn and Desbuqois, 1980	120,000	–	Decreased
		60,000	–	Decreased
	Marmont and Houslay, 1980	140,000	+	Decreased
		80,000	+	Decreased
		52,000	+	Increased
		28,000	+	Increased
		14,000	+	Increased
Insulin receptor	Kasuga et al., 1982b	95,000 (β-subunit)	–	Increased (phospho-tyrosine)
		135,000 (α-subunit)	–	Increased

(Walaas et al., 1979). This protein has been identified as a proteolipid and is soluble in acid chloroform/methanol. The phosphorylated residues reside on a subunit with mol. wt. of 3,600 (Walaas et al., 1981a). We have also found that insulin decreases phosphorylation of sarcolemma membrane protein M_r 95,000. This effect of insulin appears to be due to an increased rate of dephosphorylation (unpublished).

Direct addition of insulin to adipocyte plasma membranes decreased phosphorylation of one protein (M_r 120,000) (Seals et al., 1979) and increased phosphorylation of another protein (M_r 60,000) (Belsham et al., 1980). In adipocytes insulin was found to decrease the extent of phosphorylation of the $Ca^{2+} + Mg^{2+}$- ATPase subunit (M_r 110,000) (Chan and McDonald, 1982). Multiple effects by insulin on protein phosphorylations in liver plasma membranes have been reported. These include decreased phosphorylation of a protein with a mol. wt. of 120,000 and increased phosphorylation of a protein with mol. wt. of 60,000 (Tran and Desbuquois, 1980). It has also been reported that direct addition of insulin to liver plasma membranes inhibits cyclic AMP-dependent phosphorylation of two integral proteins (M_r 140,000 and M_r 80,000) (Marchmont and Houslay, 1980). In addition, insulin in the presence of cyclic AMP increased phosphorylation of three peripheral proteins (M_r 14,000, M_r 28,000 and M_r 52,000), the latter protein being identified as cyclic AMP-phosphodiesterase (Marchmont and Houslay, 1981).

The diverse results reported may be explained by insulin-mediated influence on protein kinase and/or phosphoprotein phosphatase activity and perhaps through structural modifications resulting from phosphorylation of substrate proteins. However, the physiological significance of the membrane proteins which undergo phosphorylation and dephosphorylation must be understood before major progress can be made in this field.

3.   Recently Proposed Messengers of Insulin Action

Recent investigations have given evidence that interaction of insulin with its receptor generates material in the plasma membrane which mimicks the action of insulin on specific enzymes. Larner and co-workers (Larner et al., 1979) isolated a material from skeletal muscle which appeared

to control the glycogen synthase system. The material, which
could be extracted from rat and rabbit skeletal muscle, inhibited cyclic AMP-dependent protein kinase and stimulated
phosphoprotein phosphatase in a dose dependent manner. The
activity of this material was increased by pretreatment of
the muscle with insulin. Simultaneously Jarett and Seals
(1979) demonstrated that the material increased the activity
of pyruvate dehydrogenase. The activity of their preparation
increased by treatment of adipocytes or adipocyte membranes
with insulin. From the work of Larner and of Jarett it was
tentatively concluded that interaction of insulin with its
specific receptor results in release of "second messenger"
from the plasma membrane which mediate the action of insulin
on hormone sensitive enzymes. Subsequent work has shown that
the material also acts on low K_m phosphodiesterase (Kiechle
and Jarett, 1981) and $Ca^{2+} +Mg^{2+}$-ATPase (McDonald et al.,
1981). This material has been isolated from insulin target
tissues such as muscle (Larner et al., 1979), adipocytes
(Kiechle et al., 1980), adipocyte plasma membranes (Seals and
Czech, 1981) and liver cell membranes (Saltiel et al., 1981).
It has also been extracted from hepatoma cells (Parker et
al., 1982) and from lymphocytes (Jarett et al., 1980).
Insulin pretreatment of the tissues increases the activity of
the material. Incubation of lymphocyte plasma membranes with
Concanavalin A leads to release of a substance which stimulates pyruvate dehydrogenase. The effect of this material
shows characteristics identical to the material released
following exposure of adipocyte plasma membranes to insulin.

Stimulation of pyruvate dehydrogenase by material
isolated from adipocytes and hepatoma cells has been attributed to activation of phosphoprotein phosphatase. This
theory is based upon experiments where stimulation of pyruvate dehydrogenase by the released substance(s) was eliminated
in the presence of the protein phosphatase inhibitor sodium
fluoride. Other experiments demonstrated that the material
was active in the absence of ATP in the system indicating
that a protein kinase was not involved (Kiechle et al.,
1981). The influence of these preparations on pyruvate
dehydrogenase and glyeogen synthase phosphatase is biphasic
i.e., stimulation is observed at low concentrations and
inhibitory effects at higher concentrations. Further purification of the muscle material has revealed two antagonistic
fractions which could be separated (Cheng et al., 1980). In
addition to an activation of a protein phosphatase a fraction
which inhibited the enzyme was also seen. Similarly two

different fractions with opposing actions on pyruvate dehydrogenase have been separated from liver membranes.

Isolation of the material has been accomplished by gel filtration of extracts on Sephadex G-25 as well as by anion exchange chromatography. The molecular weight of the material as estimated by gel filtration on Sephadex G-25 is 1,000 - 4,000 (Seals and Czech, 1981; Kiechle et al., 1981). The wide variations in estimated molecular weight have been ascribed to differences in the eluting buffer systems. The chemical nature of the material is not yet known. There is agreement that the material is heat stable and stable in acid solution while activity is destroyed in alkaline solutions.

Evidence has been obtained that the material which stimulates pyruvate dehydrogenase is a small peptide (Seals and Czech, 1980). The conclusion was reached that insulin, in plasma membranes, activates a protease whose action releases a soluble peptide into the medium. This was based upon the observation that pretreatment of plasma membranes with protease inhibitors blocked release of the enzyme regulator under the influence of insulin. The possibility exists that different types of enzyme regulators are being investigated. After incubation of adipocyte membranes with insulin, enzyme regulator has been detected in the water phase (Seals and Czech, 1982) as well as in chloroform-methanol extracts of the medium (Kiechle et al., 1982). In the latter case several different phospholipid fractions were detected. It was further demonstrated that phosphatidyl serine mimicked the action of the enzyme regulator in stimulating the activities of pyruvate dehydrogenase and low K_m phosphodiesterase while phosphatidylinositol-4-phosphate had an inhibitory action (Macaulay et al., 1982).

In our laboratory we are investigating the possibility that subunits released from the sarcolemma membrane proteolipid M_r 15,000 may control enzyme activities. In these experiments membranes have been incubated with ^{35}S-γ-ATP giving thio-phosphorylated proteins which are resistant to phosphatase activities. The ^{35}S-labeled subunit of the proteolipid was solubilized with the non-ionic detergent Nonidet P-40 and chromatographed by HPLC on a LKB 2135 Ultrapac TSK column. As shown in Fig. 1, four different radioactive peaks were identified. The radioactivity of fraction 1 and 4 were markedly increased after incubation of the membranes with insulin. We have observed that the

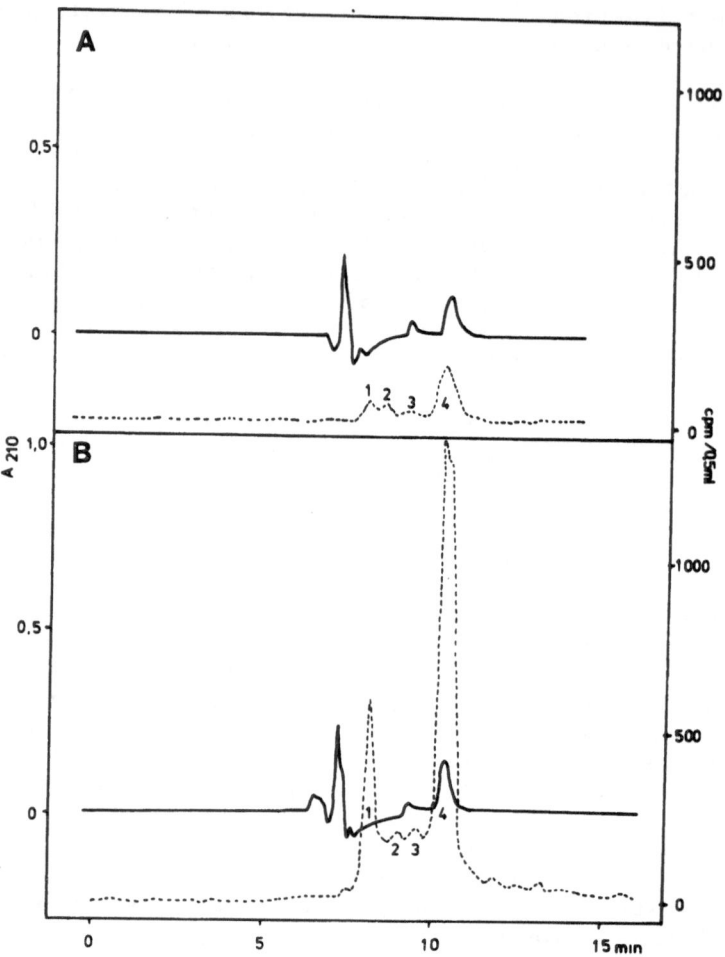

Figure 1. The effect of insulin on thio-phosphorylation of subunits of sarcolemma membrane proteolipid. Sarcolemma membranes isolated as described previously (Walaas et al., 1979) were suspended in a medium containing 50 μM ATP, 50 μCi ^{35}S-γ-thio ATP, 10 mM MgCl$_2$, 0.2 mM EDTA, 50 mM Tris HCl pH 7.4 and incubated for 3 min at 30°. Incubations were carried out in the absence and presence of insulin (500 μU/ml). After 50 × dilution with ice-cold buffer the membranes were recovered by centrifugation at 10,000 × g for 30 min. They were washed twice, lyophylized, extracted with acid chloroform/methanol and the extract was subjected to chromatography on Sephadex LH-20 as previously described (Walaas et al.,

detergent solubilized proteolipid stimulated the activity of cyclic AMP-dependent protein kinase. The curve was biphasic and the stimulatory effect has been identified with fraction 4 obtained by HPLC (unpublished). The incubation medium from this experiment was subjected to HPCL as shown in Fig. 2. In addition to $^{35}S-\gamma-ATP$ and $^{35}S-P_i$ six different radioactive fractions were identified. It is[1] of interest that fraction 6 is only seen after the membrane had been incubated with insulin. Investigation on the effect of this fraction on enzyme activities is in progress.

4.   Conclusions

The changes in the phosphorylation states of enzymes and other proteins promoted by insulin are extremely complex (Table II). Insulin mediates decreased phosphorylation of important metabolic enzymes such as glycogen synthase, pyruvate dehydrogenase, triacylglycerol lipase (Belfrage et al., 1981), and hydroxymethylglutaryl CoA reductase (Ingebritsen and Gibson, 1980). In addition, phosphorylation of some membrane proteins is decreased by insulin. The degree of phosphorylation of these enzymes and proteins is determined by the balance between the activities of protein kinases and phosphoprotein phosphatases. Insulin can influence both of these enzyme groups. Several examples can be given. There is strong evidence that the insulin mediated dephosphorylation of pyruvate dehydrogenase is brought about by increased activity of a Ca^{2+}-activated protein phosphastase. However, this effect by insulin may be secondary to an unknown action which releases mitochondrial Ca^{2+}. The dephosphorylation of glycogen synthetase induced by insulin is the result of an extremely complex regulatory system. Differing explanations of this effect have been proposed including decreased cyclic

───────────────────────────────────────

1981a). The ^{35}S-labeled fraction was evaporated to dryness in N_2 and solubilized by adding a solution containing 1% Nonidet P-40,200 mM KCl in 50 mM acetic acid. After removal of the phospholipids by centrifugation the water phase was chromatographed by HPLC on an LKB Ultrapac TSK SW column using 20 mM ammonium acetate pH 4.0 as the mobile phase. cpmx 10^3------ $A_{210}nM$————
A: Control. B: Insulin.

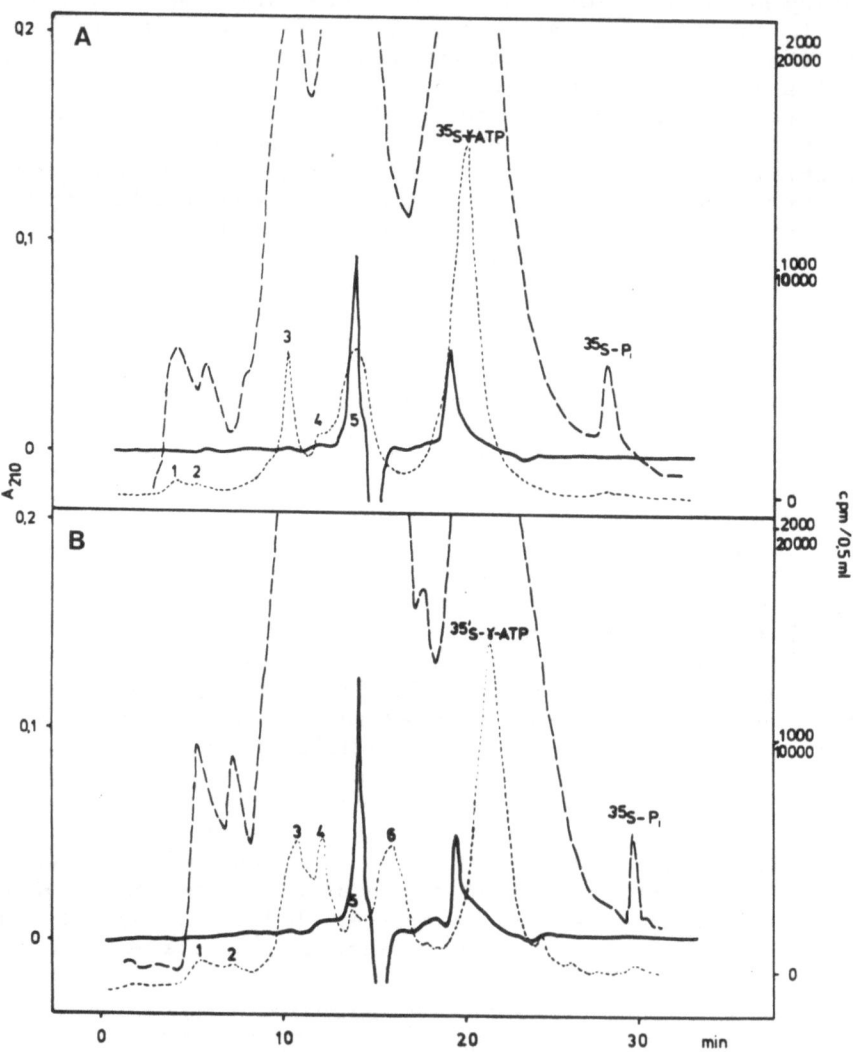

Figure 2. Isolation of thio-phosphorylated fractions released
from sarcolemma membranes. The sarcolemma had been incubated
in the absence and presence of insulin as described in legend
to Fig. 1. The incubation medium was lyophylized and subjected to HPLC as described in legend to Fig. 1.
cpmx 10^3------ cpmx 10^4------, A_{210} nM:———
A: Control. B: Insulin.

Table II. The Effect of Insulin on Phosphorylation of
Enzymes and Other Proteins

Enzyme (protein)	Phosphorylation	Activity	Proposed mechanism(s) for insulin effect on phosphorylation
Glycogen synthase	Decreased (sites 3a, 3b, 3c)	Increased	a. Decreased cyclic AMP-dependent protein kinase b. Decreased synthase kinase 3 c. Increased protein phosphatase-1
Inhibitor-1	Decreased	Decreased	a. Decreased cyclic AMP-dependent protein kinase b. Increased protein phosphatase-1
Hormonsensitive triacylglycerol lipase	Decreased	Decreased	Decreased cyclic AMP protein kinase?
Pyruvate dehydrogenase	Decreased (42,000 subunits)	Increased	Increased Ca^{2+} activated protein phosphatase
Acetyl-CoA carboxylase	Increased (specific site)	Increased	Increased membrane protein kinase
ATP-citrate lyase	Increased	-	Increased protein kinase
Ribosomal protein S6	Increased	-	Increased protein kinase

AMP-dependent activity, decreased activity of glycogen synthase kinase 3 as well as increased protein phosphatase 1. The latter enzyme is under control of inhibitor 1 which is subject to phosphorylation by cyclic AMP-dependent protein kinase and is dephosphorylated by protein phosphatase 1.

Insulin increases phosphorylation of acetyl-CoA carboxy-lase, ATP-citrate lyase and ribosomal protein S6. In plasma membranes insulin increases phosphorylation of the β-subunit of its specific receptor, a proteolipid M_r 15,000 and other proteins of unknown identity.

Enhanced phosphorylation due to the hormone might be explained by a stimulatory effect of insulin on specific membrane protein kinases dependent neither upon cyclic AMP nor increases in intracellular Ca^{++}. Support for this has been obtained by the work on acetyl-CoA carboxylase. It was shown that this enzyme can be phosphorylated at a specific site by a membrane bound protein kinase (Brownsey and Denton, 1982). In sarcolemma membranes we have identified an insulin sensitive protein kinase which phosphorylates exogenous added histones. Histone phosphorylation was increased by addition of insulin to membrane preparations and this effect was enhanced by GTP and GMP-P(NH)P (Walaas et al., 1979). After ADP-ribosylation of a membrane protein M_r 56,000 in the presence of cholera toxin the insulin effect was abolished and protein kinase activity inhibited (Walaas et al., 1981b). It seems that insulin activates this membrane protein kinase by a complex mechanism probably involving a GTP-dependent regulatory protein.

Work on identification of the second messenger of insulin action is in progress in several laboratories. A promising result obtained in this field is identification of material released from membranes in response to insulin and which is able to mimic effects of insulin on some enzymes. It has been proposed that small peptides as well as phospholipids are components of the active material. An alternative hypothesis has been set forth in which it is suggested that interaction of insulin with its receptor releases a specific membrane protein kinase which can phosphorylate intracellular enzymes without the need of a specific second messenger (Brownsey and Denton, 1982). It seems clear that the important problem of insulin action cannot be solved until the mediator system of this hormone has been identified.

ACKNOWLEDGMENTS. The work presented in this chapter was supported by Nordic Insulin Foundation.

REFERENCES

Alexander, M. C., Kowaloff, E. M., Witters, L. A., Dennihy, D. T., and Avruch, J., 1979, Purification of a hepatic 123,000-dalton hormone-stimulated ^{32}P-peptide and its identification as ATP-citrate lyase, J. Biol. Chem. 254:8052.

Alexander, M. C., Palmer, J. L., Pointer, R. H., Kowaloff, E. M., Koumjian, L. L., and Avruch, J., 1982, Insulin-stimulated phosphorylation of ATP-citrate lyase in isolated hepatocytes, J. Biol. Chem., 257:2049.

Avruch, J., Leone, G. R., and Martin, D. B., 1976, Effects of epinephrine and insulin on phosphopeptide metabolism in adipocytes, J. Biol. Chem. 251:1511.

Belfrage, P., Fredrikson, G., Nilsson, N. O., and Stalfors, P., 1981, Regulation of adipose tissue lipolysis by phosphorylation of hormone-sensitive lipase, Int. J. Obes., 5:635.

Belsham, G. J., Denton, R. M., and Tanner, J. A., 1980, Use of a novel rapid preparation of fat-cell plasma membranes employing Percoll to investigate the effects of insulin and adrenaline on membrane protein phosphorylation within intact fat-cells, Biochem. J., 192:457.

Benjamin, W. B., and Singer, I., 1974, Effect of insulin on the phosphorylation of adipose tissue protein, Biochim. Biophys. Acta 351:28.

Brownsey, R. W., and Denton, R. M., 1979, Role of phosphorylation in the short-term regulation of acetyl-CoA carboxylase by insulin and adrenaline, Les Colloques de l'INSERM, Obesity - cellular and molecular aspects, INSERM 87:185.

Brownsey, R. W., and Denton, R. M., 1982, Evidence that insulin activates fat-cell acetyl-CoA carboxylase by increased phosphorylation at a specific site, Biochem. J. 202:77.

Brownsey, R. W., Belsham, G. J., and Denton, R. M., 1981, Evidence for phosphorylation and activation of acetyl-CoA carboxylase by a membrane-associated cyclic AMP-independent protein kinase, FEBS Lett. 124:145.

Chan, K. -M., and McDonald, J. M., 1982, Identification of an insulin-sensitive Calcium-stimulated phosphoprotein in rat adipocyte plasma membranes, J. Biol. Chem. 257:7443.

Cheng, K., Galasko, G., Huang, L., Kellogg, J., and Larner, J., 1980, Studies on the insulin mediator. II. Separation of

two antagonistic biologically active materials from fraction II, Diabetes, 29:659.

Cohen, P., Recently discovered systems of enzyme regulation, in:
"Molecular Aspects of Cellular Regulation," Vol. 1 pp. 255-
268, P. Cohen, ed., Elsevier, Amsterdam (1980).

Cohen, P., 1982, The role of protein phosphorylation in neuronal
and hormonal control of cellular activity, Nature, 296:613.

Cohen, P., Yellowlees, D., Aitken, A., Donella-Deana, A.,
Hemmings, B. A., and Parker, P. J., 1982, Separation and
characterization of glycogen synthase kinase 3, glycogen
synthase kinase 4 and glycogen synthase kinase 5 from
rabbit skeletal muscle, Eur. J. Biochem. 124:21.

Cushman, S. W., and Wardzala, J., 1980, Potential mechanism of
insulin action on glucose transport in the isolated rat
adipose cell, J. Biol. Chem., 255:4758.

Czech, M. O., Massaque, J., and Pilch, P. F., 1981, The insulin
receptor: Structural features, Trends Biochem. Sci.,
6:222.

Foulkes, J. G., Jefferson, L. S., and Cohen, P., 1980, The
hormonal control of glycogen metabolism: Dephosphorylation
of protein phosphatase inhibitor-1 in vivo in response to
insulin, FEBS Lett., 112:21.

Hughes, W. A., Brownsey, R. W., and Denton, R. M., 1980, Studies
on the incorporation of [^{32}P]phosphate into pyruvate dehydrogenase in intact rat fat-cells, Biochem. J., 192:469.

Ingebritsen, T. S., and Gibson, D. M., Recently discovered
systems of enzyme regulation by reversible phosphorylation
of hydroxymethylglutaryl CoA reductase, in: "Molecular
Aspects of Cellular Regulation," Vol. 1, pp. 63-93.
P. Cohen, ed., Elsevier, Amsterdam (1980).

Jarett, L., and Seals, J. R., 1979, Pyruvate dehydrogenase
activation in adipocyte mitochondria by an insulin-gener-
ated mediator from muscle, Science, 206:1407.

Jarett, L., Kiechle, F. L., Popp, D. A., Kotagal, N., and Gavin,
R. G., 1980, Differences in the effect of insulin on the
generation by adipocytes and IM-9 lymphocytes of a chemical
mediator which stimulates the action of insulin on pyruvate
dehydrogenase, Biochem. Biophys. Res. Comm. 96:735.

Kasuga, M., Karlsson, F. A., and Kahn, C. R., 1982a, Insulin
stimulates the phosphorylation of the 95,000 Dalton subunit
of its own receptor, Science, 215:185.

Kasuga, M., Zick, Y., Blithe, D. L., Crettaz, M., and Kahn,
C. R., 1982b, Insulin stimulates tyrosine phosphoryla-
tion of the insulin receptor in a cell-free system,
Nature, 298:667.

Kiechle, F. L., and Jarett, L., 1981, The effect of an insulin-sensitive chemical mediator from rat adipocytes on low K_m and high K_m cyclic AMP phosphodiesterase, FEBS Lett., 133:279.

Kiechle, F. L., Jarett, L., Popp, D. A., and Kotagel, N., 1980, Isolation from rat adipocytes of a chemical mediator for insulin activation of pyruvate dehydrogenase, Diabetes, 29:852.

Kiechle, F. L., Jarett, L., Kotagal, N., and Popp, D. A., 1981, Partial purification from rat adipocyte plasma membranes of a chemical mediator which stimulates the action of pyruvate dehydrogenase, J. Biol. Chem., 256:2945.

Kiechle, F. L., Strauss, J. F., Tanada, T., and Jarett, L., 1982, Phospholipids as possible chemical mediators of insulin action of pyruvate dehydrogenase, Fed. Proc. 41:1082.

Larner, J., Galasko, G., Cheng, K., Depaoli-Roach, A. A., Huang, L., Daggy, P., and Kellogg, J., 1979, Generation by insulin of a chemical mediator that controls protein phosphorylation and dephosphorylation, Science, 206:1408.

Macaulay, S. L., Kiechle, F. L., and Jarett, L., 1982, Phospholipids as possible chemical mediators of insulin action on low K_m cAMP phosphodiesterase, Fed. Proc. 41:1082.

Marchmont, R. J., and Houslay, M. D., 1980, Insulin controls the cyclic AMP-dependent phosphorylation of integral and peripheral proteins associated with the rat liver plasma membrane, FEBS Lett., 118:18.

Marchmont, R. J., and Houslay, M. D., 1981, Characterization of the phosphorylated form of the insulin-stimulated cyclic AMP phosphodiesterase from rat liver plasma membranes, Biochem. J., 195:653.

Mor, M. A., Vila, J., Ciudad, C. J., and Guinovart, J. J., 1981, Insulin inactivation of rat hepatocyte cyclic AMP-dependent protein kinase, FEBS Lett., 136:131.

Parker, J. C., Kiechle, F. L., and Jarett, L., 1982, Partial purification from hepatoma cells of an intracellular substance which mediates the effects of insulin on pyruvate dehydrogenase and low K_m cyclic AMP phosphodiesterase, Arch. Biochem. Biophys, 215:339.

Parker, P. J., Embi, N., Cauwell, F. B., and Cohen, P., 1982, Glycogen synthase from rabbit skeletal muscle. State of phosphorylation of the seven phosphoserine residues in vivo in the presence and absence of adrenaline, Eur. J. Biochem. 124:47.

Picton, C., Aitken, A., Bilham, T., and Cohen, P., 1982, Multi-
    site phosphorylation of glycogen synthase from rabbit
    skeletal muscle. Organization of seven sites in the poly-
    peptide chain, Eur. J. Biochem., 124:37.
Ramakrishna, S., and Benjamin, W. B., 1981, Phosphorylation of
    ATP-citrate lyase by a cyclic AMP-independent protein
    kinase from rat liver, FEBS Lett., 124:140.
Ramakrishna, S., Pucci, D. L., and Benjamin, W. B., 1981, ATP-
    citrate lyase kinase and cyclic AMP-dependent protein
    kinase phosphorylate different sites on ATP-citrate lyase,
    J. Biol. Chem., 256:10213.
Rosen, O. M., Rubin, C. R., Cobb, M. H., and Smith, C. J., 1981,
    Insulin stimulates the phosphorylation of ribosomal protein
    S6 in a cell-free system derived from 3T3-L1 adipocytes, J.
    Biol. Chem., 256:3630.
Sale, G. J., and Randle, P. J., 1980, Incorporation of [^{32}P]-
    phosphate into the pyruvate dehydrogenase complex in rat
    heart mitochondria, Biochem. J., 188:409.
Saltiel, A., Jacobs, S., Siegel, M., and Cuatrecasas, P., 1981,
    Insulin stimulates the release from liver plasma membranes
    a chemical modulator of pyruvate dehydrogenase, Biochem.
    Biophys. Res. Commun., 102:1041.
Schlessinger, J., 1980, The mechanism and role of hormone-
    induced clustering of membrane receptors, Trends Biochem.
    Sci., 5:210.
Seals, J. R., and Czech, M. P., 1980, Evidence that insulin
    activates an intrinsic plasma membrane protease in gene-
    rating a secondary chemical mediator, J. Biol. Chem.,
    255:6529.
Seals, J. R., and Czech, M. P., 1981, Characterization of a
    pyruvate dehydrogenase activator released by adipocyte
    plasma membranes in response to insulin, J. Biol. Chem.,
    256:2894.
Seals, J. R., and Czech, M. P., 1982, Extraction of insulin-
    dependent regulator from intact adipocytes, Fed. Proc.,
    41:1081.
Seals, J. R., McDonald, J. M., and Jarett, J., 1979a, Insulin
    effect on protein phosphorylation of plasma membranes and
    mitochondria in a subcellular system from rat adipocytes,
    J. Biol. Chem., 254:6991.
Seals, J. R., McDonald, J. M., and Jarett, L., 1979b, Insulin
    effect on protein phosphorylation of plasma membranes and
    mitochondria in a subcellular system from adipocytes, J.
    Biol. Chem., 254:6997.

Shen, L. C., Villar. Palasi, C., and Larner, J., 1970, Hormonal
    alteration of protein kinase sensitive to 3',5'-cyclic AMP,
    Physiol. Chem. Phys., 2:536.
Smith, C. J., Rubin, C. R., and Rosen, O. M., 1980, Insulin-
    treated 3T3-L1 adipocytes and cell-free extracts derived
    from them incorporate ^{32}P into ribosomal protein S6, Proc.
    Natl. Acad. Sci. USA, 77:2641.
Smith, C. J., Weiksnora, P. J., Warner, J. B., Rubin, C. S., and
    Rosen, O. M., 1979, Insulin-stimulated protein phosphoryla-
    tion in 3T3-L1 preadipocytes, Proc. Natl. Acad. Sci. USA,
    76:2725.
Suzuki, K., and Kono, T., 1980, Evidence that insulin causes
    translocation of glucose transport activity to the plasma
    membrane from an intracellular storage site, Proc. Natl.
    Acad. Sci. USA, 77:2542.
Swergold, G. D., Rosen, O. M., and Rubin, C. S., 1982, Hormonal
    regulation of the phosphorylation of ATP-citrate lyase in
    3T3 L1 adipocytes, J. Biol. Chem., 257:4207.
Tran, P. L., and Desbuqois, B., 1980, Protein phosphorylation in
    rat liver plasma membranes. In vitro and in vivo inhibi-
    tion by insulin, FEBS Lett., 116:149.
Ushiro, H., and Cohen, S., 1980, Identification of phosphotyro-
    sine as a product of epidermal growth factor-activated
    protein kinase in A-431 cell membranes, J. Biol. Chem.,
    255:8363.
Vandenheede, J. R., Yang, S. -D., and Merlevede, W., 1981,
    Rabbit skeletal muscle protein phosphatase. Identity of
    phosphorylase and synthase phosphatase and interconversion
    to the ATP-Mg-dependent enzyme form, J. Biol. Chem., 256:
    5894.
Walkenbach, R. J., Hazen, R., and Larner, J., 1978, Reversible
    inhibition of cyclic AMP-dependent protein kinase by
    insulin, Mol. Cell. Biochem., 19:31.
Walkenbach, R. J., Hazen, R., and Larner, J., 1980, Hormonal
    regulation of glycogen synthase. Insulin decreases protein
    kinase sensitivity to cyclic AMP, Biochim. Biophys. Acta,
    629:421.
Walaas, O., and Horn, R. S., 1981, The controversial problem of
    insulin action, Trends Pharmacol. Sci., 2:196.
Walaas, O., Walaas, E., and Grønnerød, O., 1973, Hormonal regula-
    tion of cyclic AMP-dependent protein kinase of rat dia-
    phragm by epinephrine and insulin, Eur. J. Biochem.,
    40:465.
Walaas, O., Walaas, E., Rye Alertsen, Aa., Horn, R. S., and

Fossum, S., 1977, A stimulatory effect of insulin on phosphorylation of a peptide in sarcolemma-enriched membrane preparation from rat skeletal muscle, FEBS Lett., 80:417.

Walaas, O., Walaas, E., Rye Alertsen, Aa., and Horn, R. S., 1979, The effect of insulin and guanosine nucleotides on protein phosphorylations in sarcolemma membranes from skeletal muscle, Mol. Cell. Endocrinol., 16:45.

Walaas, O., Sletten, K., Horn, R. S., Lystad, E., Adler, A., and Rye Alertsen, Aa., 1981a, Insulin-dependent phosphorylation in membranes. Isolation and characterization of a phosphorylated proteolipid from sarcolemma, FEBS Lett., 128:137.

Walaas, O., Horn, R. S., Lystad, E., and Adler, A., 1981b, ADP-ribosylation of sarcolemma membrane proteins in the presence of cholera toxin and its influence on insulin-stimulated membrane protein kinase activity, FEBS Lett., 128:133.

DISCUSSION

Answer to question from Wells:

WALAAS: We have examined hydrolysed membrane protein samples using high-volt electrophoresis at both pH 3.5 and pH 1.9. We observed only one radioactive spot and this corresponded to phosphoserine. We have also subjected extracts of phosphorylated membranes to thin sheet chromatography performed according to Hauser et al., 1981, Biochim. Biophys. Acta, 248, 87-95. This procedure, which resulted in good separation of polyphosphoinositide standards gave no indication of ^{32}phosphate in such materials in our membrane extracts.

INSULIN REGULATION OF NUCLEAR ENVELOPE FUNCTIONS:

RELATIONSHIP TO mRNA METABOLISM

I. D. Goldfine, F. Purrello and R. Vigneri

Cell Biology Research Laboratory,
Harold Brunn Institute
Mount Zion Hospital and Medical Center
San Francisco, California 94120 and
Departments of Medicine, Physiology
University of California, San Francisco

1. Introduction

Insulin is a major anabolic hormone for most mammalian species. The hormonal potency of insulin results, to a large extent, from its ability to regulate target cells at a variety of cellular sites. The effects of insulin on membrane transport, enzyme activity, and protein synthesis have been studied extensively. Most likely many of these effects result from the direct interaction of insulin with its plasma membrane receptor. Insulin also regulates nuclear functions such as DNA and RNA synthesis, but how insulin influences these processes is unknown. The presence of specific binding sites for insulin on nuclei and nuclear envelopes has been documented and characterized. These binding sites have biochemical characteristics that are different from insulin binding sites on the plasma membrane. Moreover, direct in vitro effects of insulin on messenger RNA (mRNA) metabolism have now been reported. These effects include: (1) stimulation of mRNA efflux from intact nuclei; (2) stimulation of nuclear envelope nucleoside triphosphatase (NTPase), the enzyme that regulates mRNA efflux; and (3) inhibition of ^{32}P incorporation into nuclear envelopes. Thus, significant insight is now being gained concerning the actions of insulin on nuclear function.

183

2.   Actions of Insulin on DNA and RNA Synthesis

Insulin in vitro stimulates the growth of cells in tissue culture (Gey and Thalhimer, 1924). In most studies, however, higher than physiological concentrations of insulin are necessary for this effect (Rechler et al., 1974; Smith and Temin, 1974) and it is likely that in many instances insulin is interacting with receptors for the various insulin-like growth factors, such as somatomedin, MSA, or non-suppressible insulin-like activity (NSILA-s) (Rechler et al., 1974; Smith and Temin, 1974; Chochinov and Daughaday, 1976). In a few instances, however, physiological concentrations of insulin increase cell division. It has been shown that insulin is necessary for the regeneration of liver that follows partial hepatectomy in rats and other animals (Bucher and Weir, 1976; Price, 1976). Also, in cultured cells from regenerating rat liver, there is evidence indicating that insulin stimulates DNA synthesis (Richman et al., 1976). Finally, physiological concentrations of insulin stimulate DNA synthesis in H35 hepatoma cells (Koontz and Iwahashi, 1980).

Insulin regulates RNA levels in many tissues. It is possible that insulin has multiple effects on RNA metabolism, including the regulation of transcriptional and post-transcriptional events. Effects of insulin on transcription have been reported in liver, pancreas, adipose tissue, and mammary gland. Insulin, in vivo, increases both RNA polymerase activity and template activity of liver (Steiner, 1966; Morgan and Bonner, 1970). Inhibition of RNA synthesis by actinomycin D has been reported to block the insulin-stimulated synthesis of several enzymes in diabetic rats, including fatty acid synthetase, glycogen synthetase, hexokinase, phosphofructokinase, and pyruvate kinase (Steiner and King, 1964; Steiner, 1966; Weber, 1972; Krahl, 1974). In liver of diabetic rats, insulin administration inhibits the activities of glucose-6-phosphatase, fructose-1,6-diphosphatase, pyruvate carboxylase, and phosphoenolpyruvate carboxykinase; actinomycin D pretreatment of animals also blocks this inhibition (Steiner and King, 1964; Steiner, 1966; Weber, 1972; Krahl, 1974).

Insulin also influences mRNA levels (Table I). Recent studies have indicated that the production of mRNA for tyrosine aminotransferase (Hill et al., 1981) is decreased in the liver of adrenalectomized rats, and albumin (Peavy et al., 1978), fatty acid synthetase (Pry and Porter, 1981) and α_{2u} globulin (Roy et al., 1980) are decreased in the liver of diabetic rats. These diminished levels of mRNA can be restored by insulin administration in vivo. In the adrenal-ectomized rat, insulin causes a generalized increase in mRNA content (Hill et al., 1981).

Table I. Influence of Insulin on mRNA Levels in Liver and Other Tissues[a]

Liver

    1. Albumin

    2. TAT (tyrosine aminotransferase)

    3. Fatty acid synthetase

    4. α_{2u} globulin

Pancreas

    1. Amylase

Mammary gland

    1. Casein

---

[a]Peavy et al., 1978; Roy et al., 1980; Bolander et al., 1981; Hill et al., 1981; Korc et al., 1981b; Pry and Porter, 1981.

Administration of insulin to diabetic rats both restores diminished pancreatic acinar cell amylase levels (Söling and Unger, 1972; Korc et al., 1981a) and reduces increased tryp-sinogen levels; actinomycin D treatment blocks this effect (Söling and Unger, 1972). Further, amylase mRNA levels fall dramatically in the pancreas of diabetic rats and this fall is rapidly reversed by insulin administration (Korc et al., 1981b) (Fig. 1).

In adipose tissue, insulin in vivo stimulates the synthesis of hexokinase II via the formation of new RNA (Hansen et al., 1967; Hansen and Pilkis, 1970; Krahl, 1974). Moreover, insulin stimulates the activity of glucose-6-P-dehydrogenase, phosphofructose kinase, and pyruvate kinase (Hansen et al., 1967; Hansen and Pilkis, 1970; Krahl, 1974); these effects are blocked by the administration of actinomycin D. It has been reported that insulin in vitro increases lipoprotein lipase activity in 3T3-L$_1$ fibroblasts (Spooner et al., 1979) in part by nuclear regulation.

In mammary glands, insulin in vitro activates RNA synthesis, stimulates RNA polymerase activity, the phosphorylation of histone and nonhistone proteins (Stockdale and Topper, 1966; Turkington, 1968; Topper et al., 1970; Terry et al., 1977), and increases mRNA levels (Bolander et al., 1981).

3. Binding Sites for Insulin on Nuclear Envelopes and
    Plasma Membranes

Specific binding sites for insulin on purified liver plasma membranes were first demonstrated by Freychet et al. (1971) and have now been described in many cell types (Goldfine, 1978a). The major characteristics of insulin binding to these receptors are listed in Table II. In addition to these cell surface binding sites, other insulin binding sites have also been described on intracellular

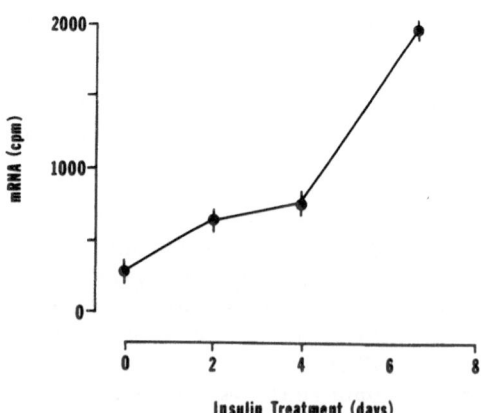

Figure 1. Effect of insulin injections on pancreatic amylase mRNA levels from diabetic rats. Adapted from Korc et al., 1981b.

structures, including nuclei (Horvat et al., 1975; Goldfine and Smith, 1976; Vigneri et al., 1978a; Brisson-Lougarre and Blum, 1979; Goidl, 1979; Brisson-Lougarre and Blum, 1980) and nuclear membranes (Goldfine et al., 1977; Horvat, 1978; Vigneri et al., 1978a), smooth and rough endoplasmic reticulum (Horvat et al., 1975; Vigneri et al., 1978a) and Golgi apparatus (Bergeron et al., 1973).

Table II.   Characteristics of Insulin Binding to
Cellular Membranes

	Plasma	Nuclear
High salt optimum	yes	no
Alkaline pH optimum	yes	no
Negative cooperativity	yes	no
Antireceptor antibody	yes	no
Low temperature stability	yes	no
Insulin degradation	yes	no
Regulation by exogenous insulin	yes	yes

Specific binding sites for insulin on purified rat liver nuclei free of other cellular components were first described by Horvat and coworkers (1975) and then confirmed both in our laboratory (Goldfine and Smith, 1976; Vigneri et al., 1978a) and that of Goidl (1979). In addition, specific nuclear binding sites have been detected in thyroid nuclei (Brisson-Lougarre and Blum, 1979, 1980). The major site of insulin binding to the nucleus is the nuclear envelope (Goldfine et al., 1977; Horvat, 1978; Vigneri et al., 1978b). When whole nuclei are incubated with native insulin followed by an immunofluorescence procedure, fluorescence is detected only on the nuclear surface (Horvat, 1978). Further, when nuclei are first incubated with ^{125}I-labeled insulin and then subfractionated, most of the specific hormone binding is seen with the nuclear envelope fractions (Vigneri et al., 1978b).

In addition, when nuclei are incubated with high concentrations of detergent to remove both layers of the nuclear envelope, binding is either reduced or eliminated. Finally, insulin does not bind directly to DNA or histones, but does bind directly to purified nuclear envelopes (Horvat, 1978; Vigneri et al., 1978b).

The binding of insulin to nuclear envelopes, like its binding to plasma membranes, fulfills the requirements of a hormone receptor. It is rapid, reversible, of high affinity and hormone-specific (Fig. 2). Two insulin analogues with decreased biological potencies, proinsulin and desoctapeptide insulin, were less effective in both nuclear and plasma membranes. The characteristics of insulin binding to the nuclear envelope differ, however, in a number of respects from the characteristics of insulin binding to plasma membranes (Table II). Studies of insulin binding to liver plasma membranes have revealed two classes of binding sites (Goldfine, 1978a). In our studies of insulin binding sites on nuclear envelopes prepared by the method of Kashnig and Kasper (1969), two orders of binding sites were seen with lower affinities (K_d 5.6 nM, 65 nM) than that seen on plasma membranes (K_d 0.5 nM, 10 nM). Both plasma membranes and nuclear envelopes, however, have similar total insulin binding capacities (approx. 2 nmol/mg protein). Horvat (1978), studying nuclear envelopes prepared by RNAase and DNAase digestion, reported only one class of binding sites for insulin having a K_d of 3 nM. In liver and other tissues, the binding of insulin to plasma membranes has three distinctive characteristics (Goldfine, 1978a; Horvat, 1978; Vigneri et al., 1978b): a sharp pH optimum of 8.0, enhanced binding in the presence of high concentrations of NaCl, and enhanced dissociation of labeled insulin in the presence of unlabeled insulin, which may be due to negative cooperativity. When the characteristics of insulin binding to nuclear envelopes were examined, we found that the pH optimum was between 7.0 and 7.5, that there was no enhanced binding in the presnece of NaCl, and that addition of unlabeled insulin did not enhance the dissociation rate of labeled insulin. Horvat also did not find any indication for negative cooperativity with insulin binding to nuclear envelopes (1978).

In the serum of patients with severe insulin resistance and acanthosis nigricans, there are antibodies to the plasma membrane insulin receptor, and preincubation of plasma

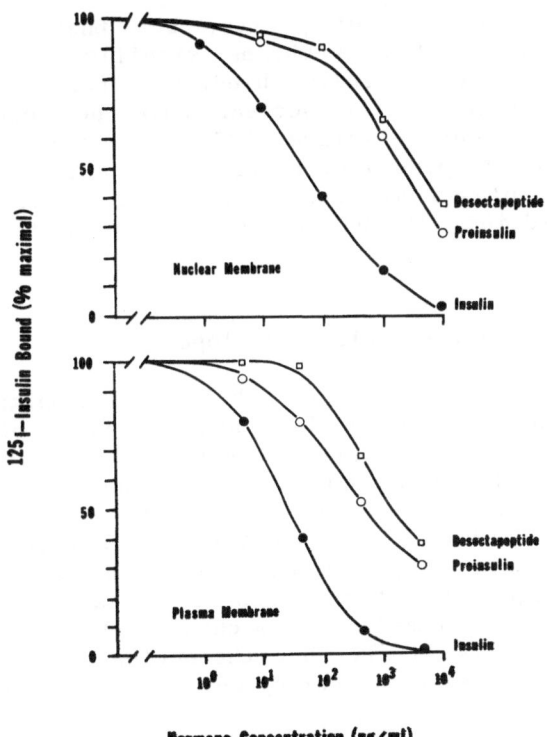

Figure 2. Inhibition of ^{125}I-insulin binding to nuclear (top) and plasma membranes (bottom) by native insulin, pro-insulin and desoctapeptide insulin.

membranes with these antibodies blocks the subsequent binding of insulin (Fig. 3) (Goldfine et al., 1977). This inhibition of binding by these antibodies can be demonstrated with insulin receptors from a variety of species and tissues. These antibodies, however, do not bind to receptors for other hormones, such as glucagon and growth hormone (Goldfine et al., 1977). When we preincubated this antiserum with nuclei, there was little inhibition of the subsequent binding of labeled hormone (Goldfine et al., 1977). This finding suggested that the insulin binding sites in the nuclear envelope are proteins different from the insulin binding sites on the plasma membrane. Another possibility is that they are the same binding site, but that the different milieu of the nuclear membrane significantly alters the characteristics of insulin binding. For instance, the lipid composition of the nuclear envelope, especially the cholesterol content (Goldfine, 1978b), is markedly different from that of the plasma membrane. Since the lipid environment of the plasma membrane causes alterations in insulin binding (Goldfine, 1978b), there is support for the latter hypothesis.

4.   Structure of the Nuclear Envelope

The nuclear envelope is a bilayered membrane structure that separates the nucleoplasm and cytoplasm of eukaryotic cells. The outer nuclear envelope is associated with the endoplasmic reticulum and the inner nuclear membrane is intimately associated with the peripheral heterochromatin (Franke, 1974; Harris and Agutter, 1976) (Fig. 4). It is known that small molecules can freely enter into and exit from the nucleus but the transport of large molecules may proceed via a more complicated mechanism (Harris and Agutter, 1976). Thus it is likely that the nuclear envelope has more than a passive role in nuclear cytoplasmic interactions.

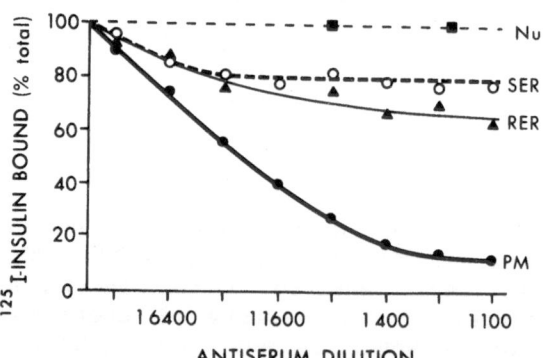

Figure 3.   The effect of preincubation with an antiserum to the plasma membrane insulin receptor on the subsequent specific binding of ^{125}I-labeled insulin to isolated nuclei (Nu), rough (RER) and smooth (SER) endoplasmic reticulum, and plasma membranes (PM). Adapted from Goldfine et al. (1977).

Pores filled with a unique structure termed the nuclear pore complex are dispersed throughout the nuclear envelope (Fig. 4). The nuclear pore complex has a double annulus, each annulus having eight peripheral subunits of approximately 250 Å in diameter (Franke, 1974; Harris and Agutter, 1976). In addition, there is a central granule between the double annuli (Fig. 4). The nuclear pore complex is attached to both the inner and outer nuclear envelope, but the nuclear pore complex is not covered on its inner surface by hetero-chromatin. Further, it has been postulated that both the central granule and peripheral subunits are hollow tubes. Thus the nuclear pore complex could play a role in the nuclear cytoplasmic translocation of mRNA.

5.   Relationship Between mRNA Efflux and Nuclear Membrane NTPase

In order to understand the mechanism of mRNA transport from the nucleus, rats have been injected with radiolabeled orotic acid or uridine and the efflux of labeled RNA from isolated nuclei into a surrogate cytoplasm studied (Ishikawa et al., 1978; Schumm and Webb, 1978; Agutter et al., 1979a; Clawson et al., 1980). Most investigators have employed nuclei from liver. Many criteria suggest that the nature of the transported RNA (including size, base and poly A content, activity in directing protein synthesis, incorporation into

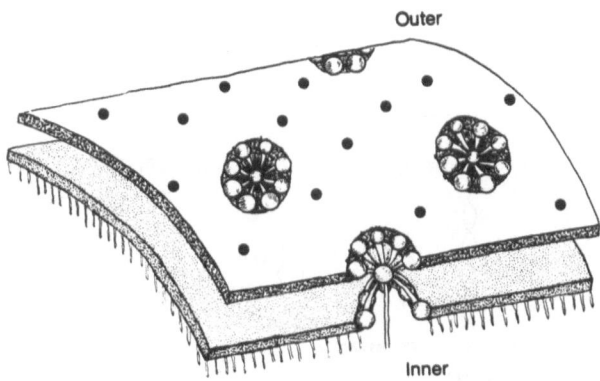

Figure 4. Schematic drawing of the nuclear envelope. Nuclear pores can be seen joining the two layers of the nuclear envelope.

polysomes, and inclusion into specific RNP particles) under the conditions studied is mRNA (Schumm and Webb, 1978; Agutter et al., 1979a; Clawson et al., 1980).

RNA transport in vitro involves both intranuclear RNA processing and subsequent efflux (Fig. 5). A source of high energy phosphate is necessary for transport, but not processing (Schumm and Webb, 1978; Agutter et al., 1979a; Clawson et al., 1980). One high energy phosphate bond is hydrolyzed to transport one nucleotide of mRNA. Studies indicate that the high energy phosphate specificity is not highly selective since ATP, UTP, CTP, and GTP are all effective (Schumm and Webb, 1978; Agutter et al., 1979a; Clawson et al., 1980).

There is considerable evidence suggesting that a nuclear membrane triphosphatase (NTPase) provides the energy for the transport of mRNA. For instance, the activation energy for RNA transport is 13 kcal/mol and for NTPase activity is 13.3-13.8 kcal/mol (Clawson et al., 1980). Further, the affinities of ATP for both NTPase activity and facilitated RNA transport are similar. Also, cyclic AMP stimulates both functions whereas NaF inhibits both of them (Schumm and Webb, 1978; Agutter et al., 1979a; Clawson et al., 1980). Finally, trypsin treatment of nuclei inactivates both functions (Agutter et al., 1979a). Histocytochemical studies indicate that this enzyme is located throughout the nuclear envelope (Clawson et al., 1980). Others, however, have suggested that this enzyme resides in the nuclear pore complex (Agutter et al., 1979a).

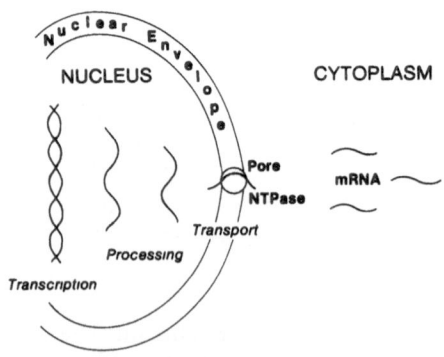

Figure 5. Major sites of mRNA processing.

6.   Insulin Action in Isolated Nuclei and Nuclear Envelopes

In view of the influence of insulin on mRNA levels in liver, several studies have been carried out in vitro with isolated nuclei and nuclear envelopes. Schumm and Webb measured mRNA transport from liver nuclei of normal rats prelabeled 30 min in vivo with [^{14}C]orotic acid and found that the direct addition of insulin in vitro to these nuclei markedly enhanced mRNA transport (1978). In these studies, however, higher than physiological levels of insulin were needed (100 nM). We have modified their methods by both eliminating liver cytosol and using diabetic rats. We now find that in vitro an effect of insulin is seen at 10 pM and at higher insulin levels the hormonal effect is diminished.

In light of the observations that insulin may directly stimulate nuclear mRNA efflux and that nuclear membrane NTPase activity is necessary for this function, we investigated whether insulin directly influenced nuclear membrane NTPase activity. Highly purified nuclear membranes were prepared by the method of Monneron et al. (1973). In these membranes we found that basal nuclear membrane NTPase activity was higher in liver of normal rats than in liver from hypo-insulinemic diabetic rats (Purrello et al., 1982). Moreover, the direct addition of insulin to purified nuclear envelopes of liver from diabetic rats stimulated NTPase activity. As with stimulation of mRNA efflux, an effect was detectable at 1 pM and maximal effects were seen at 10-100 pM. Other studies indicated that insulin increased the Vmax of the enzyme (Purrello et al., 1982).

Several groups have reported the presence of protein kinase and phosphatase activity in isolated nuclear envelopes (Agutter et al., 1979b; Lam and Kasper, 1979; Steer et al., 1979a,b) and it has been proposed that these reactions may have a regulatory role in nucleocytoplasmic transport (Agutter et al., 1979b; Lam and Kasper, 1979; Steer et al., 1979a,b). Moreover, it has been proposed that phosphorylation reactions regulate nuclear envelope NTPase activity (Agutter et al., 1979b). Accordingly we investigated whether insulin has direct effects on the phosphorylation of nuclear envelopes from rat liver. The direct addition of insulin to highly purified nuclear envelopes decreased ^{32}P incorporation into trichloroacetic acid precipitable proteins. As with stimulation of mRNA efflux and NTPase activity, an effect was

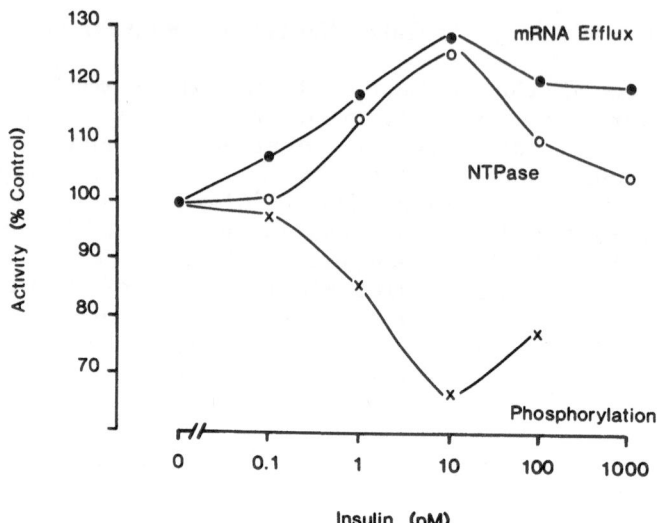

Figure 6. Effect of insulin on: (1) stimulation of [^{14}C]RNA release from isolated liver nuclei obtained from diabetic rats, (2) NTPase activity in isolated nuclear envelopes, and (3) ^{32}P incorporation into nuclear envelope proteins.

detectable at 1 pM. The dose response curve was biphasic and was a mirror image of the curves for regulation of mRNA efflux and NTPase activity. Other studies suggested that insulin was acting via stimulation of phosphatase activity.

These data suggest, therefore, a model of how insulin may regulate mRNA efflux. Nuclear envelope NTPase, the enzyme that regulates mRNA efflux, may be in either phosphorylated (inactive) or dephosphorylated (active) states (Fig. 7). When dephosphorylated, the enzyme has an increased affinity for both mRNA and ATP and as a result the nucleocytoplasmic transport of mRNA is enhanced and the hydrolysis of ATP is accelerated.

7.   Conclusion

The nuclear envelope and its pore complex play a major role in the transport of mRNA from the nucleus. It had been documented that the nuclear envelope contains specific high affinity binding sites for insulin but until recently the significance of these binding sites was unknown. Current studies now indicate that insulin not only directly stimulates the release of mRNA from isolated nuclei but also increases the activity of nuclear envelope NTPase, the ezyme that regulates mRNA efflux. Moreover, insulin inhibits ^{32}P incorporation into nuclear envelope proteins. These observations raise the possibility, therefore, that one mechanism whereby insulin regulates nuclear functions is by acting directly at the nuclear surface.

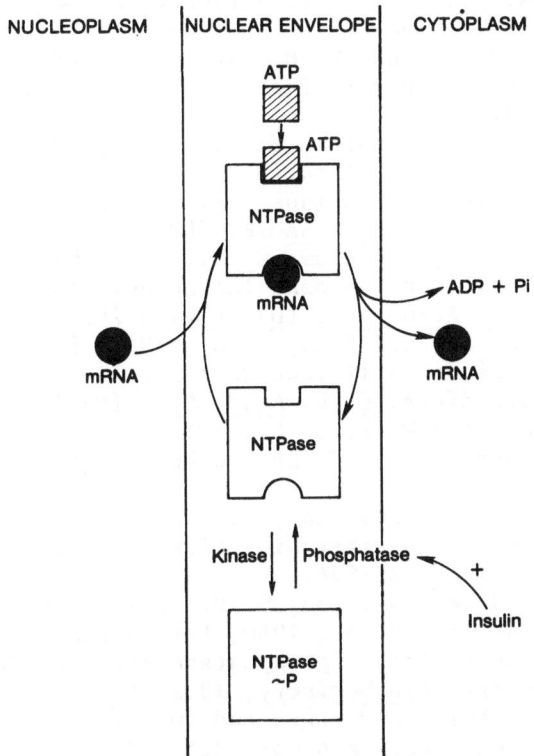

Figure 7. Proposed model of insulin stimulation of mRNA release from nuclei. Insulin first stimulates phosphoprotein phosphatase activity which in turn activates NTPase activity. NTPase then hydrolyzes ATP and promotes mRNA efflux.

ACKNOWLEDGMENTS: This research was supported by NIH grant
no. AM26667 and the Elise Stern Haas Research Fund, Harold
Brunn Institute, Mount Zion Hospital and Medical Center.

REFERENCES

Agutter, P. S., McCaldin, B., and McArdle, H. J., 1979a,
    Importance of mammalian nuclear-envelope nucleoside
    triphosphatase in nucleo-cytoplasmic transport of
    ribonucleoproteins, Biochem. J. 182:811.
Agutter, P. S., Cockrill, J. B., Lavine, J. E., McCaldin, B.,
    and Sim, R. B., 1979b, Properties of mammalian nuclear-
    envelope nucleoside triphosphatase, Biochem. J. 181:647.
Bergeron, J. J. M., Evans, W. H., and Geschwind, I. I., 1973,
    Insulin binding to rat liver Golgi fraction, J. Cell
    Biol. 59:771.
Bolander, F. F. Jr., Nicholas, K. R., Van Wyk, J. J., and
    Topper, Y. J., 1981, Insulin is essential for accumula-
    tion of casein mRNA in mouse mammary epithelial cells,
    Proc. Natl. Acad. Sci. USA 78:5682.
Brisson-Lougarre, A., and Blum, C. J., 1979, Sites de liaison
    nucléaire á l'insuline dans les noyaux isolés de thyoïde
    bovine, C. R. Acad. Sci. (D) (Paris) 289:129.
Brisson-Lougarre, A., and Blum, C. J., 1980, Spécificité et
    reversibilité de la liaison de l'insuline aux noyaux
    isolés thyroidïens, C. R. Acad. Sci. (D) (Paris) 209:889.
Bucher, N. L. R., and Weir, G. C., 1976, Insulin, glucagon,
    liver regeneration, and DNA synthesis. Metab. Clin. Exp.
    25:1423.
Chochinov, R. H., and Daughaday, W. H., 1976, Current concepts
    of somatomedin and other biologically related growth
    factors, Diabetes 25:994.
Clawson, G. A., James, J., Woo, C. H., Friend, D. S., Moody,
    D., and Smuckler, E. A., 1980, Pertinence of nuclear
    envelope nucleoside triphosphatase activity of ribonucleic
    acid transport, Biochemistry, 19:2748.
Feldherr, C. M., 1972, Structure and function of the nuclear
    envelope. Adv. Cell and Mol. Biol. 2:273.
Franke, W. W., 1974, Structure, biochemistry, and functions of
    the nuclear envelope, in: "International Review of
    Cytology", G. H. Bourne, and J. F. Danielli, eds., p. 71,
    Academic Press, New York.
Freychet, P., Roth, J., and Neville, D. M. Jr., 1971, Insulin
    receptors in the liver: specific binding of (^{125}I) insulin
    to the plasma membrane and its relation to insulin bio-
    activity, Proc. Natl. Acad. Sci. USA 68:1833.

Gey, G. O., and Thalhimer, W. J., 1924, Observations on the effects of insulin introduced into the medium of tissue cultures, J. Am. Med. Assoc. 82:1609.

Goidl, J. A., 1979, Insulin binding to isolated liver nuclei from obese and lean mice, Biochemistry 18:3674.

Goldfine, I. D., 1978a, The insulin receptor, in: "Receptors in Pharmacology", J. R. Smythies and R. J. Bradley, eds., p. 335, Marcel Dekker, New York.

Goldfine, I. D., 1978b, Insulin receptors and the site of action of insulin, Life Sci. 23:2639.

Goldfine, I. D., and Smith, G. J., 1976, Binding of insulin to isolated nuclei, Proc. Natl. Acad. Sci. USA 73:1427.

Goldfine, I. D., Vigneri, R., Cohen, D., and Pliam, N. B., 1977, Intracellular binding sites for insulin are immunologically distinct from those on the plasma membrane, Nature 269:698.

Hansen, R. J., and Pilkis, S. J., 1970, Effect of insulin on the synthesis in vitro of hexokinase in rat epididymal adipose tissue, Endocrinology 86:57.

Hansen, R. J., Pilkis, S. J., and Krahl, M. E., 1967, Properties of adaptive hexokinase isozymes of the rat, Endocrinology 81:1397.

Harris, J. R., and Agutter, P. S., 1976, The isolation and characterization of the nuclear envelope, in: "Biochemical Analysis of Membranes", A. H. Maddy, ed., p. 132, John Wiley, New York.

Hill, R. E., Lee, K.-L., and Kenny, F. T., 1981, Effects of insulin on messenger RNA activities in rat liver, J. Biol. Chem. 256:1510.

Horvat, A., 1978, Insulin binding sites on rat liver nuclear membranes: biochemical and immunofluorescent studies, J. Cell Physiol. 97:37.

Horvat, A., Li, E., and Katsoyannis, P. G., 1975, Cellular binding sites for insulin in rat liver, Biochim. Biophys. Acta 382:609.

Ishikawa, K., Sato-Odani, S., and Ogata, K., 1978, The role of ATP in the transport of rapidly-labeled RNA from isolated nuclei of rat liver in vitro, Biochim. Biophys. Acta. 521:650.

Kashnig, D. M., and Kasper, C. B., 1969, Isolation, morphology, and composition of the nuclear membrane from rat liver, J. Biol. Chem. 244:3786.

Koontz, J. W., and Iwahashi, M., 1980, Insulin as a potent, specific growth factor in a rat hepatoma cell line, Science 211:947.

Korc, M., Iwamoto, Y., Sankaran, H., Williams, J. A., and Goldfine, I. D., 1981a, Insulin action in pancreatic acini from streptozotocin-treated rats. I. Stimulation of protein

synthesis, Am. J. Physiol. 240 (Gastrointest. Liver
    Physiol. 3):G56.

Korc, M., Owerbach, D., Quinto, C., and Rutter, W. J., 1981b,
    Pancreatic islet-acinar cell interaction: amylase messen-
    ger RNA levels are determined by insulin, Science 213:351.

Krahl, M. E., 1974, Endocrine function of the pancreas, Annu.
    Rev. Physiol. 36:331.

Lam, K. S., and Kasper, O. B., 1979, Selective phosphorylation
    of a nuclear envelope polypeptide by an endogenous protein
    kinase, Biochemistry 18:307.

Monneron, A., Blobel, G., and Palade, G. E., 1973, Fractiona-
    tion of the nucleus by divalent cations. Isolation of
    nuclear membranes, J. Cell Biol. 55:104.

Morgan, C. R., and Bonner, J., 1970, Template activity of liver
    chromatin increased by in vitro administration of insulin,
    Proc. Natl. Acad. Sci. USA 65:1077.

Peavy, D. E., Taylor, J. M., and Jefferson, L. S., 1978,
    Correlation of albumin production rates and albumin mRNA
    levels in livers of normal, diabetic, and insulin-treated
    diabetic rats, Proc. Natl. Acad. Sci. USA 75:5879.

Price, J. B. Jr., 1976, Insulin and glucagon as modifiers of DNA
    synthesis in the regenerating rat liver, Metab. Clin. Exp.
    25:1427.

Pry, T. A., and Porter, J. W., 1981, Control of fatty acid
    synthetase mRNA levels in rat liver by insulin, glucagon
    and dibutyryl cyclic AMP, Biochem. Biophys. Res. Comm.
    100:1002.

Purrello, F., Vigneri, R., Clawson, G. A., and Goldfine, I. D.,
    1982, Insulin stimulation of nucleoside triphosphatase
    activity in isolated nuclear envelopes, Science 216:1005.

Rechler, M. M., Podskalny, J. M., Goldfine, I. D., and Wells,
    C. A., 1974, DNA synthesis in human fibroblasts: stimula-
    tion by insulin and by nonsuppressible insulin-like
    activity (NSILA-S), J. Clin. Endocrinol. Metab. 39:512.

Richman, R. A., Claus, T. H., Pilkis, S. J., and Friedman, D.
    L., 1976, Hormonal stimulation of DNA synthesis in primary
    cultures of adult rat hepatocytes, Proc. Natl. Acad. Sci.
    USA 73:3589.

Roy, A. K., Chatterjee, B., Prasad, M. S. K., and Unakar, J. J.,
    1980, Role of insulin in the regulation of the hepatic
    messenger RNA for alpha 2u-globulin in diabetic rats, J.
    Biol. Chem. 255:11614.

Schumm, D. E., and Webb, T. E., 1978, Effect of adenosine 3':5'-
    monophosphate and guanosine 3':5'-monophosphate on RNA
    release from isolated nuclei, J. Biol. Chem. 253:8513.

Smith, G. L., and Temin, H. M., 1974, Purified multiplica-
     tion-stimulating activity from rat liver cell conditioned
     medium: comparison of biological activities with calf
     serum, insulin, and somatomedin, J. Cell Physiol.
     84:181.
Söling, H. D., and Unger, K. O., 1972, The role of insulin in
     the regulation of α-amylase synthesis in the rat pancreas,
     Eur. J. Clin. Invest. 2:199.
Spooner, P. M., Chernick, S. S., Garrison, M. M., and Scow,
     R. O., 1979, Insulin regulation of lipoprotein lipase
     activity and release in 3T3-L1 adipocytes. Separation
     and dependence of hormonal effects on hexose metabol-
     ism and synthesis of RNA and protein, J. Biol. Chem.
     254:10021.
Steer, R. C., Wilson, M. J., and Ahmed, K., 1979a, Protein phos-
     phokinase activity of rat liver nuclear membrane, Exp. Cell
     Res. 119:403.
Steer, R. C., Wilson, M. J., and Ahmed, K., 1979b, Phosphopro-
     tein phosphatase activity of rat liver nuclear membrane,
     Biochem. Biophys. Res. Commun. 89:1082.
Steiner, D. F., 1966, Insulin and the regulation of hepatic
     biosynthetic activity, Vitam. Horm. (NY) 24:1.
Steiner, D. F., and King, J., 1964, Induced synthesis of hepatic
     uridine diphosphate glucose-glycogen glucosyltransferase
     after administration of insulin to alloxan-diabetic rats,
     J. Biol. Chem. 239:1292.
Stockdale, F. E., and Topper, Y. J., 1966, The role of DNA
     synthesis and mitosis in hormone-dependent differentiation,
     Proc. Natl. Acad. Sci. USA 56:1283.
Terry, P. M., Banerjee, M. R., and Lui, R. M., 1977, Hormone-
     inducible casein messenger RNA in a serum-free organ
     culture of whole mammary gland, Proc. Natl. Acad. Sci.
     USA 74:2441.
Turkington, R. W., 1968, Hormone induced synthesis of DNA by
     mammary gland in vitro, Endocrinology 82:540.
Vigneri, R., Pliam, N. B., Cohen, D. C., Pezzino, V., Wong, K.
     Y., and Goldfine, I. D., 1978a, In vivo regulation of cell
     surface and intracellular insulin binding sites by insulin,
     J. Biol. Chem. 253:8192.
Vigneri, R., Goldfine, I. D., Wong, K. Y., Smith, G. J., and
     Pezzino, V., 1978b, The nuclear envelope. The major site
     of insulin binding in rat liver nuclei, J. Biol. Chem.
     253:2098.
Weber, G., 1972, Integrative action of insulin at the molecular
     level, Isr. J. Med. Sci. 8:325.

DISCUSSION

SCHRADER: You showed a general effect of insulin on phosphorylation of nuclear envelope proteins. Isn't this finding in contrast with the specific effect of insulin on NTPase dephosphorylation you envision?

GOLDFINE: We did see a dephosphorylation of the 68K complex which presumably contains the NTPase. It is possible that by preparation of the envelope the phosphatase loses selectivity and acts on all proteins whereas in the intact cell it only acts on the 68K protein.

TAYLOR: Where do you envision selectivity in your model? Whereas insulin stimulates the synthesis of some proteins, apparently by increasing cytoplasmic levels of mRNA, insulin inhibits the synthesis of other proteins (e.g., PEP-CK). In its simplest form, your model predicts insulin might increase the cytoplasmic levels of all mRNA species.

GOLDFINE: Insulin may act at specific nuclear pores which in turn may increase the transport of specific mRNAs. It is also possible that at other pores insulin may act to decrease mRNA transport.

HANSSON: Have you tested whether somatomedins or other growth factors bind to your nuclear membrane receptors? Secondly, the K_d of insulin binding was approximately 5 nM, whereas your effects were in the pM range.

GOLDFINE: No, we have not tested these compounds but we plan to do so in that they are important insulin-like compounds.

Yes, there appears to be a considerable amount of spare receptors. We have not seen a higher affinity binding site in nuclear membranes but one may exist; therefore, we will repeat our binding studies to look for one. In H35 rat hepatoma cells the binding of insulin has a K_d of 30 nM, but insulin increases TAT levels at a concentration of 1 pM. This instance, in my opinion, is the most extreme case of spare receptors.

BIRNBAUMER: Have you done experiments in which you added plasma membranes together with insulin to nuclei and tested whether this might result in an increase in the effect(s) you obtain with insulin?

GOLDFINE: This is an interesting point and we plan to do
these studies.

Intracellular Modulation of
Peptide Hormone Response

THE ROLE OF THE CYTOSKELETON IN THE

RESPONSES OF TARGET CELLS TO HORMONES

Peter F. Hall

Worcester Foundation for Experimental Biology
222 Maple Avenue
Shrewsbury, Massachusetts 01545

1. Introduction

To make the best use of its organelles and macromole-
cules, the cell requires a cytoskeleton. This term is applied
to three systems of tubules found in most if not all cells,
namely microtubules (diameter, 25 nm), intermediate filaments
(diameter, 10 mn) and microfilaments (diameter 6 nm). The
basic component of microtubules is the protein tubulin;
intermediate filaments contain a variety of proteins (keratin,
desmin, and vimentin) (Lazarides, 1980) and microfilaments
are composed of actin. The term cytoskeleton is intended to
evoke analogies with the skeletal system of vertebrate organisms which provides a rigid support for the attachment of the
contractile machinery of the body. As a result of this
relationship, the muscles can both shorten and provide force
at a fixed length. The analogy has some virtue but inevi-
tably comparisons between the mechanics of one cell and those
of a whole organism cannot be taken too far. Since little is
known about the functions of intermediate filaments (Lazarides, 1980), this chapter will be confined to the consideration
of microtubules and microfilaments. With respect to microfilaments, the widespread occurrence of extramuscular myosin
suggests that analogies with muscle may extend to myosin
ATPase. However, at present this idea cannot be accepted at
face value because too little is known about the functions of
extramuscular myosin.

2. Microtubules

The most striking feature of tubulin is that given the right conditions it can rapidly polymerize into long hollow tubules and can depolymerize with equal rapidity. Polymerization requires GTP (Weisenberg, 1972) and is regulated by proteins associated with tubulin - called MAPS (microtubule-associated proteins). One MAP called dynein acts as a specialized ATPase (Dentler et al., 1980). Regulation of polymerization involves Ca^{2+} (Kiehart, 1981) and since MAPS are subject to phosphorylation (Vallee, 1980), cyclic AMP may also play a regulatory role. The effects of these two regulatory agents mean that polymerization and depolymerization of tubulin can be integrated into many cellular activities influenced by one or both agents. In the case of Ca^{2+} it appears that calmodulin may be important in mediating the influence of this ion on microtubules (Means and Dedman, 1980).

The most influential theory concerning the function of microtubules is referred to as treadmilling - polymerization at one end and depolymerization at the other end (Margolis and Wilson, 1978). This process gives the illusion of movement because at steady-state the length of the tubule remains constant but it has grown at one end and has lost tubulin at the same rate from the other end. Treadmilling can, at least in theory, generate force and produce movement. Movement has been most clearly demonstrated in the mitotic spindle that draws the chromosomes towards the two poles of the spindle (McIntosh, 1979; Nicklas, 1971). In addition it has been proposed that microtubules give direction to certain intracellular processes. For example, Freed and Lebowitz (1970) showed that the pathways of saltatory movement of particles within the cell are clearly related to the organization of microtubules. The tubules appear to provide a framework for intracellular traffic. In addition, rapid polymerization and depolymerization of tubulin could result in the thrusting forth and withdrawl of rigid tubules within the cell. Such processes are likely to influence the shape and the internal organization of the cell.

3. Microfilaments

The widespread occurrence of both actin and myosin in extramuscular tissue suggests that microfilaments may provide cells with a contractile system involved in both internal and external shortening. The best studied example of such a function is seen in the constriction that takes place during cytokinesis (Schroeder, 1973; Fujiwara et al., 1978). In addition, microfilaments show polarity - both structural polarity and polarity of polymerization. When microfilaments are decorated with heavy meromyosin they reveal the classical arrowheads seen when thin filaments of muscle are similarly decorated (Ishikawa et al., 1969). Such structural polarity determins the direction of the sliding of filaments during shortening. This polarity is important in determining the direction of intracellular events involving a sliding filament mechanism. In addition, microfilaments grow by polymerization at both ends but growth at one end is more rapid than that at the other end. Rapid growth occurs towards the point of attachment of a filament to a cellular membrane (Woodrum et al., 1975). How such polymerization can proceed at an attached end is uncertain.

In addition to changes in length of microfilaments, actin is involved in striking changes in consistency of the cytoplasm of certain cells. For example, the cytoplasm of amoeba undergoes local transitions in physical state referred to as gelation (formation of a solid or gel) and solation (formation of a more fluid sol (Taylor and Condeelis, 1979). Gelation results from cross-linking of microfilaments and solation results from breakdown of microfilaments and that of interfilamentous connections. It is believed that these transitions are essential for amoeboid movement (Taylor and Condeelis, 1979). Gelation also occurs in mammalian cells (Weihing, 1977), although the functional significance of this process is not clear in such cells.

As in the case of microtubules, actin is associated with a variety of proteins that greatly influence the organization of microfilaments (Korn, 1978). This is most clearly seen when we consider the fact that G actin is present in cells above the critical concentration for polymerization - given the ionic composition of cytoplasm we would expect all cell actin to be polymerized. The presence of G actin in cells results from the presence of proteins which inhibit polymeri- zation. Profilin is one such protein (Carlsson et al., 1976). Other proteins (e.g., filamin and α-actinin) also promote polymerization (Korn, 1978). On the other hand, some proteins promote breakdown of formed microfilaments to insure that the process of filament formation is reversible (Korn, 1978).

With these fragments of information we must tread the fine line between, on the one hand, considering structure to the exclusion of function and, on the other hand, stretching what little information we have beyond safe limits into the realm of guesswork. The following generalizations represent an attempt to walk that tight rope.

(i)   The cytoskeleton appears to be important in transmitting signals from the surface of the cell to the interior and as a means of influencing the organization of the plasma membrane;

(ii)   the cytoskeleton integrates the organelles of the cell and provides a matrix for cellular activities through which productive encounters between subcellular structures are encouraged;

(iii)   microfilaments and microtubules are capable of causing shortening;

(iv)   the cytoskeleton provides support (stiffening and local rigidity);

(v)   the cytoskeleton establishes vectors within the cell - it provides direction.

In considering these functions we can appreciate the importance of the ability of monomers (G actin and tubulin) to polymerize and depolymerize because these changes enable the cell to construct new organelles and to cancel old ones. In this way the cytoskeleton can provide new vactors, new contacts between organelles and can influence new regions of the plasma membrane. The cytoskeleton is a major element in the asymmetry, in the compartmentation and in the inhomo-geneity that distinguishes the cytoplasm from an equeous solution. Such ideas were well described by Wolosewick and Porter when they defined the so-called microtrabecular system (Wolosewick and Porter, 1979).

We must now consider how hormones can influence the cytoskeleton. Before doing so however it will be well to discuss experimentally useful inhibitors of microfilaments and microtubules because, in spite of their undoubted limita-tions, these substances provide important tools for the investigation of cytoskeletal function for which there exist all too few alternatives. The most important inhibitor of

microtubules is undoubtedly colchicine which inhibits polymerization of tubulin (Borisy and Taylor, 1967). An important
control for effects of colchicine is available in the form of
lumicolchicine which does not inhibit polymerization of
tubulin. For microfilaments the preferred inhibitors are the
cytochalasins which inhibit polymerization of actin (Lin et
al., 1980). In addition, cytochalasin cleaves (Hartwig and
Stossel, 1979) and rearranges (Miranda et al., 1974) microfilaments. Unfortunately cytochalasins exert many effects
outside the microfilaments so that at best their use with
whole cells is confined to preliminary studies. If cytochalasins do not inhibit a given physiological action, microfilaments are unlikely to be involved. Unfortunately the
converse is not necessarily true. Numerous substances inhibit
microtubules and microfilaments (griseofulvin, D_2O, vinblastine, etc.) but they are too non-specific to be useful as
experimental tools to study the functions of the cytoskeleton.

4.   The Role of the Cytoskeleton in the Actions of Peptide
Hormones.

4.1   TSH

The steps in the synthesis, storage and secretion of
thyroid hormone are clearly organized in a vectorial manner

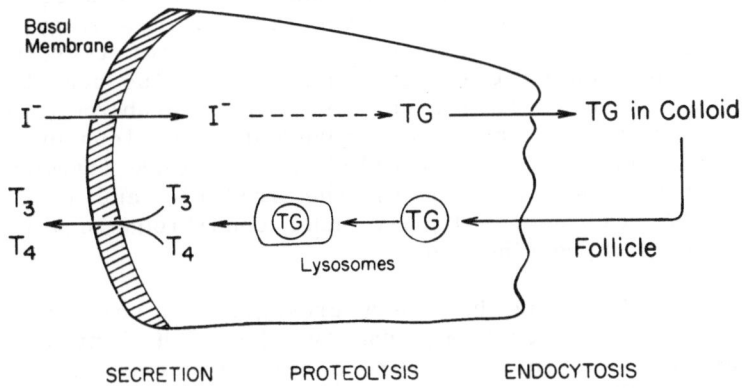

Figure 1. Organization of the synthesis, storage and secretion of thyroid hormone.

so that intermediates in the process move through the cell in specific directions.

Since these processes involve movement and direction, it would not be surprising to discover that the cytoskeleton is involved. Williams and Wolff (1970) measured secretion of ^{131}I-labeled thyroid hormones by isolated thyroid glands in vitro. The glands were prelabeled with ^{131}I in vivo. Secretion of labeled hormones by the glands was greatly increased by addition of TSH in vitro. Colchicine inhibited this response to TSH. Light microscopy showed accumulation of colloid droplets in the thyroid cells incubated with TSH in contrast to cells from unstimulated glands and those incubated with TSH plus colchicine (Williams and Wolff, 1970). These findings suggested that uptake of stored colloid into the cytoplasm of the cell (Figure 1) requires microtubules. Nève and co-workers (1972) studied this process by means of electron microscopy. The thyroid cell, under the influence of TSH, thrusts out villous processes into the colloid and appears to engulf fragments of colloid which are transported to lysosomes within the cell. Formation of these processes is prevented by treatment with colchicine and cytochalasin B. It is not difficult to consider possible mechanisms by which the cytoskeleton might participate in the uptake of colloid-thrusting out processes (polymerization of tubulin), moving the droplets within the cell (contraction of filaments), etc. However, the molecular basis of these events cannot be described at present and as so often happens in Biology, if it is true that our understanding of secretion of thyroid hormones is advanced by these findings, it is also true that we are brought face to face with the enormous problem of understanding how the formation and movement of villous processes can be so effectively controlled as to pluck fragments of colloid from the interior of the follicle and move them through the cell and that only under conditions in which the body requires thyroid hormone.

One further clue has been presented in this system of thyroid hormone secretion, namely that TSH increases the association of actin with thyroid cell lysosomes (Dickson et al., 1979). Since colloid droplets are known to be processed by thyroid cell lysosomes (Wollman, 1969), these findings suggest that actin is involved in the intracellular transport of droplets to lysosomes. While the molecular basis of these various responses cannot be described at present, the vectorial properties of the thyroid cell make it a useful system for the study of cytoskeletal function. The figure above shows the flow of raw material towards the colloid for synthesis and the flow of hormones towards the exterior of the follicle for secretion. The two membranes (basal and follicular) are different in appearance (Klinck et al., 1970), which is consistent with differences in function.

4.2 Insulin

The secretion of insulin provides an interesting example of the regulated movement of lipid droplets through a cell. The beta cell is an attractive system for studies on the mechanism of secretion, because a variety of preparations of islets are available for studies in vitro e.g. isolated islets, beta cells, etc. and because the biochemistry of the regulation of insulin secretion is well understood. Colchicine inhibits secretion of insulin in response to addition of glucose (Lacy et al., 1968). Moreover, Pipeleers et al. have shown that the response to glucose involves increase in the proportion of tubulin in the polymerized form (Pipeleers et al., 1976). Much attention has been given to a remarkable electron micrograph published by Lacy et al. (1968). This shows part of a beta cell with secretory granules apparently associated with microtubules. Only careful guantitation of such an apparent association will make the evidence convincing.' However, it must be said that these electron micrographs are provocative and give substance to vague ideas of how tubules could conceivably function in the process of secretion.

5. Stimulation of Steroid Synthesis by Trophic Hormones (ACTH and LH)

The process of steroidogenesis begins with the transport of cholesterol from the cytoplasm to mitochondria where the first step in' the biosynthetic pathway takes place. This reaction is catalyzed by an enzyme system in the inner mitochondrial membrane and results in the synthesis of prenenolone from which the other steroids are formed. The conversion of cholesterol to pregnenolone is called side-chain cleavage. Pregnenolone must leave the mitochondrion to undergo enzymatic transformation elsewhere.' In the adrenal cortex the steroid intermediate must return to the mitochondrion for the last step in the pathway (11-deoxycortisol → cortisol). The completed hormone is now ready for export by secretion.

There is much evidence that transport of cholesterol by mitochondria is the rate-limiting step in steroid synthesis (Hall et al., 1970) and is stimulated by ACTH in the adrenal cortex (Hall et al., 1979a). This process can be measured by inhibiting side-chain cleavage by means of aminoglutethimide; (Hall et al., 1979a; Mahafee et al., 1974; Nakamura et al., 1980). In the presence of this inhibitor, any cholesterol that is transported to mitochondria must accumulate in that organelle. The difference between the concentration of cholesterol in inner mitochondrial membrane (in moles/mg protein) at time t and that at time zero, provides a measure of cholesterol transport (Hall et al., 1979a; Mahaffee et al., 1974).

Some years ago we discovered that cytochalasin B added to adrenal cells, inhibits the steroidogenic response to ACTH (Mrotek and Hall, 1975) and (Mrotek and Hall, 1977). Moreover, this inhibition was exerted specifically at the step of transport of cholesterol to mitochondria (Mrotek and Hall, 1977). The fact that cytochalasin B inhibits microfilaments, suggested that these structures are involved in the response to ACTH and specifically in the transport of cholesterol to mitochondria (Mrotek and Hall, 1977). The effect of

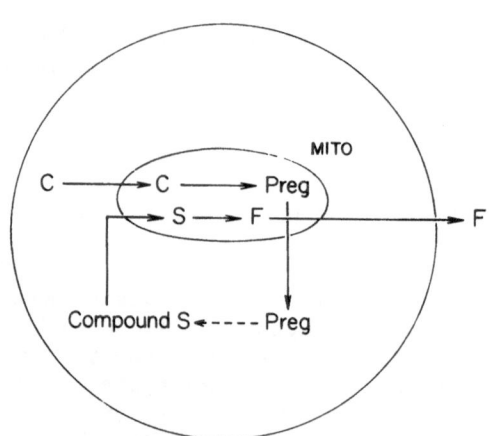

C   Cholesterol
Preg Pregnenolone
(Compound) S II-deoxycortisol
F   Cortisol
MITO Mitochondrion

Figure 2.   Cholesterol transport and steroidogenesis.

cytochalasin is rapid, reversible and apparently specific
(Mrotek and Hall, 1977). However, cytochalasin B has numerous
non-specific effects in a variety of cells. To relate inhibition by cytochalasin to its effect on microfilaments, four
members of the cytochalasin family were examined (B, D, and E
and reduced B). Values for ED_{50} were determined for inhibition of steroidogenesis and binding to purified adrenal actin
(Hall et al., 1981a). Although the four compounds inhibit
steroidogenesis at different concentrations, there was a
clear relationship between ED_{50} for inhibition and that for
binding to actin for each of the four cytochalasins (Hall et
al., 1981a).

In spite of these consistent findings, the hypothesis
that microfilaments are involved in the response to ACTH
rested on indirect evidence with a non-specific inhibitor.
When Gabbiani and co-workers reported the isolation and
characterization of highly purified anti-actin antibodies
from the sera of patients suffering from hepatitis (Gabbiani
et al., 1973), the opportunity was taken to test the hypothesis with a more specific agent. Anti-actin was incorporated
into liposomes which were then fused with adrenal cells by
incubation at 37°C for 1 hour followed by washing the cells
and a second incubation to test each of three responses to
ACTH namely: (i) production of steroids by the cells (in Y-1
adrenal tumor cells 20α-dihydroprogesterone is usually measured), (ii) transport of cholesterol to the inner mitochondrial membrane and (iii) production of pregnenolone by isolated mitochondria (Hall et al., 1979a). For the second and
third assays, cells were incubated with aminoglutethimide to
inhibit side-chain cleavage and with and without ACTH. After
a period of incubation (generally 1 hour), mitochondria were
prepared and for (ii) the inner mitochondrial membrane was
prepared and the cholesterol content was measured; for (iii)
mitochondria were washed to remove aminoglutethimide and
isolated mitochondria were incubated at 30°C to measure
production of pregnenolone. It can be seen from Fig. 3 that
fusion of adrenal cells with liposomes containing anti-actin
inhibits the increased production of 20α-dihydroprogesterone
produced by ACTH. Fig. 3 also shows inhibition of the response
to cyclic AMP and the third panel of the figure shows that
fusion of cells with liposomes containing buffer does not
influence the subsequent response to ACTH. Figure 4 shows a
number of important control studies. Normal human IgG and
boiled anti-actin do not inhibit the response to ACTH. When
anti-actin is added "free" i.e. not entrapped in liposomes,

it shows little or no effect. The serum from which the anti-actin is prepared is inhibitory but most important when anti-actin is mixed with a four-fold molar excess of the antigen (smooth muscle actin), the antibody is not inhibitory

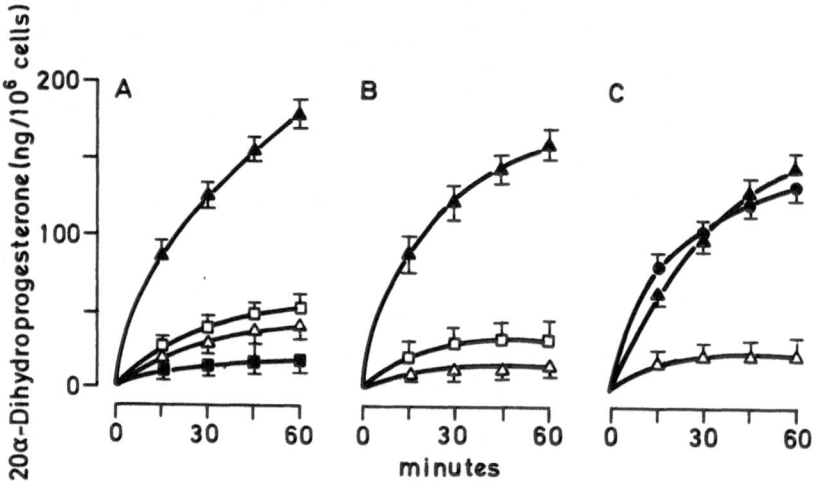

Figure 3. Effect of Anti-actin in liposomes on the steroido-genic response of Y-1 cells to ACTH (A) or Bt_2cAMP (B). Y-1 cells were incubated for 1 h with liposomes containing buffer plus anti-actin (a total dose of 50 μg of antibody protein/-dish of cells) (first incubation). Medium was removed, cells were washed, and fresh medium containing albumin/saline (control), ACTH (86 millunits/ml), or Bt_2cAMP (2mM), but no liposomes (second incubation), was added. Incubation was continued for various periods of time. The reaction was stopped and production of 20α-dihydroprogesterone was measured by radioimmunoassay. C, effect of adding liposomes containing buffer only, on the response to ACTH. Values show means and ranges for duplicate determinations. Open triangles, lipo-somes with buffer; no ACTH or Bt_2cAMP. Closed triangles, liposomes with buffer; ACTH or Bt_2cAMP. Open squares, lipo-somes with anti-actin; ACTH or Bt_2cAMP. Closed squares, liposomes with anti-actin; no ACTH or Bt_2cAMP, closed circles, no liposomes; ACTH. In these symbols, the additions for the first incubation are shown to the left of the semicolon and those for the second incubation, to the right. In C, values for no liposomes and no ACTH are so similar to those for liposomes and no ACTH that they have been omitted for the sake of clarity (Hall et al., 1979a).

Evidently the anti-actin acts as an antibody and not non-spec-
ifically.   Figure 5 shows that fusion of adrenal cells with
liposomes containing anti-actin. inhibits the stimulatory
effect of ACTH on transport of cholesterol to mitochondria.
It can be seen from Fig. 6 that anti-actin also inhibits the
increased production of pregnenolone ·by isolated mitochondria
following treatment with ACTH and cyclic AMP.

These studies strongly support the hypothesis that ACTH,
acting by way of the second messenger, cyclic AMP, stimulates
transport of cholesterol to mitochondria by a mechanism which
involves microfilaments and that this increased transport is
at least partly responsible for the increased production of
steroids characteristic of the action of ACTH.   Such findings
illustrate the role of microfilaments in regulating vectorial
transport through the cytoplasm.   Crivello and Jefcoate (1980)

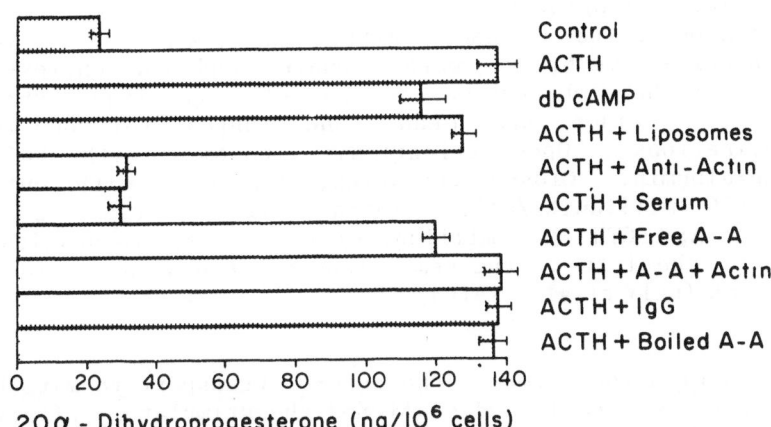

Figure 4.   The experimental details are given under Fig. 3.
Liposomes refers to liposomes containing only buffer.
"Free" anti-actin means that the protein was not entrapped in
liposomes, but was added to the mixture of liposomes, buffer
and cells, and + actin refers to cases in which liposomes
contained anti-actin previously mixed with a 5-fold molar
excess of actin.   Hepatitis serum was added in amounts of 15
µl/ml of medium and proteins other than ACTH were present in
a concentration of 10 µg/ml.   ACTH was added to 86 milliunits-
/ml and the concentration of Bt_2cAMP was 2 mM.   Values are
means and ranges of duplicate determinations. A-A: anti-actin.

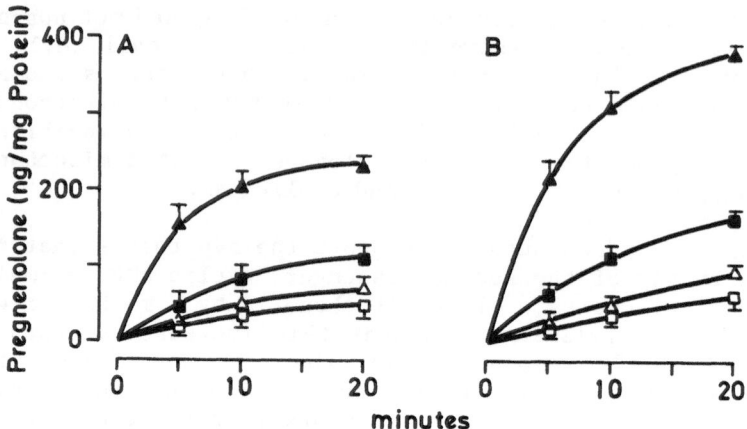

Figure 5. Effect of anti-actin on the response of cholesterol levels in mitochondrial membranes to ACTH. Cells were
incubated for 1 h with liposomes containing buffer and
anti-actin. The cells were washed twice and fresh medium
containing aminoglutethimide (0.76 mM) and either ACTH or
saline/albumin was added. After the times shown, inner
mitochondrial membranes were prepared and the cholesterol
content of the membranes was determined by gas liquid chromatography. Values are means and ranges for duplicate
determinations. Open triangles, liposomes with buffer;
saline/albumin. Closed triangles, liposomes with buffer;
ACTH (86 milliunits/ml). Closed squares, liposomes with
anti-actin; ACTH (86 milliunits/ml). First incubation is
shown to the left of the semicolon and second incubation, to
the right (Hall et al., 1979a).

have measured the rates of cholesterol transport to mitochondria in adrenal cells and confirmed the stimulatory effect of
ACTH and the involvement of microfilaments in this process.
Similar studies with Leydig cells gave essentially the same
results - anti-actin inhibits cholesterol transport to mitochondria and hence steroid production in response to LH and
cyclic AMP in these cells (Hall et al., 1979b; Hall et al.,
1980). Evidently the proposed mechanism for the regulation
of steroid synthesis is applicable to both testis and adrenal.

For some years it has been known that the responses to
ACTH and cyclic AMP require Ca^{2+}. Unfortuantely, chelating
agents and Ca^{2+} ionophores (all of which show numerous non-

specific effects in cells), have not established the basis for involvement of Ca^{2+} in steroidogenesis. More recently it has become apparent that many of the biological effects of Ca^{2+} are directed to specific regions or to specific activities within the cell by the calcium-binding protein calmodulin (Means and Dedman, 1980). Calmodulin is therefore seen as focusing the effects of a general increase in (for example) cytoplasmic Ca^{2+} to certain molecules within the cell. To approach the question of whether calmodulin is involved in the trophic regulation of steroidogenesis or not, we used trifluoperazine as an inhibitor of calmodulin (Fertel and Weiss, 1976). It can be seen from Fig. 7 that trifluoperazine

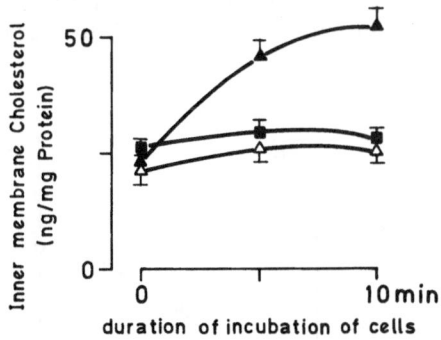

Figure 6. The effect of anti-actin on side-chain cleavage of cholesterol by mitochondria. Cells were incubated with liposomes containing buffer or buffer plus anti-actin (a total of 50 μg of antibody protein in liposomes added to each flask) (first incubation). One hour later, medium was changed, cells were washed, and fresh medium was added containing ACTH (86 milliunits/ml), cyclic AMP (2 mM), or saline/albumin and, in every flask, aminoglutethimide PO$_4$ (0.76 mM) (second incubation). After 30 min, mitochondria were prepared in medium containing aminoglutethimide, but without ACTH and cyclic AMP. Mitochondria were washed twice without aminoglutethimide and incubated at 30°C for the times shown to measure production of pregnenolone. Values are means and ranges for duplicate determinations. Open triangles, liposomes with buffer; no ACTH or Bt$_2$cAMP. Closed triangles, liposomes with buffer; ACTH or Bt$_2$cAMP. Open squares, liposomes with anti-actin; no ACTH or Bt$_2$cAMP. Closed squares, liposomes with anti-actin; ACTH or Bt$_2$cAMP. First incubation is shown to the left of the semicolon and the second, to the right (Hall et al., 1979a).

(50 μM) inhibits the stimulation of testosterone production by adrenal cells <u>in vitro</u> which results from addition of either ACTH or cyclic AMP to the cells <u>in vitro</u>. Panel C shows that a sulfoxide derivative of trifluoperazine does not inhibit this response to LH: the sulfoxide of trifluoperazine is a weak inhibitor of calmodulin effects (Weiss et al., 1974). Figures 8 and 9 show that trifluoperazine inhibits two other steriodogenic responses to ACTH and cyclic AMP, namely increased transport of cholesterol to the inner mitochondrial membrane (Fig.8) and increased production of pregnenolone by isolated mitochondria (Fig. 9). Moreover, panel C of Fig. 9 shows that addition of trifluoperazine to isolated mitochondria (as opposed to cells), does not inhibit the increased production of pregnenolone caused by ACTH - presumably cholesterol has already

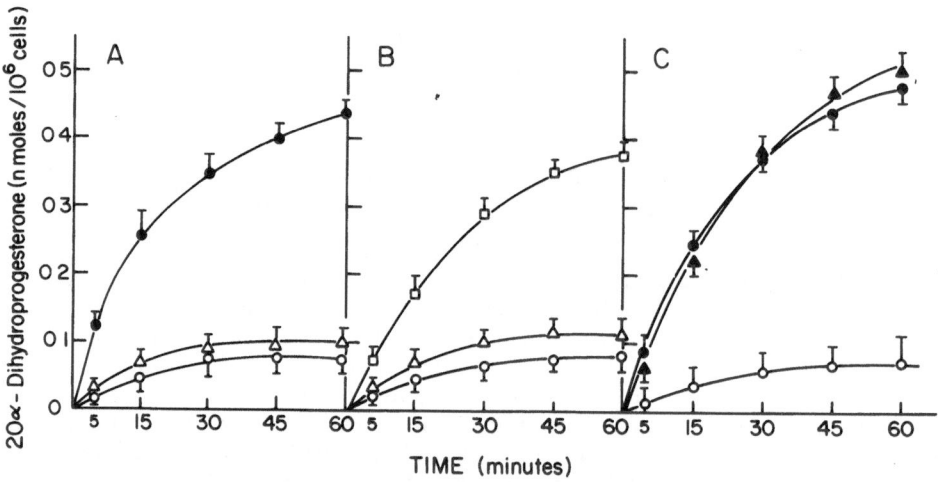

Figure 7. Effect of trifluoperazine on the steroidogenic response of Y-1 cells to ACTH (A) and db cyclic AMP (B). Cells were incubated in EMEM with and without ACTH (40 mU/ml (A) or db cyclic AMP (1mM) (B) and trifluoperazine (50 μM) for the times shown. After incubation, the concentration of 20α-dihydroprogesterone in the medium was determined by radioimmunoassay. Values shown are means and ranges for duplicate determinations. In C, trifluoperazine sulfoxide (50 μM) was used in place of trifluoperazine. Open circles, control; closed circles, ACTH; open squares, db cyclic AMP; open triangles, ACTH (or db cyclic AMP) plus trifluoperazine; closed squares, ACTH plus trifluoperazine sulfoxide (Hall et al., 1981b).

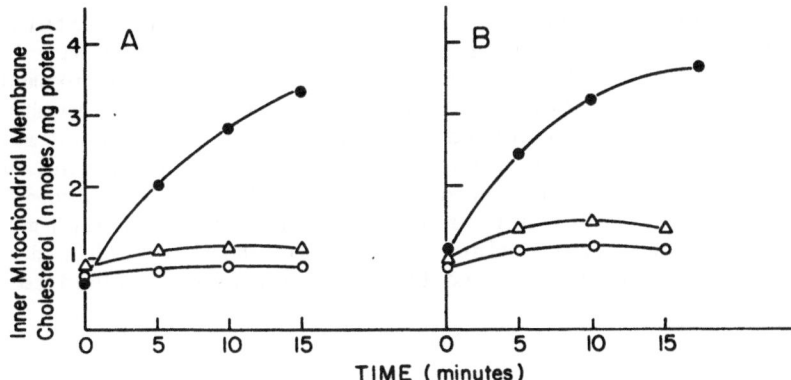

Figure 8. Influence of trifluoperazine on the increase in intracellular transport of cholesterol produced by ACTH (A) and by db cyclic AMP (B). Side-chain cleavage was inhibited by incubation of Y-1 cells with aminoglutethimide PO_4 (0.76 mM) for 15 min before addition of ACTH (40 mU) or db cyclic AMP (1 mM) with and without trifluoperazine (50 μM). After incubation inner mitochondrial membrane was prepared. The cholesterol content of the membrane was measured by gas/liquid chromatography. Open circles, control; closed circles, ACTH or db cyclic AMP; and open triangles, ACTH or db cyclic AMP plus trifluoperazine (Hall et al., 1981b).

reached the mitochondria before the cells were disrupted to prepare these organelles. The metabolism of mitochondrial cholesterol (conversion to pregnenolone), is evidently not influenced by trifluoperazine - it is the transport of the steroid to the mitochondrion that is affected.

These findings suggested that calmodulin may be involved in the response of adrenal cells to ACTH and cyclic AMP and that the protein may be important in cholesterol transport. However, trifluoperazine is not entirely specific so that a more direct approach to this problem was necessary. For this purpose calmodulin was purified from rat testis (Dedman et al. 1977) and incorporated into liposomes which were fused with adrenal cells (Hall et al., 1981b). Figure 10 shows that calmodulin stimulated the production of 20α-dihydroprogesterone by adrenal cells. This effect is abolished by dialysis of calmodulin against EGTA. On the other hand, Ca^{2+} incorporated

into liposomes is without effect, but calmodulin saturated
with Ca^{2+} causes striking stimultion that is inhibited by
trifluoperazine. Figure 11 shows that calmodulin promotes
transport of cholesterol to the inner mitochondrial membrane
(A) and increased production or pregnenolone by isolated mitochondria (B). Panel B also shows a number of important controls. Once again trifluoperazine inhibits the response if it
is added to cells but not if it is added to the isolated mitochondria. The figure also shows that aminoglutethimide is
necessary for the resonse and that calmodulin-Ca^{2+} added to

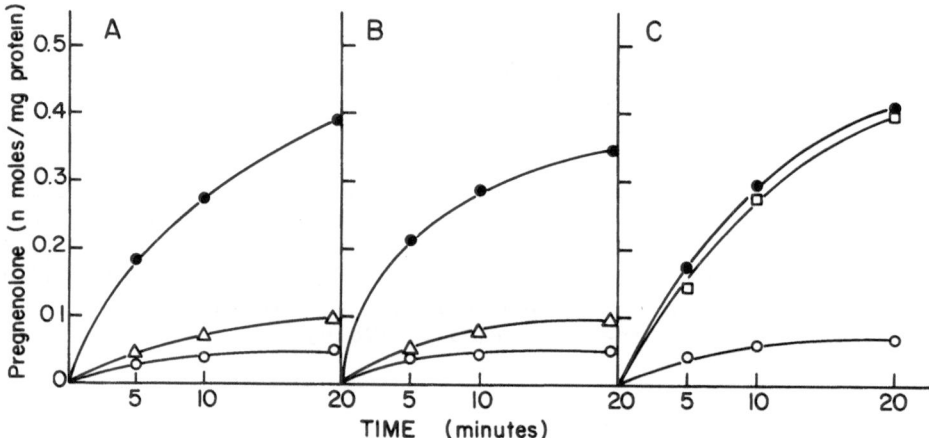

Figure 9. The influence of trifluoperazine on the production
of pregnenolone by mitochondria isolated from Y-1 cells
previously incubated with aminoglutethimide. Y-1 cells were
incubated for 60 min with aminoglutethimide PO_4 (0.76 mM)
with and without ACTH (40 mU) or db cyclic AMP (1 mM) with
and without trifluoperazine (50 µM). After incubation,
mitochondria were prepared from the cells in the presence of
aminoglutethimide (0.76 mM) at 0°C for the times shown. The
mitochondria were then washed twice to. remove animoglutethi-
mide and incubated at 39°C for the times shown. Pregnenolone
was measured in samples of medium by radioimmunoassay. In C,
cells were incubated with ACTH and aminoglutethimide; trifluoperazine (50 µM) was added to the isolated mitochondria.
Open circles, control; closed circles, ACTH, or db cyclic AMP;
open triangles, ACTH or db cyclic AMP plus trifluoperazine;
and, open squares ACTH; trifluoperazine added to mitochondria
(Hall et al., 1981b).

the isolated mitochondria is without effect on side-chain cleavage.

These studies show that Ca^{2+} and calmodulin are involved in the transport of cholesterol to mitochondria - the same step in steroidogenesis in which actin is involved. It is not clear at present, how these two agents (actin and calmodulin) are involved in the transport of cholesterol but they are both necessary for the responses to ACTH and cyclic AMP.

These results were strikingly confirmed by analogous studies with isolated Leydig cells stimulated by LH (Hall et al., 1981c).

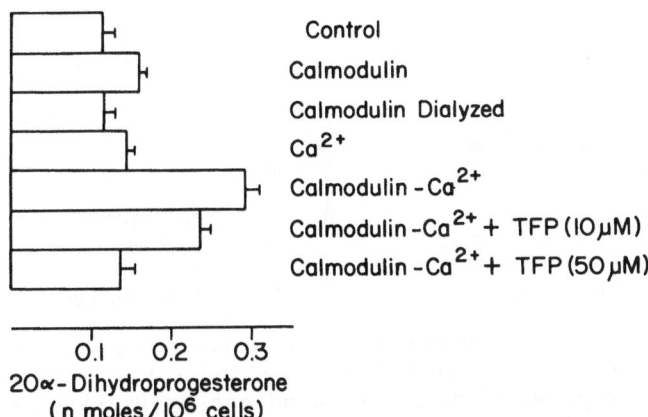

Figure 10. The influence of calmodulin and Ca^{2+} on steriodogenesis by Y-1 cells. Cells were incubated for 60 min with liposomes containing buffer or buffer plus the additions shown. At the end of this time, medium was removed, cells were washed twice with PBS at 0°C, and fresh medium was added with liposomes (200 µl; 10 nmol of phospholipid/dish) containing buffer (control) or the additions shown. Incubation was continued for 30 min and 20α-dihydroprogesterone was measured in samples of medium. Calmodulin dialyzed refers to calmodulin extensively dialyzed against EGTA (1 mM). Trifluoperazine was added to the medium "free", i.e. not in liposomes. The values shown represent means and ranges for duplicate determinations. Ca^{2+} refers to $CaCl_2$ (5 mM) incorporated into liposomes (Hall et al., 1981b).

6.   Other Hormones

6.1   Antidiuretic Hormone

The action of ADH on the epithelial cells of the toad bladder is associated with a remarkable rearrangement of

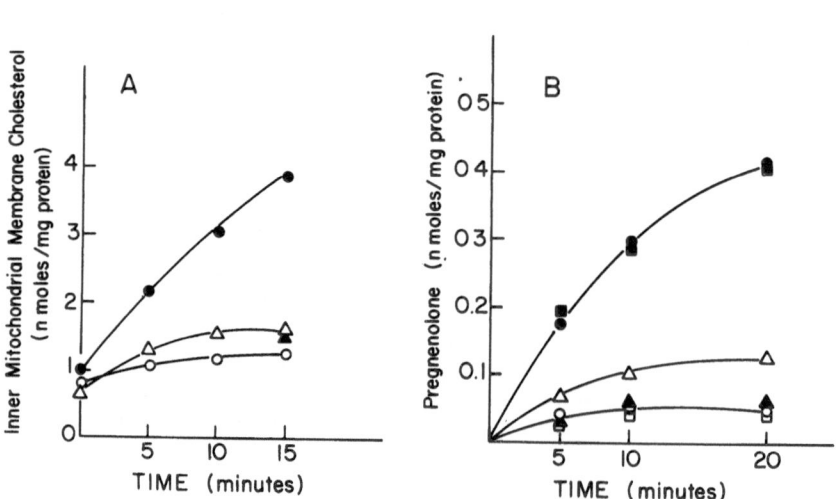

Figure 11.   The influence of calmodulin with calcium on the accumulation of cholesterol in the inner mitochondrial membrane and on production of pregnenolone by isolated mitochondria.   Y-1 cells were incubated with liposomes containing buffer (control) or buffer with calmodulin and Ca^{2+} (200/dish) as described under Figure 10. The incubation medium contained trifluoperazine (50 μM) where indicated and aminoglutethimide (0.76 mM).   After incubation for the times shown in A, inner mitochondrial membrane was prepared and the cholesterol content was measured.   In B, pregnenolone production was determined after removal of aminoglutethimide as described under Figure 9.   open circles, control; closed circles, calmodulin-Ca^{2+}; open triangles, calmodulin-Ca^{2+} plus trifluoperazine; open squares, control plus calmodulin-Ca^{2+} added to mitochondria; closed triangles, calmodulin-Ca^{2+} and no aminoglutethimide; closed square, calmodulin - Ca^{2+}; trifluoperazine (50 μM) added to isolated mitochondria; closed triangles, calmodulin - Ca^{2+} and no aminoglutethimide (Hall et al., 1981b).

particles in the plasma membranes of these cells. The particles, which originate from membranes within the cells, aggregate in the plasma membrane (Bourquet et al., 1976). The processes by which particles are transported to the plasma membrane in vesicles which fuse with the membrane, are inhibited by colchicine and cytochalasin B which also inhibit the response to the hormone (Muller et al., 1980; Kathadorian et al., 1979). These findings suggest a number of experimental approaches to explore the possibility that microtubules and microfilaments are involved in the response to ADH.

6.2   The secretion of·Parathyroid Hormone

It appears that destruction of microtubules by colchicine inhibits the secretion of parathyroid hormone (Reaven and Reaven, 1975). Moreover, the same inhibitor presents the conversion of proparathyroid hormone to parathyroid hormone (Kemper at al., 1975); in contrast, cytochalasin B is without effect. Since the prohormone is made on rough endoplasmic reticulum and cleaved by proteolysis in the Golgi apparatus, it is reasonable to propose that transport from ER to Golgi is mediated by microtubules. This intriguing idea warrants further investigation in an attempt to establish some quantitative relationship between the rate of production of the completed hormone and some parameter related to the function of microtubules.

6.3 Miscellaneous Hormones. Secretion of growth hormone and prolactin by pituitary cells is inhibited by colchicine (Gautwik and Tashjian, 1973; Labrie et al., 1973). This inhibitor also decreases the secretion of catecholamines from the adrenal medulla (Poisner and Cooke, 1975; Unsicker et al., 1979).

REFERENCES

Borisy, G. G., and Taylor, E. W., 1967, The mechanism of chol-
      chicine, J. Cell Biol. 34:535-548.
Bourquet, J., Chevalier, J., and Hugon, J. S., 1976, Altera-
      tions in membrane-associated particle distribution during
      antidiuretic challenge in frog urinary bladder epithelium,
      Biophysical J. 16:627-639.
Carlsson, L., Mystrom, L. E., Lindberg, U., Kannan, K. K.,
      Cid-Dresdner, H., Lovgren, S., and Jornvall, H., 1976,

Crystallization of a non-muscle actin, J. Mol. Biol.
105:353-366.

Crivello, J. F., Jefcoate, C. R., 1980, Intracellular movement
of cholesterol in rat adrenals, J. Biol. Chem. 255:
8144-8151.

Dedman, J. R., Porter, J. D., Jackson, R. L., Johnson, J. D.,
and Means, A. R., 1977, Physiochemical properties of rat
testis regular protein of cyclic nucleotide phosphodie-
terase, J. Biol. Chem. 252:8415-8422.

Dentler, W. L., Pratt, M. M., and Stephens, R. E., 1980, Mic-
rotubulemembrane interactions in cilia. II: Identification of a membrane-associated dyneine-like ATPase, J.
Cell. Biol. 84:381-403.

Dickson, J. G., Malan, P. G., and Ekins, R. P., 1979, The
association of actin with a thyroid lysosomal fraction,
Europ. J Biochem. 97:471-479.

Fertel, R. M., and Weiss, B., 1976, Properties and drug
responsiveness of cyclic nucleotide phosphodiesterases
of rat lung, Molec. Pharmacol. 12:678-687.

Freed, J. J., and Lebowitz, M. M., 1970, The association of a
class saltatory movements with microtubules in cultured
cells, J. Cell Biol. 45:334-354.

Fujiwara, K., Porter, M. E., and Pollard, T. D., 1978, Alpha-
actinin localization in the cleavage furrow during cytokinesis, J. Cell Biol. 79:268-275.

Gabbiani, G., Ryan, G. B., Lamelin, J. P., Vassalli, P., Majno,
G., Bouvier, C., Rimchaud, A., and Luscher, E. F., 1973,
Human smooth muscle autoantibody, Amer. J. Pathol.
72:473-488.

Gautwik, K. M., and Tashjian, A. H., 1973, Effects of cholchicine on release of prolactin and growth hormone by pituitary tumor cells in vitro, Endocrinology 93:793-799.

Hall, P. F., 1970, Gonadotrophic regulation of testicular
function, in: "Androgens of the Testis," K. B. Eik-Nes,
ed., Marcel Dekker Inc., New York, pp. 73-115.

Hall, P. F., Charponnier, C., Nakamura, M., and Gabbiani, G.,
1979, role of microfilaments in the response of adrenal
tumor cells to ACTH, J. Biol. Chem. 254:9080-9084.

Hall, P. F., Charponnier, C., Nakamura, M., and Gabbiani, G.,
1979b, The role of microfilaments in the responses of
Leydig cells to LH, J. Steroid Biochem. 11:1361-1366.

Hall, P. F., Charponnier, C., and Gabbiani, G., 1980, Role
of actin in the response of Leydig cells to LH, in:
"Testicular Development Structure and Function," A.
Steinberger and E. Steinberger, eds., p. 229, Raven
Press, New York.

Hall, P. F., Nakamura, M., and Mrotek, J. J., 1981a, The actions of various cytochalasins on mouse adrenal tumor cells in relation to trophic stimulation of steroidogenesis, Biochim. Biophys. Acta. 676:338-344.

Hall, P. F., Osawa, S. and Thomasson, C. L., 1981b, A role for calmodulin in the regulation of steroidogenesis, J Cell Biol. 90:402-407.

Hall, P. F., Osawa, S., and Mrotek, J. K., 1981c, Influence of calmodulin on steroid synthesis in Leydig cells from rat testis, Endocrinology 109:1677-1682.

Hartwig, J. H., and Stossel, T. P., 1979, Cytochalasin B and the structure of actin gels, J. Mol. Biol. 134:539-553.

Ishikawa, H., Bischoff, R., and Holtzer, H., 1969, Formation of arrowhead complexes with heavy meromyosin in a variety of cell types, J. Cell Biol. 43:312-328.

Kathadorian, W. A., Ellis, S. J., and Muller, J., 1979, Possible role for microtubules and microfilaments in ADH action, Amer. J. Physiol. 236:F_{14}-F_{20}.

Kember, B., Habener, J. F., Rich, A., and Potts, J. T., 1975, Microtubules and the intracellular conversion of proparathyroid hormone to parathyroid hormone, Endocrinology 96:903-912.

Kiehart, D. P., 1981, Studies on in vivo sensitivity of spindle microtubules to Ca^{2+}, J. Cell Biol. 88:604-617.

Klinck, G. H., Oertel, J. E., and Winship, T., 1970, Ultrastructure of normal human thyroid, Lab. Invest. 22:2-22.

Korn, E. D., 1978, Biochemistry of actomycin-dependent cell motility, a review, Proc. Natl. Acad. Sci. 75:588-599.

Labrie, F., Pelletier, G., Gauthier, M., Borgeat, P., Lemay, A., and Gouge, J. J., 1973, Role of microtubules in basal and stimulated release of growth hormone and prolactin in rat adenohypophysis in vitro, Endocrinology 93:903-914.

Lacy, P. E., Howell, S. L., Young, D. A., and Fink, C. J., 1968, New hypothesis of insulin secretion, Nature 219:1177-1179.

Lazarides, E., 1980, Intermediate filaments as mechanical integrators of cellular space, Nature 283:249-256.

Lin, D. C., Tobin, K. D., Grumet, M., and Lin, S., 1980, Cytochalasins inhibit nuclei-induced actin polymerization by blocking filament elongation, J. Cell Biol. 84:455-460.

Mahafee, D., Reitz, R. C., and Ney, R. L., 1974, The mechanism of action of ACTH. The role of mitochondrial cholesterol accumulation in the regulation of steroidogenesis, J. Biol. Chem. 249:227-233.

Margolis, R. L., and Wilson, L., 1978, Opposite end assembly and disassembly of microtubules at steady state in vitro, Cell 13:1-8.

McIntosh, J. R., 1979, Cell division, in: "Microtubules," K.
    Roberts and J. S. Hyams, eds., p. 381, Academic Press,
    New York.
Means, A. R., and Dedman, J. R., 1980, Calmodulin - an intra-
    cellular calcium receptor, Nature 285:73-77.
Means, A. R., and Dedman, J. R., 1980, Calmodulin - an intra-
    cellular calcium receptor, Nature 285:73-84.
Miranda, A. F., Godman, G. G., and Tanenbaum, S. W., 1974,
    Action of cytochalasin D on cells of established lines,
    J Cell Biol. 62:406-423.
Mrotek, J. J., and Hall, P. F., 1975, The influence of cyto-
    chalasin B on the response of adrenal tumor cells to ACTH
    and cyclic AMP, Biochem. Biophy. Res. Commun. 64:891-896.
Mrotek, J. J., and Hall, P. J., 1977, Response of adrenal tumor
    cells to ACTH: site of inhibition by cytochalasin B,
    Biochemistry 16:3177-3181.
Muller, J., Kachadorian, W. A., and DiScala, V. A., 1980,
    Evidence that ACTH-stimulated intramembrane particle
    aggregates are transferred from cytoplasmic to luminal
    membranes in toad bladder epithelial cells, J. Cell Biol.
    85:83-95.
Nakamura, M., Watanuki, M., Tilley, B., and Hall, P. J., 1980,
    Effect of ACTH on intracellular cholesterol transport, J.
    Endocrinol. 84:179-188.
Neve, P., Keyelbant-Balasse, P., Willems, C., and Dumont, J. E.,
    1972, Effect of inhibitors of microtubules and microfila-
    ments on dog thyroid slices in vitro, Exper. Cell Res.
    74:227-244.
Nicklas, R. B., 1971, Chromosomal movement during cell division,
    in: "Advances in Cell Biology," D. M. Prescott, L.
    Goldstein and E. McConkey, eds., Appleton, Century, Crofts,
    New York, Vol. 2, pp. 225-297.
Pipeleers, D. G., Pipeleers-Marichal, M. A., and Kipnis, D. M.,
    1976, Microtubule assembly and intracellular transport of
    secretory granules in pancreatic islets, Science 191:88-89.
Poisner, A. M., and Cooke, P., 1975, Microtubules and the
    adrenal medulla, Ann. N. Y. Acad. Sci. 253:653-668.
Reavan, E. P., and Reaven, G. M., 1975, A quantitative ultra-
    structural study of microtubule content in parathyroid
    gland, J. Clin. Invest. 56:29-55.
Schroeder, T. R., 1973, Actin in dividing cells: contractile
    ring filaments bind heavy meromyosin, Proc. Natl. Acad.
    Sci. 70:1688-1692.
Taylor, D. L., and Condeelis, J. S., 1979, Cytoplasmic struc-
    ture and contractility in amoeboid cells, International
    Review of Cytology 56:57-144.

Unsicker, K., Limmeroth-Everet, B., Otten, U., Lindmar, R., Loffel-holz, K., and Wolff, U., 1979, Effects of vinblastine on rat adrenal medulla, Cell Tissue Res. 196:271-288.

Vallee, R. B., 1980, Structure and phosphorylation of MAPS. Proc. Natl. Acad. Sci. 77:3206-3210.

Weihing, R. R., 1977, Effect of myosin and heavy meromyosin on actin-related gelation of HeLa cell extract, J. Cell Biol. 75:95-103.

Weisenberg, R. C., 1972, Microtubule formation in vitro in solutions containing low calcium concentrations, Science 177:1104-1105.

Weiss, B., Fertel, R., Tichn, R., and Uzunov, P., 1974, Selective alteration of the activity of the multiple forms of AMP phosphodiosterase of rat cerebum, Molecular Pharmacology 12:581-589.

Williams, J. A., and Wolff, J., 1970, Possible role of microtubules in thyroid secretion, Proc. Natl. Acad. Sci. 67:1901-1908.

Wollman, S. H., 1969, Lysosomes in Biology and Pathology, ed. J. T. Dingle and H. B. Fell, North-Holland, Amsterdam, Vol. 2, p. 483.

Wolosewick, J. J., and Porter, K. R., 1979, Microtrabecular lattice of the cytoplasmic ground substance - artifact or reality, J. Cell. Biol. 82:114-139.

Woodrum, D. T., Rich, S. A., Pollard, T. D., 1975, Evidence for biased bidirectional polymerization of actin filaments using heavy meromysin prepared by an improved method, J. Cell Biol. 67:231-237.

DISCUSSION

ROMMERTS: There is no doubt that the amount of cholesterol can regulate cholesterol side-chain cleavage activity and regulation of transport within the cell is therefore important. However, the question is whether this transport constitutes the rate-limiting step in the control of steroidogenesis. It has been shown with normal adrenal cells and Leydig cells that after stimulation with hormones, activated mitochondria (activated for side-chain cleavage), can be isolated and mitochondria from control cells can also be activated by cytosols from stimulated cells. That suggests that microfilaments are not required. In addition it has been shown that cycloheximide inhibits steroid production and that cytosols from animals treated with ACTH (LH) and cycloheximide cannot stimulate isolated mitochondria. My question is how these observations can be incorporated in your model?

HALL: The activation of mitochondrial side-chain cleavage by prior treatment with ACTH results from anaerobic mitochondria-low O_2 tension inhibits side-chain cleavage and allows accumulation of cholesterol in the inner mitochondrial membrane just as eliptèn does. With cultured cells mitochondria are easier to maintain in an aerobic state. If mitochondria are exposed to low oxygen tension during incubation or preparation, side-chain cleavage can be inhibited and cholesterol accumulates. When the mitochondria are incubated, the accumulated cholesterol is used to produce pregnenolone at an accelerated rate compared to mitochondria from control cells where no accumulation of cholesterol occurs. The effects of cycloheximide are complex and include inhibition of side-chain cleavage as reported by Kimura et al. As far as addition of cytoplasm from stimulated cells is concerned, the added cytoplasm contains microfilaments.

STRAUSS: I have two questions. First, could you comment on the reported stimulation of steroidogenesis by inhibitors of microtubular function when applied to Y-1 cells? How do you fit these observations into your scheme? Second, in what form do you envision cholesterol being transported to the mitochondria (i.e. in the form of lipid droplets containing sterol ester or as free sterol associated with sterol carrier proteins)?

HALL: First. The work of Wolff shows that under some conditions, colchicine stimulates steroidogenesis. It has been proposed that this response results from the fact that cholesterol droplets are bound to microtubules which thereby prevent transport of cholesterol to mitochondria. Disruption of microtubules by colchicine permits escape from this restraint and allows spontaneous transport of cholesterol to mitochondria. These studies were not primarily directed at the action of tropic hormones. Second. Cholesterol is probably transported to mitochondria as free cholesterol - because esterase activity (stimulated by ACTH) is required to mobilize cholesterol from depots of cholesterol ester. Incidentally, cytochalasin-β and anti-actin do not inhibit the esterase. Hence inhibition of esterase could not account for our results with these agents. Saez and coworkers have isolated an adrenal cytoplasmic protein (MW 30,000) which specifically binds cholesterol. I would presume that cholesterol transport takes place bound to this protein. The free cholesterol may be transported as individual molecules of cholesterol - carrier or in large numbers of molecules within vesicles.

HANSSON: I was surprised to see that Ca^{2+}-calmodulin added in liposomes to whole adrenal cells gave an increase in steroidogenesis. I would have thought that these cells would have excess calmodulin and further addition of calmodulin should not give any further effect. I would like your comments on that.

HALL: Presumably in the resting adrenal, the Ca^{2+} and calmodulin are either separated or are not present where they are required to stimulate steroidogenesis. For this reason the cell shows a low level of steroid synthesis. ACTH can evidently change this situation - although we don't know how. Perhaps calmodulin moves or Ca^{2+} moves or increases under the influence of ACTH and cAMP. Calmodulin-Ca^{2+} enters the cell from the liposomes and presumably floods the cytoplasm to provide enough calmodulin-Ca^{2+} in those locations in the cell where it is needed to trigger increased steroidogenesis.

AAKVAAG: Do you know whether there is an effect of prostaglandins on microfilaments of ovarian cells?

HALL: I am not aware of any effect of prostaglandins on microfilaments.

NAOR: If I remember correctly, Zor's group has demonstrated involvement of cytoskeletal elements in prostaglandin stimulation of cAMP production in ovarian granulosa cells.

CALMODULIN - A RECEPTOR FOR CALCIUM MODULATING HORMONE

RESPONSIVITY

A. R. Means and J. G. Chafouleas

Department of Cell Biology
Baylor College of Medicine
Houston, TX 77030

1. Introduction

In order to survive in a dynamic environment all living cells must be able to identify and respond to variation in specific extracellular signals. The action of peptide hormones on mammalian cells is a specific case in point. Target cells recognize the hormone through specific receptors on the outer surface of their plasma membrane. The binding of hormone to receptor initiates a series of rapid events which eventually translates this external signal into a specific cellular response mediated by a selective alteration of the intracellular metabolism. The mechanism by which the extracellular event is transduced to an intracellular event is still not totally understood. The effect of adrenergic agents on cAMP metabolism led Sutherland to propose that cAMP was the second messenger responsible for this transduction through the activation of a cAMP-dependent protein kinase. While this mechanism explains many hormonal events, it does not explain the studies of Hutson et al. (1976) and Cherrington et al. (1976), who demonstrated that cAMP metabolism or activation of cAMP-dependent protein kinase was not involved in the α-adrenergic activation of glycolysis and gluconeogenesis in rat liver. In fact, Keppens et al. (1977) and Assimacopoulos et al. (1977) presented data which supported the concept that the α-adrenergic response was mediated through Ca^{++}. It is now apparent that Ca^{++} plays a major role in the regulation of cellular activity. Berridge (1975) and Rassmussen et al. (1976) have written extensive reviews delineating the involvement of Ca^{++} in the regulation of cell

231

metabolism. The extent to which calcium is involved in cellular processes has led Rassmussen to propose that calcium be classed with the cyclic nucleotides as a second messenger to external stimuli. Indeed, the relationship between the cyclic nucleotides and calcium has been alluded to in several reviews on the subject (Rassmussen, 1970; Rasmussen et al., 1976; Berridge, 1975; Rebhun, 1977). Although the involvement of Ca^{++} in the transduction of external stimuli into cellular responses has been well documented, the biochemical mechanisms mediating the Ca^{++} effects have yet to be elucidated. Kretsinger (1976, 1979) has pointed out the importance of the cytosolic Ca^{++}-binding proteins, and has suggested that the intracellular targets for Ca^{++}, functioning as second messenger, are these proteins. Because of the multitude of enzymatic systems which are known to be Ca^{++}-regulated, Ca^{++} would have to interact with either a great many different proteins, each with one specific function or one or several proteins, each with multiple functions. This latter group of proteins could be viewed as intracellular Ca^{++} receptors.

2.   Calmodulin as the Ca^{++} Receptor

Several criteria must be met before a protein may be classified as a Ca^{++} receptor: (1) It must specifically bind Ca^{++} with high affinity; (2) The binding of Ca^{++} to the protein must be mandatory to its regulatory role; (3) It must regulate vital intracellular processes common to all eucaryotic cells; (4) It must be ubiquitous; and (5) Because of its critical role in cell survival it must be highly conserved.

Calmodulin is a heat-stable, 17,000 M_r multifunctional Ca^{++} binding protein which meets all the criteria set forth for a Ca^{++} receptor (Means and Dedman, 1980). It contains four equivalent Ca^{++} binding sites with a K_d of $2.4 \times 10^{-6}M$ which do not bind Mg^{++} under physiological conditions (Dedman et al., 1977). Ca^{++} binding induces a more α-helical conformation of the protein which preceeds activation of the calmodulin-dependent phosphodiesterase (Ho et al., 1975; Klee, 1977; Dedman et al., 1977). In further investigating this confomational transition accompanied by Ca^{++} binding, Richman (1979) has examined the microenvironment of the two tyrosine residues of the protein. In the absence of free Ca^{++}, both tyrosine residues 99 and 138 are accessible to acetylation by N-acetylimidazole whereas in the presence of Ca^{++}, only residue 99 can be acetylated. These findings suggest that

Ca^{++} binding alters the microenvironment of tyrosine residue 138 and could play a role in the biological activity of the protein.

This protein has been shown to mediate the calcium regulation of a large number of fundamental intracellular enzyme systems. These enzymes include a calcium-dependent form of phosphodiesterase (Kakiuchi et al., 1970; Cheung, 1970), brain adenylyl cyclase (Brostrom et al., 1977; Lynch et al., 1976), human erythrocyte membrane Ca^{++}, Mg^{++}-ATPase (Gopinath and Vincenzi, 1977; Luthra et al., 1977; Jarrett and Penniston, 1977), myosin light chain kinase (Yagi et al., 1978; Dabrowska et al., 1977; Hathaway and Adelstein, 1979) skeletal muscle phosphorylase kinase (Cohen et al., 1978), glycogen synthase kinase (Srivastava et al., 1979; Soderling et al., 1979), human phospholipase-A_2 (Wong and Cheung, 1979) and pea and sea urchin NAD kinase (Anderson and Cormier, 1978; Epel et al., 1981). Calmodulin has also been reported to be the calcium-binding protein regulating calcium transport in the sarcoplasmic reticulum (Katz and Remtulla, 1978; LePeuch et al., 1979) and autophosphorylation of membrane proteins (Schulman and Greengard, 1977, 1978; DeLorenzo et al., 1979). In addition, immunofluorescence studies on a variety of cultured cells have demonstrated that calmodulin is localized on the actomyosin-containing stress fibers in interphase and is a dynamic component of the mitotic apparatus (Welsh et al., 1978, 1979; Dedman et al., 1978; Andersen et al., 1978). In this regard, this protein has been shown to regulate the calcium-dependent assembly-disassembly of microtubules in vitro (Marcum et al., 1978).

Calmodulin represents the major intracellular calcium receptor in all non- and smooth muscle cells (Means and Dedman, 1980; Means et al., 1982). It constitutes between 0.1 and 1.0% of the total protein in all cells from the lowest to the highest order plants and animals. As might be expected for a protein so important and widely distributed, calmodulin is remarkedly conserved phylogenetically. The molecule has been sequenced from representatives of mammalian, fish, coelenterate, protozoan and plant phyla (Dedman et al., 1978a; Watterson et al., 1980; Grand and Perry, 1978; Grand et al., 1981; Jamieson et al., 1980; Yazawa et al., 1981). Of the 148 amino acids, no more than seven have been shown to be altered between species. In all cases, amino acid substitutions are of a conservative nature and could be accounted for by a single base point mutation in the genes. In addition to the conservation of the primary amino acid sequence, calmodulins appear to be immunologically identical. A radio-immunoassay developed utilizing an antibody prepared against unmodified mammalian protein has revealed identical competition curves generated by calmodulin present in extracts of tissue prepared from a wide variety of species from ameoba to man (Chafouleas et al., 1979).

3.   Recent Studies on the Calmodulin Gene

The calmodulin antibody has recently been used in an immunoprecipitation assay to monitor the purification of calmodulin mRNA (Chafouleas et al., 1979). Total poly(A)$^+$ RNA was isolated from the electroplax tissue of the electric eel and fractionated by sucrose gradient centrifugation (Munjaal et al., 1981). One fraction was demonstrated to contain approximately 39% calmodulin mRNA by in vitro translation and hybridization analysis. This partially purified mRNA was transcribed into double-stranded cDNA by reverse transcriptase and cloned in the Pst I site of pBR-322 using E. coli RRI as the host. A structural gene probe (pCM109) was identified and shown by sequence analysis to contain the nucleotides coding for amino acids 93-148 of calmodulin as well as 180 nucleotides from the 3'-nontranslated region including a AAUAAA polyadenylation signal.

pCM109 was shown to hybridize to DNA isolated from diverse animal and plant species suggesting that the calmodulin gene may also be highly conserved during evolution. Analysis of the DNA hybridization data revealed that the calmodulin gene was represented less than 3 times in both eel and chicken. The eel cDNA was also utilized to select and characterize a full-length cDNA complementary to electroplax calmodulin mRNA. DNA sequence of this recombinant molecule, pCM116, has shown it to contain 26 nucleotides of 5'-nontranslated sequence, the initiator codon AUG, the entire coding region, the terminator codon UGA, 409 nucleotides of 3'-nontranslated DNA and a poly(a) tail. Translation of the coding region revealed only a single conservative amino acid substitution compared to the published calmodulin sequence from bovine and human material. Hybridization of ^{32}P-labeled pCM116 to poly(A)$^+$ mRNA from electroplax distributed on a polyacrylamide gel and then transferred to nitrocellulose paper yielded 3 bands of approximately equal intensity at 820, 1100 and 2000 nucleotides, respectively. These data were obtained whether the RNA was isolated from total cell, cytoplasm or polyribosomes. However, when nuclear RNA was similarly analyzed an additional RNA species 5500 nucleotides in length was also observed. pCM116 was found to contain an AAUAAA sequence at 580 nucleotides and another at 873 nucleotides. The sequence of the 3' nontranslated region of pCM109 was identical to the same portion of pCM116 up to the first polyadenylation site. A DNA fragment isolated 3' from the first AAUAAA of pCM116 hybridized to the 5500 nuclear RNA species as well as to the 2000 and 1100 nucleotide cytoplasmic mRNA but not to the 820 nucleotide RNA. Together these data suggest that the 3 cytoplasmic mRNAs differ only in the 3' nontranslated region and could be derived from the 5500 nuclear molecule by differential addition of poly(A). It also apppears that pCM109 may have been generated from the 820 nucleotide mRNA whereas the 1100 nucleotide species gave rise to pCM116. Multiple species of calmodulin mRNA have been identified in poly(A)$^+$ RNA from rat, cow, chicken, baboon and human arguing for a common mechanism for processing of calmodulin mRNA.

The calmodulin cDNA probes have also been employed to screen a chicken DNA library. Two calmodulin (or calmodulin-like) genes have been isolated and characterized. The first gene was isolated as a 10.6 Kb fragment and the calmodulin DNA was found to be localized to a 1.4 Kb fragment at the extreme 5'-end. DNA sequence analysis has shown this fragment to contain all but 33 nucleotides complementary to the coding region of calmodulin mRNA (410 nucleotides) plus 481 nucleotides of 3'-nontranslated DNA, a polyadenylation site (AAUAAA), and a stretch of polyT residues. Derivation of the amino acids codes for by the structural segment illustrates that this genomic DNA begins with amino acid 12 (phe). Sixteen differences exist between this amino acid sequence and that derived from the eel cDNA (pCM116). Nine of the substitutions are nonconservative with two of the most striking being the presence of cysteine at positions 26 and 130. When this DNA was used as a hybridization probe in Northern analysis, only skeletal muscle demonstrated a positive signal (at 800 nucleotides) out of seven chicken tissues examined. Together these data suggest the possibility that this DNA represents either a processed calmodulin gene or a pseudogene.

The second chicken DNA was cloned as a 13.5 Kb fragment. EcoRI cleaved this DNA into a 5' 7.0 Kb and a 3' 6.5 Kb fragment. Sequence analysis of the 6.5 Kb fragment (5' → 3') revealed that this DNA begins with nucleotide 34 of the coding region of the calmodulin gene. Nucleotides 34-168 are identical to those of pCM116. However, restriction hybridization analysis has shown the calmodulin DNA to encompass approximately 4 Kb and to be interrupted by at least two introns; one in the structural sequence and one in the 3'-non-translated region. Whether additional introns exist in the 5' nontranslated region remains to be established. A mRNA was isolated from chicken brain poly(A)$^+$ RNA using pCM116 as a hybridization probe. This mRNA has been cloned and sequenced. It is now apparent that this mRNA is encoded by the calmodulin gene containing intervening sequences. Indeed, the sequence of the chick brain cDNA is identical to pCM116 within the entire coding segment (444 nucleotides). Poly(A)$^+$ RNA from all 8 chicken tissues examined (including skeletal muscle) contain species complementary to the second chicken gene. In all cases, the predominant mRNA is approximately 1600 nucleotides. Finally, Southern analyses under stringent hybridization conditions suggest that this calmodulin gene is unique.

4.   Calmodulin and Hormone Action

     Since calmodulin is a component of virtually every intracellular compartment as well as the plasma membrane (Lin et al., 1980), efforts have been made to determine whether cell surface acting agents promote an alteration in the distribution of calmodulin. Distinct anatomical regions of the central nervous system such as the corpus striatum contain dopamine receptors which seem to be coupled to adenylyl cyclase (Hanbauer et al., 1979a). Calmodulin has been suggested to mediate dopamine action since phosphorylation of membrane proteins promotes the apparent release of calmodulin from membrane-bound to soluble form (Gnegy and Lau, 1980; Hanbauer et al., 1979). Since a soluble calmodulin-dependent phosphoriesterase exists, it has been proposed that long-term stimulation of dopamine receptors is associated with an increase in the soluble calmodulin content thereby activating PDE and decreasing receptor responsiveness. Similar data suggest interneuronal pathways also exist where opiates increase soluble calmodulin via a release of dopamine and thus act as indirect dopamine agonists (Hanbauer and Phyall, 1980). Smoake and Solomon (1980) have reported altered

calmodulin distribution in liver cells from rats with strepto-
zotocin-induced diabetes. These authors conclude that such
changes might play a role in the alteration of cAMP metabolism
known to exist in such pathological states.

The difficulties with interpretation of most calmodulin
distribution studies is that the protein is assayed by its
ability to stimulate a calmodulin-dependent enzyme. Since
all such assays are Ca^{++}-dependent and other calmodulin-
binding proteins are likely to be present in each subcellular
fraction, it is difficult to obtain quantitative values for
calmodulin. This difficulty is circumvented when a radioimmunoassay is employed since the assay can be performed in
the presence of EGTA and is therefore Ca^{++}-independent
(Chafouleas et al., 1979). The radioimmunoassay has been
utilized to determine the quantity and subcellular distribution of calmodulin in the rat pituitary gonadotrops before
and during GnRH-induced LH release (Conn et al., 1981).
Indeed, the distribution of calmodulin does change in response
to GnRH. There is an initial rise in the percentage of
calmodulin associated with the plasma membrane which appears
concomitantly with the depletion of cytoplasmic calmodulin.
These changes occur temporally in concert with secretion of
LH. As the calmodulin begins to be cleared from the plasma
membrane, its level increases first in the secretory granule
and microsomal fractions before finally replenishing the
cytoplasm. The magnitude of the changes that occur between
plasma membrane and cytoplasmic content of calmodulin are
related to the dose of GnRH. Calmodulin redistribution is
also hormone specific since analogs such as des[1] GnRH (2-10)
which has no efficacy in promoting LH secretion did not alter
intracellular changes in calmodulin. Finally, a budget of
calmodulin content in all subcellular fractions revealed that
GnRH did not increase total calmodulin and greater than 95%
of the cellular calmodulin was recovered.

The data presented above suggest that calmodulin may be
important in the regulation of protein secretion, but provide
little information concerning the mechanism. At this juncture
it is impossible to predict whether calmodulin redistribution
is a cause or consequence of the secretory process. In the
red blood cell (Hinds et al., 1978), pancreatic islet
(Pershadsingh et al., 1980b) and adipocyte (Pershadsingh et
al., 1980a), calmodulin-activated ATPases are found in the
plasma membrane and, at least in the adipocyte, the enzyme

appears to be hormonally regulated. Plasma membranes from
islet cells also have been reported to contain a calmodulin-
stimulated adenylyl cyclase activity (Valverde et al., 1979).
Calmodulin is also a major component of postsynaptic membranes
(Grab et al., 1979; Lin et al., 1980; Wood et al., 1980), has
been proposed to mediate the Ca^{++} effects on synaptic transmission (Gregy and Lau, 1980; Hanbauer et al., 1978a,b), and
accordingly, may play a role in neurotransmitter release
(DeLorenzo et al., 1979). Finally, trifluoperazine and
naphthalenesulfonamides are drugs that bind to calmodulin and
inhibit many of its actions. These drugs also inhibit the
receptor-mediated secretory process in a variety of systems.

   Receptor-mediated endocytosis is also a Ca^{++}-dependent
process and also involves clathrin-coated vesicles (Goldstein
et al., 1979; Salisbury et al., 1980). Although internalization of GnRH does not appear to be required for the LH release
process, the response of the gonadotrops to this releasing
hormone does include the pattern of patching, capping and
internalization observed for many cell surface-mediated
ligand systems (Conn et al., 1980). This receptor redistribution pattern in the gonadotrops is mimicked by changes found
in calmodulin associated with the plasma membrane when
assessed by indirect immunofluorescence microscopy. Recruitment of clathrin-coated vesicles to the plasma membrane of
human lymphoblastoid cells occurs following stimulation with
multivalent anti-IgM antibodies (Salisbury et al., 1980).
This recruitment is inhibited by the presence of anti-calmodulin drugs and calmodulin is a component of such vesicles.
Thus, the appearance of calmodulin at the plasma membrane may
be associated with the accumulation of coated pits involved
in the receptor internalization process. Insulin, which also
is internalized following cap formation, promotes the translocation of glucose transport activity from the microsomal or
Golgi fractions to the plasma membrane (Cushman and Wardzala,
1980; Suzuki and Kono, 1980). Actin and myosin have also
been reported to co-cap with several cell surface receptors
(Bourguignon et al., 1978; Flanagan and Koch, 1978) and
actin-containing matrices have been isolated from D.
discoideum (Condeelis, 1979), murine tumor cells and lymphocyte plasma membranes (Mescher et al., 1981) associated with
various receptors. Thus, the phenomenon of redistribution of
new activities to the plasma membrane may be a generalized
occurance for plasma membrane receptor-mediated events. This
redistribution suggests a mechanism by which calmodulin-
regulated events could be affected without the requirement

for new protein synthesis. It is likely that calmodulin redustribution is secondary to alterations in the net flux or distribution of Ca^{++} within the cell.

5.   Mechanism of Action of Calmodulin

    Although calmodulin is involved in the regulation of a variety of enzyme systems, it appears to mediate this regulation in most cases by activating specific protein kinases. Calmodulin plays a major role in mediating the Ca^{++} regulation of glycolysis as the calcium binding subunit of phosphorylase kinase. Of extreme interest is that this regulation occurs in two ways, for not only does phosphorylase kinase activate phosphorylase through phosphorylation in the presence of Ca^{++}, it also inactivates the antagonistic enzyme, glycogen synthase, through the same mechanism. As reported by Blackmore et al. (1981), these data explain the manner by which α-adrenergic agonists regulate glycogen metabolism in hepatocytes in the absence of cAMP metabolism.

    The possibility that calmodulin mediated phosphorylation may be a major mechanism for intracellular regulation is suggested by the work of Yamauchi and Fujisawa (1979), who have demonstrated that most of the Ca^{++}-dependent endogenous phosphorylation of rat brain cytosolic proteins requires calmodulin. More specifically, calmodulation-directed protein phosphorylation may be a major regulatory mechanism in stimulus-secretion coupling. This indeed has been demonstrated in the release of neurotransmitter in brain. DeLorenzo and Freedman (1978) observed that Ca^{++} stimulation of endogenous release of norepinephrine from isolated synaptic vesicles was associated with a rapid increase in phosphorylation of specific vesicle proteins. Schulman and Greengard (1978) demonstrated that an endogenous heat stable cytosolic protein was required for the calcium-dependent phosphorylation of synaptosomal membrane fractions from rat cerebral cortex. They also observed that authentic calmodulin could substitute for the endogenous protein. The authors therefore suggested that the calcium-dependent phosphorylation was mediated through calmodulin. That such a heat-stable protein (most likely calmodulin) regulates neurotransmitter release was demonstrated by DeLorenzo et al. (1979). They showed that removal of the endogenous heat-stable protein from purified synaptic vesicles caused these vesicles to become refractory to Ca^{++} stimulation. The Ca^{++} stimulation of norepinephrine release and membrane protein phosphorylation could be restored to these depleted vesicles in a dose-dependent manner by the addition of authentic calmodulin. Schulman and Greengard (1978) have demonstrated that the Ca^{++} dependent phosphorylation of membrane proteins is not restricted to neuronal tissues, but also occurs in many non-neuronal tissues. However, while these membrane phosphorylations all required Ca^{++} and calmodulin, tissue-specific endogenous substrates for the kinases were observed.

The possibility of a coordinate regulation of brain membrane protein phosphorylation by both cAMP and Ca^{++} is suggested by the study of Sieghart et al. (1979). They observed that the phosphorylation of the brain-specific proteins Ia and Ib are regulated by both Ca^{++} and cAMP. However, while both kinases phosphorylate these two proteins, they do so at different amino acid residues. LePeuch et al. (1979) have demonstrated that this coordinated regulation is not limited to these two brain proteins. They have shown that the rate of Ca^{++} uptake by cardiac sarcoplasmic reticulum is regulated by cAMP and Ca^{++}-calmodulin-dependent phosphorylation of the membrane protein phospholamban. cAMP mediates its regulation through cAMP-dependent protein kinase, while the Ca^{++}-dependent phosphorylation is mediated through a membrane-bound protein kinase which requires both Ca^{++} and calmodulin for activity. Both kinases phosphorylate different sites on the protein and it is the Ca^{++}-dependent phosphorylation which is mandatory for Ca^{++} uptake. The cAMP-dependent phosphorylation, while incapable by itself to stimulate Ca^{++} uptake, does however, amplify uptake when Ca^{++}-dependent phosphorylation has taken place. The possibility that this membrane-bound calmodulin-dependent protein kinase may be similar to phosphorylase kinase or in fact a form of phosphorylase kinase devoid of its δ-subunit (calmodulin) is suggested by the fact that it is capable of phosphorylating exogenous phosphorylase in the presence of calmodulin. Conversely, exogenous phosphorylase kinase is capable of phosphorylating phospholamban. These findings are intriguing when taken with the work of Browning et al. (1979). They have shown that the preferential phosphorylation of a 40,000 Mr protein in synaptic-plasma membranes following electrical stimulation can be minicked by exogenous phosphorylase kinase, but not only by cAMP-dependent protein kinase. These studies would suggest that the calmodulin regulation of protein phosphorylation mediated through phosphorylase kinase may be more extensive than previously thought. Of equal interest is the coordinated regulation of protein phosphorylation exhibited by calmodulin, since calmodulin in fact is involved in both processes. While calmodulin plays a direct role in Ca^{++}-dependent phosphorylation, it also plays an indirect role in cAMP-dependent phosphorylation by regulating cAMP metabolism through activation of both adenylyl cyclase and cyclic nucleotide phosphodiesterase.

Whether calmodulin mediates its regulatory function solely through protein phosphorylation or through other mechanisms, its ability to regulate is entirely dependent on the intracellular free Ca^{++} concentration. Since calmodulin controlled systems would either be constitutively turned on or off in the presence of a constant intracellular free Ca^{++} concentration, it is apparent that true regulation must be mediated through the control of these intracellular levels. This, in fact, may be the mechanism by which external signals are transduced into intracellular responses in hormone action. Indeed, the most characteristic aspect of hormone action is the occurrence of Ca^{++} fluxes (Berridge, 1975; Rassmussen et al., 1976).

Although Ca^{++} fluxes are observed as a consequence of hormone action in target cells, it may not be a true increase or decrease in the intracellular levels of Ca^{++}, but a mobilization and redistribution of membrane-bound Ca^{++} that is essential. This is suggested by studies employing chlorotetracycline to monitor the shifts in membrane-bound calcium. LeBreton et al. (1976) demonstrated that the ADP- or ionophore A23187-induced shape change in human platelets was temporarily associated with a decrease in membrane-bound calcium. A similar phenomenon was also observed in rabbit neutrophils following stimulation with chemotactic factors (Naccache et al., 1979). In fact, the redistribution of Ca^{++} is so rapid that the authors have suggested this mobilization may represent one of the initial molecular events following the binding of chemotatic factor to its membrane receptor. Recent studies by Chafouleas et al. (1980) and Conn et al. (1981) have suggested that this redistribution of intracellular Ca^{++} may, in fact represent a redistribution of the intracellular Ca^{++}-calmodulin complex.

6.   Immunologic Techniques for the Study of Calmodulin

It became apparent early on that the data derived by any of the biological assays for calmodulin might be inaccurate due to the multifunctional aspect of the protein. Since each assay was dependent on the presence of Ca^{++}-dependent binding by a "biologically active" calmodulin molecule, it was probable, that such assays could yield lower values for the protein due to competition by other calmodulin binding proteins. No such restrictions would be imposed, however, by immunological probes since these assays are predicted on the highly specific antigen-antibody interaction and would not require Ca^{++}-dependent binding.

Interestingly, those aspects which made calmodulin exciting to study - its highly conserved and ubiquitious nature as well as low M_r and pI proved to be deterents in production of antisera to the protein. Initial attempts to produce antibody against native protein in rabbits were negative. However, Dedman et al. (1978a) were able to elicit antibody to the native protein in goat. Chafouleas et al. (1979) subsequently reported antibody toward native calmodulin produced in sheep which was used in development of an RIA. Detection of these antibodies, however, required affinity chromatography on a calmodulin affinity column. While these two reports are the only ones dealing with antibody against the native protein, other investigators have reported on the production of antisera to calmodulin modified by alum precipitation (Andersen et al., 1978), dinitrophenylation (Wallace and Cheung, 1979) or performate oxidation (Van Eldik and Watterson, 1981).

6.1. Calmodulin and Microfilaments

Antibodies developed against native rat testis calmodulin have been employed to localize the protein in a variety of tissue culture cells by indirect immunofluorescence microscopy. In cells in interphase, calmodulin predominantly decorates the actin-containing stress fibers (Dedman et al., 1978b), whereas in skeletal muscle, the protein is preferentially associated with the I-bands. The logic of these distributions becomes readily apparent when considering the biochemical reactions involved in contractility. In all types of cells, an enzyme termed myosin light chain kinase (MLCK) is present that phosphorylates one of the myosin light chains (LC_{20}) (see Stull, 1980 for review). This enzyme was found to be calmodulin-dependent (Dabrowska et al., 1977; Yagi et al., 1978). Myosin light chain kinase has been purified from smooth (Adelstein and Klee, 1981; Dabrowska et al., 1977; Guerriero et al., 1981), skeletal (Pires and Perry, 1977; Blumenthal and Stull, 1980; Crouch et al., 1981), and cardiac muscle (Wolf and Hofmann, 1980; Walsh et al., 1979). The reported molecular weights of the enzymes from these tissues range from 80,000 to 130,000 depending on both the tissue and procedure used for purification. It has been suggested that either there are multiple forms of MLCK in these tissues (Yamauchi and Fujisawa, 1980; Stull, 1980) or the smaller molecular weight proteins are proteolytic fragments of the native enzyme (Walsh et al., 1980). A recent study by Guerriero et al. (1981) addressed this question by producing an antibody against chicken gizzard MLCK. Using this probe and the protein transfer technique of Towbin et al. (1979), the molecular weight of the enzyme in a variety of chicken tissues was found to be 130,000. These data suggest that some proteolysis of the native enzyme may occur during purification.

In non- and smooth muscle cells LC_{20} phosphorylation is positively correlated with tension development and contractility (Stull, 1980). Thus, Ca^{++} binds to calmodulin which promotes the association of this complex with an inactive myosin light chain kinase (MLCK). Activation of MLCK results in LC_{20} phosphorylation. This modification promotes a conformational change in myosin that allows actin binding and consequent stimulation of the myosin ATPase. Hydrolysis of ATP provides the energy required for contraction. Indeed myosin, tropomyosin and myosin light chain kinase have also been revealed to be components of the stress fibers in non-muscle cells (Guerriero et al., 1981; deLanerolle et al., 1981). Contractility of skeletal muscle is primarily controlled by the troponin system and LC_{20} phosphorylation does nothing to enhance the primary contractile response. Rather, this calmodulin-dependent alteration seems to be involved in post-tetanic potentiation of the action potential. In order for this to occur, actin, MLCK and calmodulin should all be present on the I-band (which they are). Only following contraction would the I-band be in register with myosin to allow LC_{20} phosphorylation and the post-tetanic response. Enzymes that dephosphorylate the regulatory light chain of myosin have been purified from skeletal (Morgan et al., 1976) and smooth muscle (Pato and Adelstein, 1980). Dephosphorylation of smooth muscle myosin results in a form of myosin ATPase that cannot be activated by actin. The removal of the phosphate from the regulatory light chain, then, leads to smooth muscle relaxation.

6.2. Calmodulin and Microtubules

In mitotic cells, calmodulin was determined to be localized in the half-spindle (Welsh et al., 1978, 1979; Andersen et al., 1978). In metaphase, calmodulin was observed in association with the mitotic spindle. In anaphase, calmodulin was found only in the region of the spindle between the centrioles and the chromosomes and was completely absent from the interzonal region. This initial study suggested a similarity between calmodulin localization and that of the microtubules. In order to further evaluate this, Welsh et al. (1979) compared the immunofluorescence localization of calmodulin and tubulin in several mammalian tissue culture cells throughout mitosis. Although calmodulin was always restricted to the half-spindles, tubulin was found throughout the mitotic apparatus.

The cytoskeletal component in the mitotic apparatus to which calmodulin was associated was evaluated by a series of drug studies (Welsh et al., 1979). Treatment with cytochalasin B, a drug known to disrupt microfilaments, caused no change in either the concentration of localization of calmodulin or tubulin. However, when cells were treated with agents known to disrupt microtubules (i.e., colcemid), spindle structure was altered and tubulin and calmodulin-specific fluorescence were equally affected. Colcemid treatment completely disrupted the spindle as reflected by tubulin immunofluorescence and equally abolished calmodulin localization in the mitotic apparatus. Treatment of cells with nitrous oxide, which causes disorganization of the spindle, but does not cause disassembly of spindle microtubules, disrupted spindle structure as visualized by tubulin-specific fluorescence. However, calmodulin was still concentrated in the cell center in the same region as the microtubules of the disorganized spindle. Finally, Brinkley and Cartwright (1971) had shown that two types of microtubules exist in the mitotic apparatus. The microtubules from pole to chromosome are known to be stable to cold temperatures whereas lowering the tempreature of 4°C disrupts those microtubules present in the interzone region that extend from pole to pole. In order to substantiate the premise that calmodulin was associated with the former, cells were subjected to 4°C and immunofluorescence staining performed. As expected, treatment of cells at 4°C resulted in the disruption of the pole-to-pole microtubules as visualized by antibutulin immunofluorescence. However, the pole-to-chromosome tubules were intact. No

change in the distribution of calmodulin was found upon exposure of the cells to cold temperatures suggesting that if
calmodulin is associated with microtubules during mitosis,
the most likely components are the pole-to-chromosome microtubules which comprise the half spindles. Subsequent studies
by Andersen et al. (1978) confirmed this localization pattern
using an antibody that had been prepared against alum-precipi-
tated calmodulin. In addition, Lin et al. (1980) as well as
deMey et al. (1980) have localized calmodulin in mitotic
mammalian cells by an electron microscopic method. Again,
the distribution pattern described above was shown to be the
case. Thus, a gradient of calmodulin concentration was seen
in which the greatest concentration of calmodulin was present
at the poles and the least at the chromosomes.

Although the intracellular distribution of calmodulin
appears to be very elaborate, one consistant theme does
arise. During mitosis there is a striking correlation between
the location of calmodulin staining and the area in which
microtubules are undergoing depolymerization. These experiments suggested that the calcium lability of microtubules may
be mediated by calmodulin. In order to test this hypothesis,
microtubules were isolated by four cycles of polymerization/
depolymerization as described by Borisy et al. (1975).
Microtubule formation was monitored by a change in absorbancy
at 320 nanometers and polymerization was initiated by the
addition of GTP (Marcum et al., 1978). 0.3 micromolar calcium
had no effect on microtubule polymerization. Increasing the
concentration to 11 micromolar caused only about a 10%
reduction in the extent of microtubule polymerization. When
calmodulin was added to the mixture in buffer containing 0.3
micromolar free Ca^{++}, little effect on polymerization was
observed. However, elevating the Ca^{++} concentration to 11
micromolar calcium in the presence of calmodulin completely
prevented microtubule polymerization. Similarly, addition of
11 micromolar calcium plus calmodulin to polymerized microtubules resulted in a complete depolymerization of these
structures. Further examination of this effect revealed that
calmodulin caused a shift in the concentration of calcium
required for microtubule polymerization (Dedman et al., 1980).
Thus, in the absence of calmodulin, the amount of calcium
required for depolymerization was approximately 10^{-3} M.
However, in the presence of calmodulin the concentration of
calcium required for complete depolymerization of microtubules
was 10^{-5} molar. Therefore, a 100-fold change in sensitivity
of calcium was achieved by the addition of calmodulin.

While the experiments demonstrated the involvement of calmodulin on the calcium sensitivity of microtubule depolymerization, the molar ratios of calmodulin to tubulin required to elicit these effects was 6:1. Since calmodulin has been shown to interact with its other regulated systems in 1:1 stoichiometry, these experiments were less than ideal. In order to further substantiate these data in a more in situ situation, a detergent-permeabilized cell system was used as described by Brinkley et al. (1980). In this system, isolated tissue culture cells are incubated with colcemid to disrupt the cytoplasmic microtubule complex. The cells are then permeabilized by treatment with Triton X-100 and washed to remove depolymerized 6S tubulin and the colcemid. Visualization of these cells by indirect immunofluorescence microscopy using anti-tubulin reveals that the only fluorescent structure present in each interphase cell is the single organizing center associated with the centrosomal region. Addition of 6S tubulin to this preparation results in the specific nucleation of microtubule assembly from the single nucleating site. Incubation of these lysed cells with 11 micromolar free calcium produces no difference in the degree of microtubule polymerization. However, if calmodulin is added in the presence of 11 micromolar calcium, complete abolition of microtubule polymerization is achieved. Brinkley et al. (1980) established that the optimal concentration of tubulin for microtubule assembly was 1 milligram per ml. Assuming a molecular weight of 110,000 for the 6S dimer, this results in a tubulin concentration of approximately 10 micromolar. The optimal concentration of CaM in this system was 6 micromolar. Thus, the ratio of calmodulin/tubulin required for optimal effects was much closer to 1:1 than the concentrations required in the in vitro microtubule polymerization experiments.

Taken together, these experiments suggest that there should be an inverse relationship between the concentration of calmodulin in the cell and the number of polymerized microtubules. Several systems have been developed to examine this possibility. The first was achieved by first determining the distribution of anti-calmodulin in mitotic cells by immunofluorescence microscopy and then serially sectioning them for electron microscopy (Dedman et al., 1980). Each of the sections was evaluated for the number of microtubule profiles as described by Brinkley and Cartwright (1971). In metaphase, when high concentrations of calmodulin were found at the poles, no polymerized microtubules were counted in those sections. However, as the gradient of calmodulin decreased from the poles toward the chromosomes, the number of polymerized microtubules increased, reaching the highest numbers at the kinetochore plates of the chromosomes. On the other side of the chromosomes an inverse relationship was again observed where high concentrations were observed close to the kinetochore followed by a decreasing gradient towards the opposite pole. This relationship held throughout mitosis even in late anaphase where calmodulin was found to be transiently associated on both sides of the chromosomes. In such cells, the only polymerized microtubules were found in the middle of the cell corresponding to the position of the developing cleavage furrow. Once again, therefore, there was an inverse relationship between the concentration of calmodulin and the number of polymerized microtubules.

The second approach was to isolate mitotic spindles from sea urchin eggs as described by Salmon and Segall (1980). These spindles demonstrate micromolar sensitivity to calcium and were found to contain calmodulin by radioimmunoassay (Dedman et al., 1980). Staining of the metaphase mitotic spindle by anti-tubulin demonstrated that the entire mitotic spindle contained tubulin, including the asters at each pole. Examination of the immunofluorescence pattern of calmodulin revealed localization only in the region of the centrioles. Serial sections of the mitotic spindles revealed that no polymerized microtubules were found in association with the poles. As the distance between the pole and chromosome increased, the number of polymerized microtubules increased. Again, in this system, there is an association between the calmodulin concentration and the number of polymerized microtubules. Finally, Cande and Wolniak (1978) have developed a eucaryotic mammalian cell system in which the rate of metaphase-anaphase chromosome movement can be studied. This movement is markedly enhanced by the addition of micromolar calcium. In collaborative experiments, we have recently shown that this movement can be blocked by incubation of the mitotic spindles with calmodulin antibody or the anticalmodulin agent, W13, described by Hidaka et al. (1980). It seems reasonable to assume, therefore, that calmodulin may be involved in the regulated depolymerization of microtubules that occurs during metaphase-anaphase chromosome movement. It should also be pointed out that in those systems where calcium concentration has been measured, micromolar concentrations of calcium are not achieved in the spindle. Therefore, high concentrations of calmodulin as observed by immunofluorescence would be required in order to assure proper depolymerization of micro-tubules. However, the exact mechanism by which calmodulin affects microtubule depolymerization remains to be determined.

6.3. Radioimmunoassay of Calmodulin

The next major use for the calmodulin antibody was in the development of a RIA for calmodulin. Since the antibody had been successfully prepared, the only major hurdle to cross was radiolabeling the tracer calmodulin. In that the sensitivity of the assay would be directly related to the specific activity achieved, the procedure of radiolabeling was very important. Calmodulin contains only two tyrosine residues, one of which is inaccessible to the exterior of the protein. In addition, calcium binding to calmodulin poten-tiates a dramatic change in the tyrosine fluorescence of the molecule. These observations, therefore, would suggest that labeling procedures which were directed to the tyrosine residues might result in low specific activity as well as reduced biological activity. Indeed, when the lactoperoxidase and chloramine T procedures were utilized to radioiodinate calmodulin, low specific radioactivity and significant loss in biological activity was observed (Chafouleas et al., 1979). Calmodulin does, however, contain 8 lysine residues and so the procedure of Bolton and Hunter (1975), in which the iodine is conjugated to the ε amino side groups of lysine was used. Calmodulin labeled by this procedure had high specific radioactivity (2400 Ci/mmol) and retained complete biological activity (Chafouleas et al., 1979). The resultant radioimmunoassay was shown to have an interassay variability of less than 5% and an intraassay variability of less than 3%. The statistical assay sensitivity was 150 pg whereas the limit of detection was 15 pg (Chafouleas et al., 1979).

The radioimmunoassay was first used to confirm the highly conserved nature of calmodulin. When pure calmodulin isolated from bovine brain, rat testis, Renilla reniformis and the peanut plant (Arachis hypogea) were used to obtain standard dilution curves, it was found that all 4 proteins described the same curve (Chafouleas et al., 1979). On the other hand, troponin C from rabbit skeletal muscle required 660-fold greater protein concentration to achieve 50% competi-tion and demonstrated a statistically different slope. Again, this emphasized the fact that although troponin C and calmodulin are homologous, they are not identical. Another small molecular weight calcium-binding protein, paravalbumin, demonstrated no cross reactivity even at 50,000-fold protein excess.

The radioimmunoassay was also used to evaluate calmodulin levels in heat-treated supernatant solutions from highly diverse sources. Cell samples tested, regardless of source, demonstrated immunological identity to the rat testis calmodulin standard (Chafouleas et al., 1979). Tissues and organisms examined to date include rat, eel, rabbit, bovine, human, amphibian, reptile, slime mold, plants, algae, coelenterate, paramecium, tetrahymena and amoeba. These data once again illustrate the fact that the immunologic nature of calmodulin is highly conserved between the most primitive unicellular organism and man.

The radioimmunoassay was utilized to illustrate another very interesting point regarding the nature of calmodulin's interaction with its various binding proteins. The most usual assays to determine the amount of calmodulin in a sample are based on its ability to stimulate a partially purified preparation of bovine brain cyclic AMP phosphodiesterase or chicken gizzard myosin light chain kinase. When the amount of calmodulin found in various tissues and species by radioimmunoassay was compared to those determined by the phosphodiesterase assay, it was found that in all instances, the radioimmunoassay yielded higher values (Chafouleas et al., 1979). In fact, in organisms such as <u>Dictyostelium</u> and <u>Chalamydomonas</u>, no calmodulin could be detected by the phosphodiesterase assay, whereas significant concentrations were found by radioimmunoassay. The discrepencies observed between the two types of assays can be explained when the procedures employed for the biological assay are compared. The assay for calmodulin by enzyme activation depends upon the ability of "biologically active" calmodulin to activate the enzyme through Ca^{++}-dependent binding. There are many calmodulin-binding proteins present in cells. These proteins can be found in both the heat-treated samples to be assayed as well as the enzyme preparation itself. Therefore, these calmodulin-binding proteins could interfere in the assay by competing for the calmodulin and effectively resulting in a lower measured level of this protein. Since the RIA is not dependent on Ca^{++}-dependent activation, the results from this assay would not be so influenced. Indeed, when purified calmodulin is quantitated by both assays, the values obtained are in close agreement. These observations would suggest that the radioimmunoassay is the assay of choice when evaluating calmodulin levels in tissue extracts.

7.   Regulation of Calmodulin in Transformed Cells

The experiments performed using calmodulin in microtubule polymerization would suggest that there is a positive correlation between calmodulin content and microtubule depolymerization. Interestingly, Watterson et al. (1976) and LaPorte et al. (1979) had reported 2-fold elevations in calmodulin levels in chicken embryo fibroblasts transformed by Rous Sarcoma Virus when compared to the nontransformed cell. Since a diminished cytoplasmic microtubule network has been reported as one characteristic response to transformation (Brinkley et al., 1975), these reports would further substantiate the role of calmodulin in microtubule polymerization. In order to ascertain whether the elevation in calmodulin level observed in the transformed chicken embryo fibroblasts is a result of transformation in general, Chafouleas et al. (1981) compared calmodulin levels in Swiss mouse 3T3 and 3T3 cells transformed by the DNA type virus SV40, as well s normal rat kidney cells and those cells transformed by the RNA type virus, Rous Sarcoma Virus. Since the steady state concentration of a protein is a function of the rates of synthesis and degradation, these turnover parameters were determined in both the 3T3/SV3T3 and NRK/SNRK systems. In addition to calmodulin, similar determinations were performed for tubulin. In both cell systems, calmodulin levels were elevated at least 2-fold in the transformed cells compared to their appropriate nontransformed counterpart. This was in contrast to tubulin which retained the same levels in the normal and transformed cells. The rate of synthesis of calmodulin, tubulin and total protein were all increased in the transformed cells. While tubulin and total protein demonstrated about a 2-fold increase, calmodulin was synthesized three times as fast. In addition, the transformed cells also exhibited greater rates of degradation. Calmodulin and total protein exhibited similar changes. Tubulin, on the other hand, had a rate of degradation which was twice that present in the normal cell. Therefore, tubulin levels are unaltered in the transformed cells through reciprocal changes in the rates of degradation and synthesis. A net increase in the intracellular levels of calmodulin is achieved through a selective increase in the rate of synthesis which is twice as great as the change in degradation. These changes in the steady state concentrations of calmodulin and tubulin result in a 2-fold increase in the calmodulin-to-tubulin molar ratio in the transformed cells.

8.   Calmodulin and the Cell Cycle

During the growth cycle of mammalian cells in tissue culture, dramatic changes in cell shape and function occur. Non-transformed cells require rather large amounts of Ca^{++} in the media and Ca^{++} seems to be necessary both for progression from G_1 into S as well as for mitosis. On the other hand, transformed cells appear to require much less Ca^{++} for cell growth. For these reasons, Chafouleas et al. (1982) evaluated changes in calmodulin that occur during the growth cycle of CHO-K_1 cells. These Chinese hamster ovary cells were chosen because they exhibit a relatively short cell cycle (12-16 hr) and consequently, can be synchronized by mitotic shake (Terasima and Tolmach, 1961) without the need for the addition of drugs such as thymidine or cholchicine. The population of cells utilized for the initial experiments were shown to exhibit a 16 hr cell cycle distributed as follows: M = 1; G_1 = 5; S = 8; and G_2 = 2. Mitotic cells were released into the cycle by increasing the temperature from 4°C to 37°C. During the subsequent 16 hr, the % of cells in S was evaluated by 10 min pulses with ^{3}H-TdR followed by radioautography to quantitate the number of cells with labeled nuclei. Calmodulin content was monitored by radioimmunoassay and the % of mitotic cells was also scored as a measure of cell synchrony.

At mitotis, the calmodulin content was 150 ng/10^6 cells. This value fell abruptly by 50% coincident with separation of the daughter cells. Between 4 and 6 hr after initiation of cell synchrony, calmodulin values again increased to 150 ng/10^6 cells and remained at this value for at least 12 hr. The increase in calmodulin content slightly preceeded the increase in ^{3}H-TdR labeled cells suggesting that synthesis of this protein occured at the G_1/S boundary. This postulate was tested by repeating the experiments with a population of cells that exhibited a 2 hr G_1 period. Again, calmodulin values halved as cells were released from mitotic synchrony and increased again preceeding DNA synthesis. Four such experiments with cells that revealed both 2 and 5 hr G_1 periods were carried out. The data were graphed as calmodulin content (ng/10^6 cells) as a function of the % cells labeled

with ^{3}H-TdR. Linear regression analysis was performed and
these parameters were found to show a correlation coefficient
of 0.966 (slope = 1.07). Thus, CaM synthesis is coupled to
the G_1/S boundary - a fact which raises the question as to
whether the doubling in CaM content may play a role in the
G_1/S transition.

If the elevation in calmodulin concentration is important
in the progression of cells from G_1 into S, then anti-calmodulin drugs might be expected to arrest the cells at this
growth cycle boundary. The primary question was which drugs
to choose for these experiments. The most widely used anti-
calmodulin compounds are members of the phenothiazine family.
These molecules, characterized by trifluoperazine (TFP) and
chlorpromazine, bind to calmodulin in a Ca^{++}-dependent manner
(Weiss and Levin, 1978) and have been linked to inert supports
to form affinity columns (Charbonneau and Cormier, 1979;
Jamieson and Vanaman, 1979). These columns have been used to
isolate calmodulin from a wide range of cell types. Whereas
the in vitro specificity of these drugs is considerable (K_d =
10^{-6} M), the specificity in vivo is questionable. Trifluoperazine is highly lipophilic and as such will bind nonspecif-
ically to cell membranes (Seeman, 1972). Moreover, TFP has
been shown to interact with the dopamine receptor (Gnegy and
Lau, 1980) as well as receptors for α-adrenergic agonists
(Blackmore et al., 1981). Control compounds such as TFP-
sulfoxide bind much less avidly to calmodulin, but also
possess a much different hydrophobicity index (measured by
the octanol:H_2O partition coefficient). These problems are
compounded because calmodulin undergoes a conformational
change upon binding Ca^{++}. This interaction exposes a highly
lipophilic surface and it is this surface that reportedly
binds to both calmodulin dependent enzymes as well as to the
phenothiazines (LaPorte et al., 1980; Tanaka and Hidaka,
1980). The importance of these considerations can be appreciated when considering the fact that phosphodiesterase (Wolff
and Brostrom, 1976; Pichard and Cheung, 1977) and MLCK (Tanaka
and Hidaka, 1980) can be fully activated in vitro by phospholipids. This type of activation precludes the need for
calmodulin as a regulatory component. Therefore, in designing
drugs to be used as anti-calmodulin compounds, it is necessary
to separate the lipophilic nature of the drugs from their
ability to bind calmodulin.

The napthalenesulfonamides may represent a class of
drugs as described above. These "W-compounds" have been

synthesized and evaluated by Hidaka and colleagues (1979, 1980). The highest affinity W-compounds (W-7 and W-13) have a Cl- attached to $C-1$ of the A-ring. These drugs bind to calmodulin in a Ca^{++}-dependent manner and exhibit similar affinities to TFP ($K_d = 10^{-6}$ M). Removal of the Cl- decreases calmodulin binding by 5- to 10-fold, but alters the hydrophobicity index by only 10-15%. For these reasons we decided to evaluate the anti-calmodulin compound W-13 and its dechlorinated control compound W-12 for effects on the growth cycle of CHO-K_1 cells. The first series of experiments were designed to assess the fraction of cells that survived following culture in the presence of increasing concentrations of W-13 or W-12. Addition of W-12 up to 80 μg/ml did not affect survival. Similarly 30 μg/ml of W-13 (10^{-4} M) caused no lethality but did alter the shape of the cells. Increasing the W-13 concentration to 35 μg/ml resulted in 40% cell death and only 0.01% of the cells survived at 60 μg/ml.

Incubation of asynchronously growing cells with 30 μg/ml W-13 resulted, within 24 hr, in a 50% reduction in the number of cells compared to cells grown in a similar concentration of W-12 or the usual culture medium (Chafouleas et al., 1982). This growth cycle arrest was completely reversible. Following removal of W-13, the cells remained quiescent for approximately 8 hr before beginning to increase in number. The cell number doubled by 30 hr and after recovery, this population of cells continued to exhibit a cell cycle of 12.5 hr. These experiments confirmed that the anti-calmodulin drug W-13 delayed progression of cells through the cell cycle in a specific and reversible manner. The next studies were designed to question the location of cell cycle arrest.

Cell were synchronized by mitotic shake and 1 hr after release into the cell cycle W-13, W-12 or normal medium was added. W-13 was found to cause a delay in G_1 progression into S as monitored by the number of cells labeled with ^{3}H-TdR. W-12 caused no effect and these cells responded precisely as did cells incubated in normal medium. Whereas 92% of the cell nuclei became labeled by 8 hr when cultured in medium or medium containing W-12, only 60% became labeled in the presence of W-13. Thus, although W-13 appeared to exert an effect at the G_1/S boundary, the arrest was incomplete. This population of CHO/K_1 cells exhibited a G_1 of only 2 hr. Subsequent experiments with the 5 hr G_1 population demonstrated that a complete delay in G_1 to S progression could be effected by W-13. During these experiments, calmodulin content was monitored by RIA. The data revealed that W-13 did not prevent the 2-fold increase in calmodulin that occurred at the G_1/S boundary. It is likely, therefore, that the W-13 was preventing an action(s) of CaM required for progression of the cells into S.

Not only does W-13 cause a delay in the progression of synchronized cells (at mitosis) from G_1 to S, but the drug also prevents progression through S phase in cells synchronized at the G_1/S in a double TdR block. On the other hand, W-13 does not affect progression through either G_2 or M. Taken together, the data suggest that the elevation in calmodulin concentration that occurs during the cell cycle is important for the progression of cells through replicative DNA synthesis (S phase) and that W-13 must prevent one or more actions of calmodulin that are premissive for this important cellular event.

The calmodulin concentration also seems to be important for the re-entry of plateau cells (G_0) into the cell cycle. Calmodulin levels increase by 50% as cells leave G_1 and enter plateau and remain at this concentration for the duration of the G_0 phase. Upon release of the cells into the growth cycle, calmodulin decreases by 40% within the first hr and remains at this concentration for 4-5 hr. By 8 hr, the intracellular levels have again doubled and remain at this level as cells pass through S, G_2 and M. This concentration is that normally achieved after the increase in calmodulin the G_1/S boundary (Chafouleas et al., 1982). Addition of W-13 at the time of treatment with fresh medium prevented entry into S phase, but the changes in the intracellular concentration of calmodulin are unaltered. When cells were treated with W-13 at various times following release from plateau, a direct correlation was observed between the precentage of cells entering S phase and the time of drug addition (r = 0.99). The labeling index increased as the interval between drug treatment and G_0 release increased. However, although some cells entered S phase, no progression through this period was observed when W-13 was added as late as 5 hr following addition of fresh medium. Removal of the drug resulted, after a 5 hr lag period, in progression of all cells through S phase in a synchronous fashion. These data strengthen the contention that calmodulin is important for the progression of cells through DNA synthesis.

Recent experimental results can be interpreted to suggest that the increase in calmodulin at G_1/S is important for optimal DNA repair prior to replicative DNA synthesis. Bleomycin is a drug known to cause DNA damage by strand scission. Concentrations of this agent can readily be found that result in potentially lethal damage to tissue culture cells. Under these conditions, approximately 90% of the cells are killed. The remaining 10%, however, can recover from the drug by repairing DNA and will eventually repopulate the culture dish. If cells are selected for potentially lethal damage and released from Bleomycin into the presence of media containing W-13, all the cells are killed within 3 hr. The most obvious explanation of these results is that calmodulin is required for DNA repair. When calmodulin is neutralized with W-13, then the cells cannot repair the DNA damage which resulted from Bleomycin. This results in cell death during the subsequent replicative phase. If such a scenario is the case, then some of the enzymes involved in DNA repair must be regulated by calmodulin. It is known that such enzymes are induced at the G_1/S boundary as is the case for calmodulin. Studies are currently underway to determine whether the DNA repair enzymes are calmodulin-binding proteins and whether the increased calmodulin synthesis at G_1/S is transcriptionally or post-transcriptionally regulated.

9. Summary and Conclusions

Over the last five years the importance of calmodulin to the eukaryotic cell has become more evident. Initially believed to be an activator for only one enzyme, cyclic nucleotide phosphodiesterase, this protein is now known to either directly or indirectly mediate the Ca^{++} regulation of 15 key enzymatic or structural systems. These facts taken together with its amazingly conserved nature and ubiquitous distribution in all eukaryotic cells clearly qualify calmodulin as the eukaryotic intracellular Ca^{++} receptor. To date, the majority of studies on calmodulin have been directed toward an understanding of the systems regulated and the mechanisms by which this regulation occurs. However, regardless of which system is regulated or by what mechanism, the ultimate control mediated by calmodulin will be dependent upon its own regulation. Utilization of the molecular probes for calmodulin will help unravel the complexity of the structural gene as well as the genetic regulation of this protein.

REFERENCES

Adelstein, R. S., and Klee, C. B., 1981, Purification and
    characterization of smooth muscle myosin light chain
    kinase, J. Biol. Chem. 256:7501.
Andersen, B., Osborn, M., and Weber, K., 1978, Specific visual-
    ization of the distribution of the calcium-dependent regu-
    latory protein of cyclic nucleotide phosphodiesterase
    (modulator protein) in tissue culture cells by immuno-
    fluorescence microscopy: mitosis and intercellular bridge,
    Eur. J. Cell Biol. 17:354.
Anderson, J. M., and Cormier, M. J., 1978, Calcium-dependent
    regulator of NAD kinase in higher plants, Biochem. Biophys.
    Res. Commun. 84:595.
Assimacopoulos-Jeanenett, F. D., Blackmore, P. F., and Exton,
    J. H., 1977, Studies on α-adrenergic activation of hepatic
    glucose output studies on role of calcium in α-adrenergic
    activation of phosphorylase, J. Biol. Chem. 252:2662.
Blackmore, P. F., El-Refai, M. F., Dehaye, J. -P., Strickland,
    W. G., Hughes, B. P., and Exton, J. H., 1981, Blockage of
    hepatic α-adrenergic receptors and responses by chlorpro-
    mazine and trifluoperazine, FEBS. Letters 123:245.
Berridge, M. J., 1975, The interaction of cyclic nucleotides and
    calcium on the control of cellular activity, in: "Advances
    in Cyclic Nucleotide Research", Vol. 6, P. Greengard and
    G. A. Robison, eds., p. 1, Raven Press, New York.
Blumenthal, D. G., and Stull, J. T., 1980, Activation of skele-
    tal muscle myosin light chain kinase by calcium (2+) and
    calmodulin, Biochemistry 19:5608.
Bolton, A. E., and Hunter, W. M., 1973, The labeling of proteins
    to high specific radioactivities by conjugation to a [125]I-
    containing acylating agent, Biochem. J. 133:529.
Borisy, G. G., Marcum, J. M., Olmstead, J. B., Murphy, D. B.,
    and Johnson, K. A., 1975, Purification of tubulin and
    associated high molecular weight proteins from porcine
    brain and characterization of microtubule assembly in
    vitro, Ann. N. Y. Acad. Sci. 253:107.
Bourguignon, L. Y. W., Tokuyasu, K. T., and Singer, S. J., 1978,
    The capping of lymphocytes and other cells studied by an
    improved method of immunofluorescence staining of frozen
    sections, J. Cell Physiol. 95:239.
Brinkley, B. R., and Cartwright, J., 1971, Ultrastructural
    analysis of mitotic spindle elongation in mammalian cells
    in vitro. Direct microtubule counts, J. Cell Biol. 50:416.

Brinkley, B. R., Pepper, D. A., Cox, S. M., Fistel, S., Brenner, S. L., Wible, L. J., and Pardue, R. L., 1980, Characteristics of centriole- and kinetochore-associated microtubule assembly in mammalian cells, in: "Microtubules and Microtubule Inhibitors", M. DeBrabander and J. DeMey, eds., p. 281, Amsterda, Elsevier.

Brinkley, B. R., Fuller, G. M., and Highfield, D. P., 1975, Cytoplasmic microtubules in normal and transformed cells in culture: analysis by tubulin antibody immunofluorescence, Proc. Natl. Acad. Sci. USA 72:4981.

Brostrom, C. O., Brostrom, M. A., and Wolff, D. J., 1977, Calcium-dependent adenylate cyclase from rat cerebral cortex, J. Biol. Chem. 252:5677.

Browning, M., Bennett, W., and Lynch, G., 1979, Phosphorylase kinase phosphorylates a brain protein which is influenced by repetitive synaptic activation, Nature 278:273.

Cande, W. Z., and Wolniak, S. M., 1978, Chromosome movement in lysed mitotic cells is inhibited by vanadate, J. Cell. Biol. 79:573.

Chafouleas, J. G., Bolton, W. E., Hidaka, H., Boyd, A. E. III, and Means, A. R., 1982, Calmodulin and the cell cycle: involvement in regulation of cell cycle progression, Cell 28:41.

Chafouleas, J. G., Dedman, J. R., Munjaal, R. P., and Means, A. R., 1979, Calmodulin: Development and application of a sensitive radioimmunoassay, J. Biol. Chem. 254:10262.

Chafouleas, J. G., Pardue, R. L., Brinkley, B. R., Dedman, J. R., and Means, A. R., 1980, Effect of viral transformation on intracellular regulation of calmodulin and tubulin, in: "Calcium-Binding Proteins: Structure and Function", F. L. Siegel, E. Carafoli, R. H. Kretsinger, D. H. MacLennan and R. H. Wasserman, eds., p. 189, Amsterdam, Elseiver.

Chafouleas, J. G., Pardue, R. L., Brinkley, B. R., Dedman, J. R., and Means, A. R., 1981, Regulation of intracellular levels of calmodulin and tubulin in normal and transformed cells, Proc. Natl Acad. Sci. USA 78:996.

Charbonneau, H., and M. J. Cormier, 1979, Purification of plant calmodulin by fluphenazine-Sepharose affinity chromatography, Biochem. Biophys. Res. Commun. 90:1039.

Cherrington, A. D., Aassimacopoulos, F. D., Harper, S. C., Corbin, J. D., Park, C. R., and Exton, J. H., 1976, Studies on the α-adrenergic activation of hepatic glucose output, J. Biol. Chem. 251:5209.

Cheung, W. Y., 1970, Cyclic 3',5'-nucleotide phosphodiesterase:

demonstration of an activator, Biochem. Biophys. Res.
   Commun. 38:533.

Cohen, P., Burchell, A., Foulkes, J. G., Cohen, P. T. W., Nairn,
   A., and Vanaman, T., 1978, Identification of the Ca^{++}-
   dependent modulator protein as the fourth subunit of rabbit
   skeletal muscle phosphorylase kinase, FEBS Letters
   92(2):287.

Condeelis, J. S., 1979, Isolation of concanavalin A caps during
   various stages of formation and their association with
   actin and myosin, J. Cell Biol. 80:751.

Conn, P. M., Chafouleas, J. G., Rogers, D., and Means, A. R.,
   1981, Gonadotropin releasing hormone stimulates calmodulin
   redistribution in rat pituitary, Nature 292:264.

Conn, P. M., Marian, J., McMillian, M., and Rogers, D., 1980,
   Evidence for calcium mediation of gonadotropin releasing
   hormone action in the pituitary, Cell Calcium 1:7.

Crouch, T. H., Holroyde, M. J., Collins, J. H., Solaro, R. J.,
   and Potter, J. D., 1981, Interaction of calmodulin with
   skeletal muscle myosin light chain kinase, Biochemistry
   20:6318.

Cushman, S. W., and Wardzala, L. J., 1980, Potential mechanism
   of insulin action on glucose transport in the isolated rat
   adipose cell, J. Biol. Chem. 255:4758.

Dabrowska, R., Sherry, J. M. F., Aromatorio, D. K., and
   Hartshorne, D. J., 1977, Modulator protein as a component
   of the myosin light chain kinase from chicken gizzard,
   Biochemistry 17:253.

Dedman, J. R., Jackson, R. L., Schreiber, W. E., and Means, A.
   R., 1978, Sequence homology of the Ca^{++}-dependent regulator
   of cyclic nucleotide phosphodiesterase from rat testis with
   other Ca^{++}-binding proteins, J. Biol. Chem. 253:343.

Dedman, J. R., Lin, T., Marcum, J. M., Brinkley, B. R., and
   Means, A. R., 1980, Calmodulin: Its role in the mitotic
   apparatus, in: "Calcium-Binding Proteins: Structure and
   Function", F. L. Siegel, E. Carafoli, R. H. Kretsinger,
   D. H. MacLennan and R. H. Wasserman, eds., p. 181,
   Amsterdam, Elsevier.

Dedman, J. R., Potter, J. D., Jackson, R. L., and Means, A. R.,
   1977, Physicochemical properties of the Ca^{++}-dependent
   regulator proteins of cyclic AMP phosphodiesterase isolated
   from rat testis, J. Biol. Chem. 252:8415.

Dedman, J. R., Welsh, M. J., and Means, A. R., 1978, Ca^{++}-
   dependent regulator: Production and characterization of a
   monospecific antibody, J. Biol. Chem. 253:7515.

deLanerolle, P., Adelstein, R. A., Feramisco, J. R., and
   Burridge, K., 1981, Characterization of antibodies to

smooth muscle myosin kinase and their use in localizing myosin kinase in non-muscle cells, Proc. Natl. Acad. Sci. USA 78:4738.

DeLorenzo, J. R., and Freeman, S. D., 1978, Calcium-dependent neurotransmitter release and protein phosphorylation in synaptic vesicles, Biochem. Biophys. Res. Commun. 80:183.

DeLorenzo, J. R., Freeman, S. D., Yohe, W. B., and Maurer, S. C., 1979, Stimulation of Ca^{++}-dependent neurotransmitter release and presynaptic nerve terminal protein phosphorylation by calmodulin and a calmodulin-like protein isolated from synaptic vesicles, Proc. Natl. Acad. Sci. USA 76:1838.

DeMey, J., Moeremans, M., Gevens, G., Muyudens, R., VanBelle, H., and DeBrabander, M., 1980, Immunocytochemical evidence for the association of calmodulin with microtubules of the mitotic apparatus, in: "Microtubules and Microtubule Inhibitors", M. DeBrabander and J. DeMey, eds., p. 227, Amsterdam, Elsevier.

Epel, D. E., Wallace, R. W., and Cheung, W. Y., 1981, Calmodulin activates NAD kinase of sea urchin eggs: An early event of fertilization, Cell 23:543.

Flanagan, J., and Kock, G. L. E., 1978, Cross-linked surface Ig attaches to actin, Nature 273:278.

Gnegy, M. E., and Lau, Y. S., 1980, Effects of chronic and acute treatment of antipsychotic drugs on calmodulin release from rat striatal membranes, Neuropharmacology 19:319.

Goldstein, J. L., Anderson, R. G. W., and Brown, M. S., 1979, Coated pits, coated vesicles and receptor-mediated endocytosis, Nature 279:679.

Gopinath, R. M., and Vincenzi, F. F., 1977, Phosphodiesterase protein activator mimics red blood cell cytoplasmic activator of (Ca^{++} + Mg^{++}) ATPase, Biochem. Biophys. Res. Commun. 77:1203.

Grab, D. J., Berzins, K., Cohen, R. S., and Siekevitz, P., 1979, Presence of calmodulin in postsynaptic desities isolated from canine cerebral cortex, J. Biol. Chem. 254:8690.

Grand, R. J. A., and Perry, S. V., 1978, The amino acid sequence of the troponin C-like protein (modulator protein) from bovine uterus, FEBS Letters 92:137.

Grand, R. J. A., Shenolikar, S., and Cohen, P., 1981, The amino acid sequence of the δ subunit (calmodulin) of rabbit skeletal muscle phosphorylase kinase, Eur. J. Biochem. 113:359.

Guerriero, V. Jr., Rowley, D. R., and Means, A. R., 1981,

Production and characterization of an antibody to myosin light chain kinase and intracellular localization of the enzyme, Cell 27:449.

Hanbauer, I., Gimble, J., and Lovenberg, W., 1979, Changes in soluble calmodulin following activation of dopamine receptors in rat striatal slices, Neuropharmacology 18:851.

Hanbauer, I., Gimble, J., Sankaran, K., and Sherard, R., 1979a, Modulation of striatal cyclic nucleotide phosphodiesterase by calmodulin: Regulation by opiate and dopamine receptor activation, Neuropharmacology 18:859.

Hanbauer, I., and Phyall, W., 1980, Involvement of calmodulin in the modulation of dopamine receptor function, Adv. Biochem. Psychopharmacol. 24:133.

Hathaway, D. R., and Adelstein, R. S., 1979, Human platelet myosin light chain kinase requires the calcium-binding protein calmodulin for activity, Proc. Natl. Acad. Sci. USA 76:1653.

Hidaka, H., Naka, M., and Yamaki, T., 1980, Effect of novel specific myosin light chain kinase inhibitors on Ca^{++}-activated Mg^{++}-ATPase of chicken gizzard actomyosin, Biochem. Biophys. Res. Commun. 90:694.

Hidaka, H., Yamaki, T., Totsuka, T., and Asano, M., 1979, Selective inhibitors of Ca^{2+}-binding modulator of phosphodiesterase produce vascular relaxation and inhibit actin-myosin interaction, Mol. Pharm. 15:49.

Hinds, T. R., Larsen, F. L., and Vincenzi, F. F., 1978, Plasma membrane Ca^{2+} transport: Stimulation by soluble proteins, Biochem. Biophys. Res. Commun. 81:455.

Ho, H. C., Dasai, R., and Wang, J. G., 1975, Effect of Ca^{++} on the stability of the protein activator of cyclic nucleotide phosphodiesterase, FEBS Letter 50(3):374.

Hutson, N. J., Brumley, F. T., Assimacopoulos, F. D., Harper, S. C., and Exton, J. H., 1976, Studies on the α-adrenergic activation of hepatic glucose output. I. Studies on the α-adrenergic activation of phosphorylase and gluconeogenesis and inactivation of glycogen synthase in isolated rat liver parenchymal cells, J. Biol. Chem. 251:5200.

Jamieson, G. A., Hayes, A., Blum, J. J., and Vanaman, T. C., 1980, Structure and function relationships among calmodulins from divergent eukaryotic organisms, in: "Calcium Binging Proteins: Structure and Function", F. L. Siegel, E. Carafoli, R. H. Kretsinger, D. H. MacLennan and R. H. Wasserman, eds., p. 165, Amsterdam, Elsevier.

Jamieson, G. A., and Vanaman, T C., 1979, Calcium-dependent affinity chromatography of calmodulin on an immobilized phenothiazine, Biochem. Biophys. Res. Commun. 980:1048.

Jarrett, H. W. and Penniston, J. T., 1977, Partial purification of the Ca^{++}-Mg^{++} ATPase activator from human erythrocytes: Its similarity to the activator of 3',5'-cyclic nucleotide phosphodiesterase, Biochem. Biophys. Res. Commun. 77:1210.

Kakiuchi, S., and Yamagaki, R., 1970, Calcium-dependent phospho-diesterase activity and its activating factor (PAF) from brain. Studies on cyclic 3',5'-nucleotide phospodiesterse (III), Biochem. Biophys. Res. Commun. 41:1104.

Katz, S., and Remtulla, M. A., 1978, Phosphodiesterase protein activator stimulates calcium transport in cardiac micro-somal preparations enriched in sarcoplasmic reticulum, Biochem. Biophys. Res. Commun. 83:1373.

Keppens, S., Vaindenheede, J. R., and DeWolf, H., 1977, On the role of calcium as second messenger in liver for the hormonally induced activation of glycogen phosphorylase, Biochim. Biophys. Acta. 496:448.

Klee, C. B., 1977, Conformational transition accompanying the binding of Ca^{++} to the protein activator of 3',5'-cyclic adenosine monophosphate phosphodiesterase, Biochemistry 16(5):1017.

Kretsinger, R. H., 1976, Calcium-binding proteins, Ann. Rev. Biochem. 45:239.

Kretsinger, R. H., 1979, The informational role of calcium in the cytosol, in: "Advances in Cyclic Nucleotide Research", Vol. 11, P. Greengard and G. A. Robison, eds., p. 1, Raven Press, New York.

LaPorte, D. C., Gidwitz, S., Weber, M. J., and Storm, D. R., 1979, Relationship between changes in the calcium-dependent regulatory protein and adenylate cyclase during viral transformation, Biochem. Biophys. Res. Commun. 86:1169.

LaPorte, D. C., Wierman, B. M., and Storm, D. R., 1980, Calcium-induced exposure of a hydrophobic surface on camodulin, Biochemistry 19:3814.

LeBreton, G. C., Dinerstein, R. J., Roth, L. J., and Feenberg, H., 1976, Direct evidence for intracellular divalent cation redistribution associated with platelet shape change, Biochem. Biophys. Res. Commun. 71:362.

LePeuch, C., Haiech, J., and Demaille, J. G., 1979, Concerted regulation of cardiac sarcoplasmic reticulum calcium transport by cyclic adenosine monophosphate-dependent and calcium-calmodulin-dependent phosphorylations, Biochemistry 18:5150.

Lin, C. T., Dedman, J. R., Brinkley, B. R., and Means, A. R., 1980, Localization of calmodulin in rat cerebellum by immunoelectron microscopy, J. Cell Biol. 85:473.

Luthra, M. G., Au, K. S., and Hanahan, D. J., 1977, Purification of an activator of human erythrocyte membrane ($Ca^{++} + Mg^{++}$) ATPase, Biochem. Biophys. Res. Commun. 77:678.

Lynch, T. J., Tallant, E. A., and Cheung, W. Y., 1976, Ca^{++}-dependent formation of brain adenylate cyclase-protein activator complex, Biochem. Biophys. Res. Commun. 68(2):616.

Marcum, M., Dedman, J. R., Brinkley, B. R., and Means, A. R., 1978, Regulation of microtubule polymerization by rat testis calcium-dependent regulator protein, Proc. Natl. Acad. Sci. USA 75:3771.

Means, A. R., and Dedman, J. R., 1980, Calmodulin: An intracellular calcium receptor, Nature 285:73.

Means, A. R., Tash, J. S., and Chafouleas, J. G., 1982, Physiological implications of the presence, distribution and regulation of calmodulin in eukaryotic cells, Physiol. Rev. 62:1.

Mescher, M. F., Jose, M. J. L., and Balk, S. P., 1981, Actin-containing matrix associated with the plasma membrane of murine tumor and lymphoid cells, Nature 289:139.

Morgan, M., Perry, S. V., and Ottaway, J., 1976, Myosin light chain phosphatase, Biochem. J. 157:687.

Munjaal, R. P., Chandra, T., Woo, S. L. C., Dedman, J. R., and Means, A. R., 1981, A cloned calmodulin structural gene probe is complementary to DNA sequences from diverse species, Proc. Natl. Acad. Sci. USA 78:2330.

Naccache, P. H., Volpi, M., Showell, J. H., Becker, E. L., and Sha'afi, R. I., 1979, Chemotatic factor-induced release of membrane calcium in rabbit neutrophils, Science 203:461.

Pato, M. D., and Adelstein, R. S., 1980, Dephosphorylation of the 20,000-dalton light chain of myosin by two different phosphatases from smooth muscle, J. Biol. Chem. 255:5535.

Pershadsingh, H. A., McDaniel, M. L., Landt, M., Bry, C. G., Lacy, P. E., and McDonald, J. M., 1980, Ca^{2+}-activated ATPase and ATP-dependent calmodulin-stimulated Ca^{2+} transport in islet cell plasma membrane, Nature 288:492.

Pershadsingh, H. A., and McDonald, J. M., 1980, A high affinity calcium-stimulated magnesium-dependent adenosine triphosphatease in rat adipocyte plasma membranes, J. Biol. Chem. 255:4087.

Pichard, A. L., and Cheung, W. Y., 1977, Cyclic 3',5'-nucleotide phosphodiesterase stimulation of bovine brain cytoplasmic enzyme by lysophosphatidyl choline, J. Biol. Chem. 252:4872.

Pires, E. M. V., and Perry, S. V., 1977, Purification and properties of myosin light chain kinase from fast skeletal muscle, Biochem. J. 167:137.

Rasmussen, H., 1970, Cell communication, calcium ion, cyclic
    adenosine monophosphate, Science 170:404.
Rasmussen, H., Goodman, D. B. P., Friedman, N., Allen,
    J. E., and Kurvkawa, K., 1976, Ionic control of metabo-
    lism, in: "Handbook of Physiology-Endocrinology".
    Vol. VII. p. 225. American Physiological Society,
    Washington, D.C.
Rebhun, L. I., 1977, Cyclic nucleotides, calcium and cell divi-
    sion, Int. Rev. Cytol. 49:1-54.
Richman, P., 1978, Conformation-dependent acetylation and nitra-
    tion of the protein activator of cyclic adenosine 3',5'-
    monophosphate phosphodiesterase. Selective nitration of
    tyrosine residue 138, Biochemistry 17:3001.
Salisbury, J. L., Condeelis, J. S., and Satir, P., 1980, Role
    of coated vesicles, microfilaments and calmodulin in
    receptor-mediated endocytosis by cultured B lymphoblastoic
    cells, J. Cell Biol. 87:132.
Salmon, E. D., and Segall, R. R., 1980, Calcium-labile mitotic
    spindles isolated from sea urchin eggs (Lytechinus
    variepatus), J. Cell Biol. 85:355.
Schulman, H., and Greengard, P., 1977, Stimulation of brain
    membrane protein phosphorylation by calcium and an endo-
    genous heat-stable protein, Nature 271:478.
Schulman, H., and Greengard, P., 1978, Ca^{++}-dependent protein
    phosphorylation system in membranes from various tissues,
    and its activation by "calcium-dependent regulator." Proc.
    Natl. Acad. Sci. USA 75:5432.
Seeman, P., 1972, The membrane actions of anesthetics and tran-
    quilizers, Pharmacol. Rev. 24:53.
Sieghart, W., Forn, J., and Greengard, P., 1979, Ca^{++} and cyclic
    AMP regulate phosphorylation of the same two membrane-
    associated proteins specific to nerve tissue, Proc. Natl.
    Acad. Sci. USA 76:2475.
Smoake, J. A., and Solomon, S. S., 1980, Subcellular shifts in
    cyclic AMP phosphodiesterase and its calcium-dependent
    regulator in liver: Role of diabetes, Biochem. Biophys.
    Res. Commun. 94:242.
Soderling, T. R., Sheorain, V. S., and Ericsson, L. H., 1979,
    Phosphorylation of glycogen synthase by phosphorylase
    kinase, FEBS Letters 106:181.
Strivastava, A. K., Waisman, D. M., Brostrom, C. O., and
    Soderling, T. R., 1979, Stimulation of glycogen synthase
    phosphorylation by calcium-dependent regulator protein,
    J. Biol. Chem. 254:583.
Stull, J. T., 1980, Phosphorylation of contractile proteins
    in relation to muscle function, Adv. Cyclic Nucl.
    Res. 13:39.

Suzuki, K., and Kono, T., 1980, Evidence that insulin causes
    translocation of glucose transport activity to the plasma
    membrane from an intracellular storage site, J. Biol.
    Chem. 77:2542.
Tanaka, T., and Hidaka, H., 1980, Hydrophobic regions function
    in calmodulin enzyme(s) interactions, J. Biol. Chem. 255:
    11078.
Tash, J. S., Means, A. R., Brinkley, B. R., Dedman, J. R., and
    Cox, S. M., 1980, Cyclic nucleotide and Ca^{2+} regulation
    of microtubule initiation and elongation, in: "Micro-
    tubules and Microtubule Inhibitors", M. DeBrabander and
    J. DeMey, eds., p. 269, Amsterdam, Elsevier.
Terasima, T., and Tolmach, L. J., 1961, Changes in X-ray
    sensitivity of HeLa cells during the division cycle,
    Nature 190:1210.
Towbin, H., Staehelin, T. and Gordon, J., 1979, Electrophoretic
    transfer of proteins from polyacrylamide gels to nitro-
    cellulose sheets: Procedure and some applications, Proc.
    Natl. Acad. Sci. USA 76:4350.
Valverde, I., Vandermeers, A., Anjaneyulu, R., and Maliasse,
    W. J., 1979, Calmodulin activation of adenylate cyclase in
    pancreatic islets, Science 206:225.
Van Eldik, L. J., and Watterson, D. M., 1981, Reproducible pro-
    duction of anti-serum against vertebrate calmodulin and
    determination of the immunoreactive site, J. Biol. Chem.
    256:4205.
Wallace, R. W., and Cheung, W. Y., 1978, Calmodulin: Production
    of an antibody in rabbit and development of a radioimmuno-
    assay, J. Biol. Chem. 254:6564.
Walsh, M. P., Cavadore, J. C., Vallet, B., and Demaille, J. G.,
    1980, Calmodulin-dependent light chain kinase from cardiac
    and smooth muscle: A comparative study, Cancer J. Biochem.
    58:229.
Watterson, D. M., Sharief, F., and Vanaman, T. C., 1980, The
    complete amino acid sequence of the Ca^{2+}-dependent modula-
    tor protein (calmodulin) of bovine brain, J. Biol. Chem.
    255:962.
Watterson, D. M., Van Eldik, L. J., Smith, R. E., and Vanaman,
    T. C., 1976, Calcium-dependent regulatory protein of cyclic
    nucleotide metabolism in normal and transformed chick
    embryo fibroblasts, Proc. Natl. Acad. Sci. USA 73:2711.
Weiss, B., and Levin, R. M., 1978, Mechanism for selectively
    inhibiting the activation of the cyclic nucleotide phos-
    phodiesterase and adenylate cyclase by antipsychotic
    agents, Adv. Cycl. Nucl. Res. 9:285.

Welsh, M. J., Dedman, J. R., Brinkley, B. R., and Means, A. R.,
     1978, Calcium-dependent regulator protein: Localization
     in mitotic apparatus of eucaryotic cells, Proc. Natl. Acad.
     Sci. USA 75:1867.
Welsh, M. J., Dedman, J. R., Brinkley, B. R., and Means, A. R.,
     1979, Tubulin and calmodulin: Effects of microtubule and
     microfilament inhibitors on localization in the mitotic
     apparatus, J. Cell Biol. 81:624.
Wolf, H., and Hofmann, F., 1980, Purification of myosin light
     chain kinase from bovine cardiac muscle, Proc. Natl. Acad.
     Sci. USA 77:5855.
Wolff, D. J., and Brostrom, C. O., 1976, Ca^{2+}-dependent cyclic
     nucleotide phosphodiesterase from brain: Identification
     of phospholipids and calcium-independent activators, Arch.
     Biochem. Biophys. 173:720.
Wong, P. Y. K., and Cheung, W. Y., 1979, Calmodulin stimulates
     human platelet phospholipase A_2, Biochem. Biophys. Res.
     Commun. 90:473.
Wood, J. G., Wallace, R. W., Whitaker, J. N., and Cheung, W.
     Y., 1980, Immunocytochemical localization of calmodulin
     and a heat-labile calmodulin-binding protein (CaM-BP$_{80}$)
     in basal ganglia of mouse brain, J. Cell Biol. 84:66-76.
Yagi, K., Yazawa, M., Kakiuchi, S., Ohshima, M., Uenishi, K.,
     1978, Identification of an activator protein for myosin
     light chain kinase as the Ca^{++}-dependent modulator protein,
     J. Biol. Chem. 253:1338.
Yamauchi, T., and Fujisawa, H., 1979, Most of the Ca^{++}-depend-
     ent endogenous phosphorylation of rat brain cytosol pro-
     teins requires Ca^{++}-dependent regulator protein, Biochem.
     Biophys. Res. Commun. 909:1172.
Yazawa, M., Yagi, K., Toda, H., Kondo, K., Narita, K., Yamazaki,
     R., Sobue, K., Kakiuchi, S., Nagao, S., and Nozawa, Y.,
     1981, The amino acid sequence of the Tetrahymena calmodulin
     which specifically interacts with guanylate cyclase,
     Biochem. Biophys. Res. Commun. 99:1051.

DISCUSSION

WELLS: In the clipping of calmodulin by a specific
protease between MET72 and MET73 when cells reenter the
cell cycle, do you attach any physical or biological
significance to the clip occurring in domain II thus
allowing the C-terminus to be released from the cell with
intact domain III and IV?

MEANS: These MET residues have been shown by physical methods to be particularly reactive to solvation and modification. Limited exposure to proteases or oxidation clips here. Fischer's lab has isolated and sequenced "half-calmodulin" from human brain autopsy material. This molecule is the C-terminal half. Whitfield and colleagues have reported the presence of a protein called "oncomodulin". This protein will stimulate the reentry of plateau cells when added to cell culture medium. We think that the half-calmodulin and oncomodulin are the same molecule. If so this suggests an autocrine function for a proteolytically generated calmodulin fragment.

ROY: How many genes for calmodulin are present in the chicken genome and which ones are ordinarily expressed?

MEANS: There appears to be one expressed gene. We call this gene cCM 2. It contains at least three intervening sequences and is expressed in all tissues examined. There is also one pseudogene that could also be processed. It contains no intervening sequences and, if expressed at all, this appears to be restricted to skeletal muscle.

LABRIE: Have you obtained evidence for specific control of the level of the three species of calmodulin mRNA at different phases of the cell cycle?

MEANS: Dr. Lagace's preliminary data suggest the presence of all mature forms of calmodulin mRNA at all phases of the cell cycle. Since all are apparently derived from a single precursor and all code for the same protein, we presume that the multiple forms are generated by differential polyadenylation in a random fashion.

FRENCH: What are your ideas regarding the common denominator of the increased levels of calmodulin in transformed cells?

MEANS: Most likely the increased levels of calmodulin are a consequence rather than a cause of transformation. It is possible that the increase could be at least partially due to the decreased cell cycle time, since calmodulin is synthesized at the G_1/S boundary. It could also be that calmodulin is one of a cluster of host cell genes close to the site of integration of the viral genome. If so, it might be modulated by viral promoters such as that of the SRC gene of Rous sarcoma virus.

FUNCTIONAL COMMUNICATION BETWEEN THE SERTOLI AND LEYDIG CELLS

Richard M. Sharpe[a] and Focko F. G. Rommerts[b]

[a]MRC Reproductive Biology Unit
Centre for Reproductive Biology
37 Chalmers Street
Edinburgh EH3 9EW, Scotland, U. K.
[b]Department of Biochemistry
Erasmus University
Rotterdam, The Netherlands

1.   The Basis for Sertoli-Leydig Cell Communication

All organs within the body are composed of cells of
several different types which together perform the various
functions of that organ. It is obvious that if the organ is
to function normally, then the activities of the different
cell types must be co-ordinated and the most logical way in
which this could be achieved is by direct communication
between the various cell types. In this context, the idea
that the Sertoli cells should communicate with the Leydig
cells within the testis is therefore far from unique, and yet
this pathway has been all but ignored by the majority of
workers engaged on research into testicular function. This
neglect is all the more remarkable when it is considered that
fertility is critically dependent on the link between Sertoli
and Leydig cells, in that spermatogenesis is regulated by the
Sertoli cell only under the driving influence of testosterone
from the Leydig cells (Hansson et al., 1978; Ritzen et al.,
1981). Because of this dependence it seems essential that
the Sertoli cells should have some means of communicating
with the Leydig cells to ensure the optimum supply of testosterone for maintenance of spermatogenesis. This paper
assesses the possible factors that might be involved in this
communication and gives particular attention to the possibility that the Sertoli cells may locally regulate testosterone
production by the Leydig cells via secretion of a luteinizing

267

hormone-releasing hormone (LHRH)-like peptide. However, before tackling this problem directly, it is worthwhile first considering the present evidence for functional communication between the Sertoli and Leydig cells.

2.   Evidence for Sertoli-Leydig Cell Communication

This evidence is indirect and is derived from two areas of information which demonstrate changes in Leydig cell structure and/or function following treatment with follicle-stimulating hormone (FSH) or as the result of dysfunction of the seminiferous tubules.

2.1. Effects of FSH on the Leydig Cell

Although there is overwhelming evidence that FSH acts exclusively on Sertoli cells within the testis (Means et al., 1976), there is nevertheless clear evidence that FSH can exert stimulatory effects on Leydig cell function (reviewed by Sharpe, 1982a). Most of the available information comes from studies of hypophysectomized immature rats in which FSH treatment for 5 or more days results not only in seminiferous tubule enlargement but also in enhanced testosterone respon-siveness of the testis to LH and an increase in the number of testicular LH-receptors, both of which represent Leydig cell changes (e.g. Odell et al., 1973; Chen et al., 1976; van Beurden et al., 1976); similar treatment with the amounts of luteinizing hormone (LH) known to contaminate the various FSH preparations was without effect. Unfortunately, it is not known if these effects of FSH represent enhancement of the functional capacity of the Leydig cells already present or whether they reflect an FSH-induced increase in the number of Leydig cells per testis. Nevertheless, the important point is that because FSH works only through the Sertoli cell, then its effects on the Leydig cell must be due to the secretion by the Sertoli cells of one of more factors affecting the Leydig cells, and this might be important in co-ordinating the pubertal development of these two cell types.

2.2. Effects of Seminiferous Tubule Damage on the Leydig Cell

The second area of evidence for Sertoli-Leydig cell communication is based on. observations made following the induction of seminiferous tubule damage in adult rats by one of several experimental procedures (e.g. cryptorchidism, efferent duct ligation, X-irradiation, local heating,

treatment with various drugs, deprivation of vitamin A or E).
In these situations there is inhibition of spermatogenesis
and alteration of Sertoli cell structure and function (Hagenas
and Ritzen, 1976; Kerr et al., 1979a), and these changes are
associated with marked alteration of Leydig cell structure
and function. The latter include cellular enlargement and
hyperplasia, hypertrophy of the cellular organelles involved
in steroidogenesis coupled with enhancement of the steroidogenic capacity of the cells and a loss of membrane LH-receptors (e.g. Kerr et al., 1979b; de Kretser et al, 1979; Rich
et al., 1979; reviewed by Sharpe, 1982a). These changes are
typical of 'stimulated' cells and are identical to those
observed following continued treatment with LH or human
chrionic gonadotropin (hCG).

Although bilaterally-induced seminiferous tubule damage
is accompanied by a three- to four-fold increase in the serum
levels of LH, it is now believed that this increase is not
responsible for the Leydig cell changes. This is partly
because the changes in Leydig cell structure and function
precede the increase in LH levels (Risbridger et al., 1981a),
but primarily because precisely the same Leydig cell changes
are observed in rats with unilateral seminiferous tubule
damage, except that they are restricted to the 'damaged'
testis and are not associated with any major increase in the
serum levels of LH (Risbridger et al., 1981b,c). Finally,
the most convincing piece of evidence comes from a study by
Aoki and Fawcett (1978). These authors implanted threads
impregnated with anti-androgens within the rat testis and
observed seminiferous tubule damage locally around these
implants, presumably due to interruption of androgen action
on the Sertoli cells. Associated with this damage there was
massive hyperplasia of the Leydig cells, a change which
occurred only in the immediate vicinity of the implants and
which was not observed elsewhere in the implanted testis or
in the contralateral testis.

What the above findings demonstrate is that any treatment
which interferes with normal seminiferous tubule function
results in associated changes in Leydig cell structure and
function. As it is the Sertoli cells which are primarily
responsible for the maintenance of seminiferous tubule
function (Ritzen et al., 1981), it is most likely that it is
the altered function of the Sertoli cells in these situations
that is responsible for the Leydig cell changes. As the
latter are indicative of 'increased stimulation', it is

perhaps most logical to conclude that the Sertoli cells secrete more of a 'Leydig cell-stimulating factor' although as good a case can be made for decreased secretion of a 'Leydig cell inhibiting factor' by the Sertoli cells. As yet there is no evidence as to which, if either, of these possibilities is correct. But the important point that these observations make is that Sertoli and Leydig cell function are inextricably linked. Having established this point we now go on to consider what factors might be involved in this relationship.

3.   Possible Factors Involved in Sertoli-Leydig Cell
       Communication

Although the Sertoli cells secrete a wide range of proteins and other factors (e.g. Rommerts et al., 1978; DePhilip et al., 1982), the function of all but a few of these are unknown and only two have been dmeonstrated to exert an effect on the Leydig cell. These are estradiol and an LHRH-like peptide. However, it should be noted that although other Sertoli cell products such as inhibin and androgen-binding protein (ABP) are not believed to exert any direct effect on the Leydig cells there is in fact no published evidence which precludes their possible involvement.

Of the two factors secreted by the Sertoli cell and which do exert effects on the Leydig cell, only one is a serious candidate in the developed testis. For although the Sertoli cells secrete estradiol (e.g. Dorrington and Armstrong, 1975; Rommerts et al., 1978) and this steroid has a potent inhibitory effect on Leydig cell function (e.g. Nozu et al., 1982), it is now established that the ability of the Sertoli cells to secrete estradiol is restricted to the immature testis and disappears at around 20 days of age (e.g. Pomerantz, 1979; Rommerts et al., 1982). Therefore, estradiol is unlikely to be important as a means of communication between the Sertoli and Leydig cells once testicular development begins and full spermatogenesis is established. In contrast, there is now very clear evidence that 'LHRH' is a potent regulator of the Leydig cell in the adult testis, and the majority of the rest of this paper is directed towards this peptide as a possible agent in Sertoli-Leydig cell communication.

4.   'Testicular LHRH' as a Communicator between Sertoli and
      Leydig Cells

In the last three years it has been established that
LHRH and its agonists can exert direct effects on the ovary
and testis of several mammalian species (see reviews by Hsueh
and Jones, 1981; Sharpe, 1982b). These effects are mediated
via receptors which are specific for LHRH and its analogues,
and in the testis there is unequivocal evidence that these
receptors are located only on the Leydig cells (e.g. Bourne
et al., 1980: Clayton et al., 1980; Sharpe and Fraser, 1980a).
The function of these receptors is to detect an LHRH-like
peptide which is produced and secreted within the testis.
This peptide can be extracted in small amounts from seminiferous tubules or whole testes (Sharpe et al., 1981; 1982b), is
secreted into the interstitial fluid (IF) that bathes the
Leydig cells (Sharpe and Fraser, 1980b) and is produced in
small amounts by Sertoli cell cultures (de Jong et al., 1979;
Sharpe et al., 1981; 1982b). However, there is as yet no
absolute proof that the Sertoli cell is the exclusive or even
the most important source of this material in the testis.

The information available on the nature of 'testicular
LHRH' is extremely limited, but there is evidence that it
differs immunologically from hypothalamic LHRH (Dutlow and
Millar, 1981; Sharpe et al., 1982b). Unfortunately, there
are major problems in the extraction, identification and
characterization of 'testicular LHRH', primarily because it
is present in the testis in very small amounts and because it
appears to be labile and highly susceptible to enzymatic
breakdown. But in the context of the present paper, the most
significant factor is that this peptide appears to be produced
by the Sertoli cells and acts specifically on the Leydig
cells, and the important question to ask is what are the
biological consequences of this interaction? Fortunately,
because native LHRH and its synthetic and more powerful
agonistic analogues interact with Leydig cell LHRH-receptors,
we are provided with the means of studying the biological
actions of 'testicular LHRH' even in the absence of the
purified native compound.

4.1. The Biological Actions of LHRH on the Leydig Cell

Initial studies demonstrated that LHRH and its agonists
caused gross inhibitory changes in Leydig cell function

both in vitro (Hsueh et al., 1981) and in vivo in gonadotro-
pin-treated hypophysectomized rats (Hsueh and Erickson, 1979;
Bambino et al., 1980). These changes include a reduction in
testis weight, a loss of LH-receptors and a massive reduction
in testosterone responsiveness to LH and hCG. Typical
findings are shown in Table I. In this experiment, 55-day-old
male rats which had been hypophysectomized three days earlier
were treated daily for 6 consecutive days with either vehicle
(controls), 10 IU hCG or 10 IU hCG together with 1 µg LHRH
agonist (D-Ser-t-bu[6],des-Gly-NH[10]) LHRH ethylamide; Hoechst,
A. G.). It is evident that the gross stimulatory effect of
hCG on testosterone levels in testicular interstitial fluid
(IF) and in peripheral blood are reduced by 80-90% following
concomitant treatment with LHRH agonist, an effect that was
accompanied by a significant reduction in testis weight.

Table I. Changes in Testis Weight and Testosterone Levels
Following Treatment of Hypophysectomized Male Rats for 6 Days
with Either Vehicle (Controls), hCG (10 IU) or hCG Together
with LHRH Agonist (LHRH-A; 1 µg).

Daily treatment	Right testis weight (mg)	Testosterone concentration (ng/ml)	
		Testicular interstitial fluid	Peripheral serum
Vehicle	920 ± 25	24 ± 4	0.4 ± 0.1
hCG	757 ± 57	1134 ± 123	33.8 ± 5.0
hCG+LHRH-A	601 ± 48[a]	171 ± 34[b]	4.1 ± 1.4[b]

Values are the mean ± S.D. for 5 rats per group.
[a]P < 0.01
[b]P < 0.001 in comparison with rats treated with hCG alone.
Details on preparation of testicular interstitial fluid can
be found in Sharpe and Fraser (1980b).

However, to induce these inhibitory effects on Leydig
cell function in vivo, at least 2 days' continuous exposure
to LHRH agonist is required (Bambino et al., 1980), and
similarly in vitro, periods of exposure of 4 or more days to
LHRH agonist are necessary to achieve inhibitory effects
(Hsueh et al., 1981). Whether these inhibitory effects have
any physiological significance is now open to doubt, because

recent findings have demonstrated that the initial effect of LHRH on the Leydig cell is to stimulate rather than to inhibit steroidogenesis.

4.2. Stimulation of Testosterone Secretion by LHRH In Vitro

Incubation of collagenase-dispersed Leydig cells for 4 hr in the presence of increasing concentrations of either LHRH or LHRH agonist results in dose-dependent stimulation of testosterone secretion (Fig. 1). Both peptides gave comparable degrees of maximal stimulation but doses of LHRH nearly 1000 times higher than those of the agonist were required to achieve a given level of stimulation, a difference which is consistent with the affinities of the two peptides for the Leydig cell LHRH-receptor (Sharpe and Fraser, 1980a). As the cells used for these studies contained many testicular cell types in addition to Leydig cells, we also tested whether LHRH agonist stimulated testosterone secretion by Leydig cells purified on a 0-90% continuous Percoll gradient. We used essentially the same methods as those described by Cooke et al., (1981), and after fractionation identified three main bands of nucleated cells with the approximate densities shown in Table II. Aliquots of equal numbers (0.14×10^6) of nucleated cells from each of the three bands were then incubated for 4 hr in vitro in the presence or absence of an excess of LHRH agonist or hCG and testosterone production assessed. It is clear that as Leydig cell purity increased from band I to band III (as measured by hCG-receptor numbers) so did the testosterone responsiveness to LHRH agonist and hCG (Table II).

LHRH agonist can also enhance testosterone responsiveness to LH or hCG in short-term (4-20 hr) incubation or cultures of Leydig cells (Hunter et al., 1982; Sharpe and Cooper, 1982), although it should be noted that whilst this interactive effect with gonadotropins has been demonstrated repeatedly, it is inconsistent, and the reasons for this variation are not yet clear.

4.3. Stimulation of Testosterone Secretion by LHRH in Hypophysectomized Rats

In keeping with the above in vitro findings, stimulation of testosterone secretion by LHRH agonist can also be demonstrated in vivo in hypophysectomized rats (Sharpe et al., 1982a). Thus, a single injection of LHRH agonist (1 µg) into

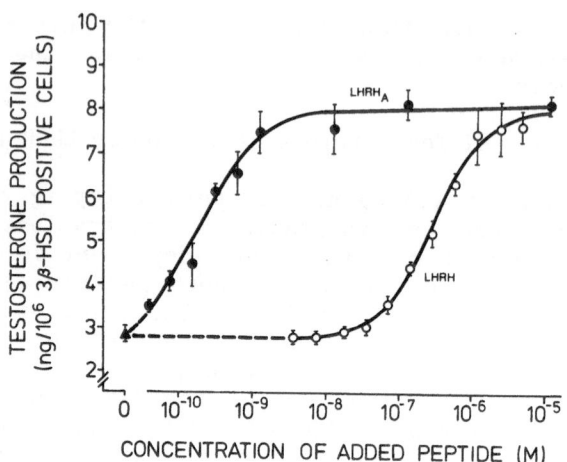

Figure 1. Dose-dependent stimulation of testosterone production by isolated Leydig cells in vitro following incubation
with LHRH or an LHRH agonist. Values are the mean ± S.D. of
triplicate incubations (reproduced with permission from
Sharpe and Cooper, 1982).

hypophysectomized 55-day-old male rats resulted 2 hr later in
a 10- to 15-fold increase in the serum levels of testosterone
when compared with vehicle-injected control rats (Fig. 2).
The magnitude of this increase was such that testosterone
levels were higher than those found in normal, untreated rats
of this age and strain. However, this stimulatory effect
disappeared with repeated exposure to LHRH agonist and by day
6 of treatment there was no increase in the serum levels of
testosterone following injection of the peptide; this loss of
responsiveness was a consequence of the peptide injections as
animals which had been treated with the vehicle for 5 days
and then injected with LHRH agonist on the sixth day showed a
large increase in testosterone levels (Fig. 2). This
'desensitization' of the Leydig cells to repeated stimulation
by LHRH agonist occurred after using a treatment schedule
similar to that used to demonstrate inhibitory effects in
vivo (see section 4.1), and it seems likely that the switch
in action of LHRH agonist from stimulatory to inhibitory is a
consequence of the duration of exposure to the peptide (see
also Hunter et al., 1982).

Table II. Stimulatory Effect of LHRH Agonist (LHRH-A, 10^{-7}M) and hCG (10^{-8}M) on Testosterone Production by Percoll-Purified Leydig Cells.

Cell band	(density)	hCG-Receptors (pg ^{125}I-hCG bound) 10^6 cells	Testosterone production (ng/10^6 nucleated cells)		
			Basal	+LHRH-A	+hCG
I	(1.05g)	195±15	1.2±0.2	0.9±0.2	5.6±0.2[b]
II	(1.06g)	711±34	5.2±0.1	6.9±0.4[a]	23.5±0.4[b]
III	(1.073-1.08g)	1632±45	17.0±0.7	32.7±1.7[b]	139.0±6.8[b]

Values are the mean ± S.D. for triplicate incubations.
[a] $P < 0.01$
[b] $P < 0.001$ compared with respective basal secretion.
hCG-receptor binding was measured as described elsewhere (Sharpe and Fraser, 1980a), following incubation of aliquots of 0.1×10^6 nucleated cells in the presence of a saturating concentration (100 ng/ml) of ^{125}I-labelled hCG. Testosterone production was assessed as described elsewhere (Sharpe and Cooper, 1982).

4.3. Stimulation of Testosterone Secretion by LHRH in Intact Rats

Under physiological conditions i.e., in the normal intact male rat, the action of LHRH agonist on the Leydig cell is also stimulatory. This was demonstrated by measuring levels of testosterone in testicular IF following intra-testicular injection of different doses of LHRH agonist. The obvious problem with this approach is that any of the injected peptide which diffuses or leaks from the site of injection into the peripheral circulation may cause release of pituitary LH and this will have a confounding effect by stimulating

steroidogenesis itself. To control for this possibility we
have injected the LHRH agonist only into the right testis and
injected the left testis with the injection vehicle alone.
Any stimulation of testosterone secretion resulting from
release of pituitary LH can thus be controlled for using the
left testis.

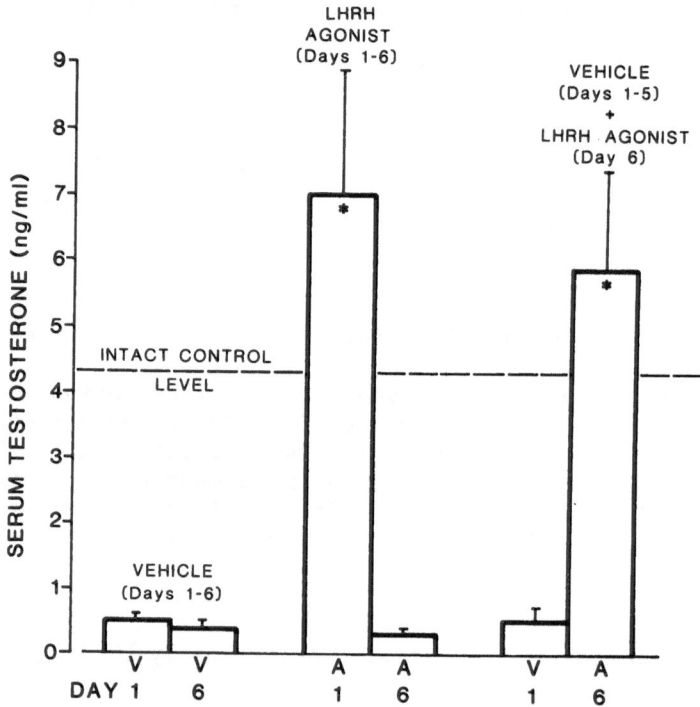

Figure 2. Serum levels of testosterone in hypophysectomized
rats following daily treatment for 1 or 6 days with either 1
μg LHRH agonist (A) or the injection vehicle (V) alone. Rats
were aged 55 days, had been hypophysectomized 3 days earlier
and were injected according to the schedules indicated above
the columns. Animals were bled from the tail vein 2 hr after
injection on days 1 and 6, and values represent the mean ±
S.D. for 4 or 5 rats per group.   *P < 0.001 compared with
vehicle-injected (control) rats.

Intra-testicular injection of doses of LHRH agonist ranging from 0.1 to 10 ng resulted 2 hr later in a significant ($P < 0.001$) increase in the IF levels of testosterone in the right testis, when compared with values for the left testis, a difference that was maintained until 4 hr for the 10 and 1 ng doses of peptide (Fig. 3). Neither of the two lower doses of LHRH agonist caused significant LH release (data not shown) and this was reflected by the fact that testosterone levels in IF from the left (control) testes of these animals did not differ from values for control animals (i.e. injected bilaterally intra-testicularly with the vehicle) at 2 hr and were slightly lowered compared with controls at 4 hr (Fig. 3). In animals injected intra-testicularly with 10 ng LHRH agonist, the serum levels of LH were raised 4- to 5-fold at both 2 and 4 hr and this was reflected in a massive increase in the levels of testosterone in IF from the left (control) testes of these rats. But despite this stimulatory effect of LH, testosterone levels in the right (LHRH agonist-injected) testis were still raised significantly (Fig. 3).

Therefore, these results confirm findings obtained with isolated Leydig cells in vitro and with hypophysectomized rats in vivo, in showing that the initial effect of LHRH and its agonists on the Leydig cell in intact rats is to stimulate testosterone secretion. But perhaps more importantly, the results in intact rats demonstrate that even when endogenous LH levels are raised considerably (following intra-testicular injection of 10 ng LHRH agonist), LHRH agonist can still cause significant stimulation of testosterone secretion via direct effects on the Leydig cell. This suggests that secretion of 'testicular LHRH' has the potential to locally regulate the testicular steroidogenic response to LH, and this has considerable implications, first with respect to the postulated attributes of a Sertoli-Leydig cell messenger (see Sections 1 and 2), and second, with respect to the physiological significance of such communication (see Section 6).

5.   Other Sertoli Cell Factors Affecting Leydig Cell Function

Because the link between the Sertoli and Leydig cells is so important with respect to maintenance of fertility, we should perhaps not be surprised if there are several pathways by which the Sertoli cells regulate the Leydig cells. We have therefore examined whether spent media from Sertoli cell

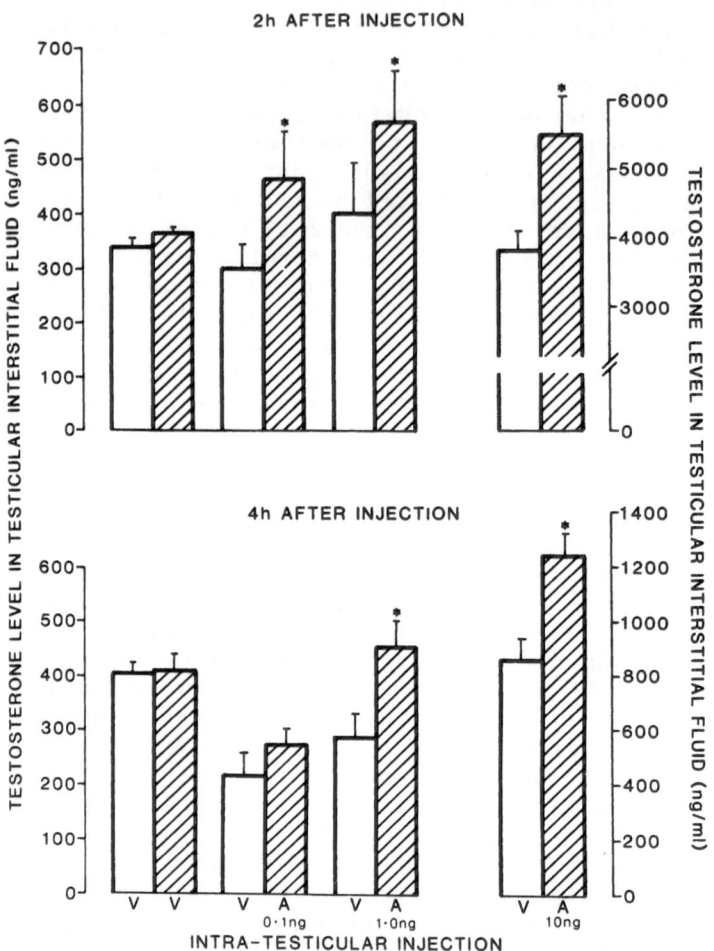

Figure 3.   Testosterone levels in testicular interstitial
fluid (IF) following unilateral intra-testicular injection of LHRH agonist (A) or the injection vehicle alone
(V = 0.05 ml saline containing 1 mg/ml gelatin and 5 mg/ml
albumin). Injections were given under light ether anaesthesia
and IF was collected as described elsewhere (Sharpe and
Fraser, 1980b). Values are shown as the mean ± S.E.M.
(N = 4) for left (open columns) and right (hatched columns)
testes.
*P < 0.001, compared with values for corresponding left
testis.

cultures (SCCM) or whether testicular IF from control and hCG-treated (i.e. stimulated) rats contains any factor(s) capable of influencing testosterone secretion by collagenase-dispersed Leydig cells in vitro. Testicular IF was used because it bathes the Leydig cells and separates them from the Sertoli cells, so that any factor secreted by the latter and acting on the Leydig cells must first be secreted into this medium. However, because IF contains steroids in high concentration together with endogenous gonadotrophins (and exogenous hCG), all of which will affect Leydig cell function, these were first removed. Thus the IF was acidified with an equal volume of IM acetic acid, boiled for 10 min, extracted four times in succession with 12 vol diethyl ether and then lyophilized and reconstituted. Furthermore, as IF is formed by capillary filtration from serum (Setchell and Sharpe, 1981), it is also possible that non-specific factors present in serum might be responsible for any effects observed, and so to control for this we used serum from hCG-treated rats which had been subjected to the same preparative procedures as described for IF. The SCCM had no hormone additions and contained no detectable testosterone (< 50 pg/ml).

Using 4 hr incubations of collagenase-dispersed Leydig cells, the effects of IF and SCCM were tested on basal testosterone secretion, maximally-stimulated testosterone secretion (i.e. in the presence of 5000 pM hCG) and on submaximally-stimulated testosterone secretion (i.e. in the presence of 0.5 pM hCG). The results are illustrated in Fig. 4. Basal testosterone secretion was unaffected by the addition of SCCM from 3 different cultures but was increased 2- to 3-fold by addition of IF from either control or hCG-treated rats. Serum from hCG-treated rats was without significant effect, thus demonstrating that the effects of IF were specific for this medium and were not derived from peripheral serum. In the presence of 0.5 pM hCG, SCCM and IF inhibited testosterone secretion when compared with the control incubation, and the IF was more potent than SCCM in this respect. In contrast, the opposite effect was obtained in the presence of 5000 pM hCG, as IF and SCCM all enhanced testosterone secretion by a similar margin (20-35%) compared with the control.

These results demonstrate that testicular IF and SCCM contain one or more heat-stable (and therefore probably low molecular weight) factors which are capable of altering the pattern of Leydig cell responsiveness to gonadotrophin stimulation. The differences between IF and SCCM in this

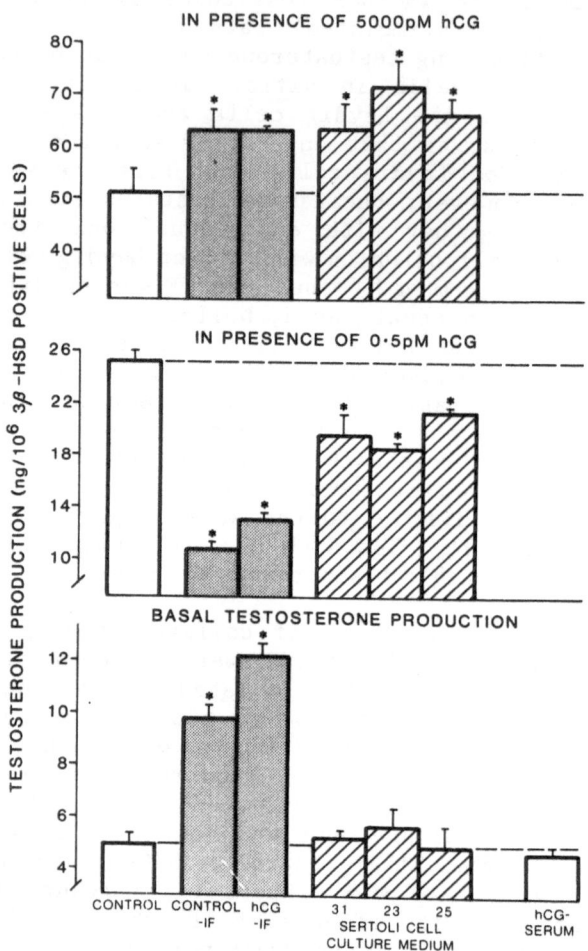

Figure 4. Effect of addition of extracted testicular interstitial fluid (IF) or serum (all 0.1 ml) or medium from
Sertoli cell cultures (0.2 ml) on basal and hCG-stimulated
testosterone secretion <u>in vitro</u> by isolated rat Leydig cells.
Sertoli cells were prepared from the testes of immature
(no. 31) or adult X-irradiated (23,25) rats and cultured for
6 days as described elsewhere (Rommerts et al., 1978) in
either the absence (23,31) or presence (25) of 1% foetal calf
serum. Serum and IF's were collected from rats treated 16 hr
previously with saline (control) or 100 IU hCG and were
extracted as described in the text. Control incubations were

respect are of some interest, because although both behaved
similarly in the presence of added hCG, SCCM was without
effect on basal testosterone secretion whilst IF was stimulatory. The obvious question is whether any of these effects
can be attributed to 'testicular LHRH', because we have
previously demonstrated LHRH-like activity in both SCCM
(Sharpe et al., 1982b) and in fresh unextracted IF from
hCG-treated rats (Sharpe and Fraser, 1980b). However,
there are three reasons for believing that the observed
activity is not due to 'testicular LHRH'. First, because
undiluted SCCM was used for these studies and we have shown
previously that SCCM contains only very low levels of 'LHRH',
and second, because LHRH-like activity in IF appears to be
extremely labile (Sharpe et al., 1982b). The third and most
conclusive piece of evidence is provided by the observation
that the effect of IF on basal testosterone secretion could
not be reversed by co-incubation with an LHRH antagonist
(D-Phe^2, Phe^3, D-Phe^6 LHRH; Hoechst, A. G.), as is illustrated
in Fig. 5. Thus, whilst addition of the LHRH antagonist was
largely able to prevent the increase in testosterone secretion
elicited by LHRH agonist, it had no such effect on testosterone secretion elicited by extracted IF from control and
hCG-treated rats. Similarly, an acid extract of rat testes
which had been boiled and extracted using the same procedures
as used for the IF was also capable of enhancing basal
testosterone production and this stimulation was not prevented
by co-incubation with the LHRH antagonist (Fig. 5).

These results suggest that a factor (or factors) which
can modulate Leydig cell testosterone production is present
within the testis, is secreted in vivo into testicular IF and
in vitro by Sertoli cell cultures. This factor(s) does not
appear to be LHRH-like and may correspond to the heat-stable,
small molecular weight compound recently reported in SCCM by
Grotjan and Heindel (1982). These authors also observed that
this factor was produced by cultures of several non-testicular
cell types, and perhpas this observation should cause us to
evaluate the present results with caution. For although our

←――

Figure 4 continued. performed as described previously
(Sharpe and Cooper, 1982) in the presence of 0.2 ml M199.
Values are the mean ± S.D. for triplicate incubations.
*P < 0.001, compared with respective control incubation.

findings demonstrate that the activity appears to be relatively testis-specific (i.e. there was no activity in serum), it
is possible that the results we have obtained are attributable
to a factor(s) which has no physiological role in vivo but
which simply improves the functional capacity or performance
of Leydig cells in our 'artificial' in vitro test system.

6.   Physiology of Sertoli-Leydig Cell Communication

As was outlined at the beginning of this paper, the most
logical reason why Sertoli cells should communicate with the
Leydig cells is to ensure that the latter provide sufficient
testosterone for the Sertoli cells to drive and maintain
spermatogenesis. We have subsequently presented biological
evidence to support this interpretation, the results demon-

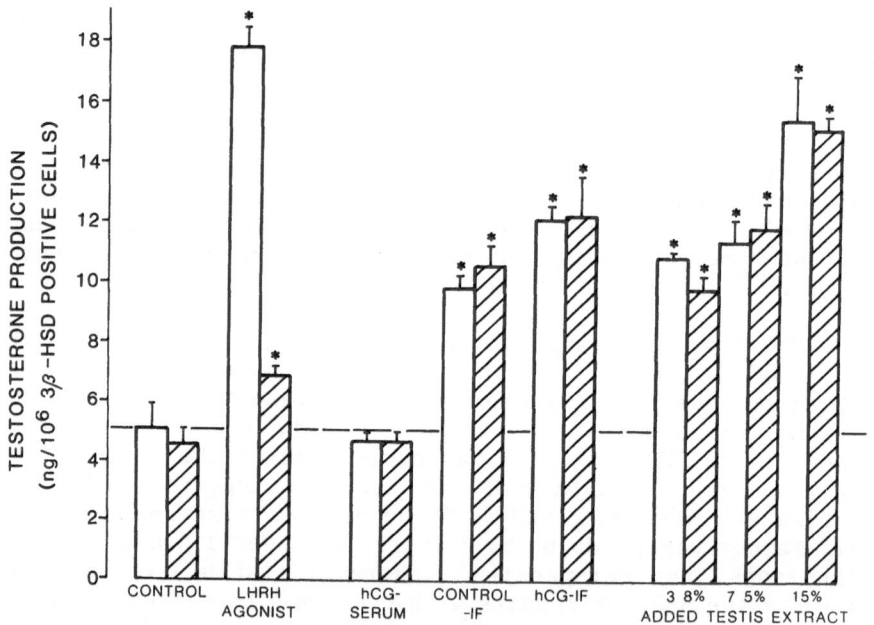

Figure 5. Effect of the addition of an LHRH antagonist (1.3
µg/ml; hatched columns) on testosterone secretion in vivo by
isolated Leydig cells incubated in the presence of LHRH
agonist (2 ng/ml) or extracts of IF (0.1 ml), serum (0.1 ml)
or whole testes. Other details are as given in the text or
in the legend to Fig. 4.

strating that the Sertoli cells probably produce one or
more factors which can influence Leydig cell steroidogenesis.
Of these there is only detailed information concerning
'testicular LHRH', because the availability of synthetic LHRH
agonists has enabled the presumed biological functions of the
endogenous peptide to be studied. But how does 'testicular
LHRH' function physiologically? When is it secreted? What
factors trigger its secretion? Unfortunately, we do not yet
have answers to these or to other questions on this subject,
although using the information available it is at least
possible to consider certain possibilities.

Perhaps the question which is central to LHRH action on
the Leydig cell is what is its basic role? There are two
obvious but distinct possiblities. First, that 'testicular
LHRH' acts as a fail-safe mechanism to ensure that
(LH-stimulated) intra-testicular levels of testosterone do
not fall below the minimum level necessary to support spermatogenesis. Second, that 'testicular LHRH' acts only within
discrete areas of the testis to enable local modulation of
Leydig cell testosterone output according to local requirements of the different stages of spermatogenesis. Implicit
in both of these possibilities is that 'LHRH' secretion is
controlled by testosterone (acting via the Sertoli cell), and
it should be emphasized that there is as yet no evidence in
support of this.

Let us first consider the possibility that 'testicular
LHRH' acts to regulate intra-testicular testosterone levels.
If this idea were correct then it would be expected that the
overall testosterone level in IF within the testis would be
increased by LHRH agonist, and that perhaps Leydig cell
responsiveness to LHRH agonist might increase when intra-
testicular testosterone levels were subnormal and decrease
when testosterone levels were supranormal. In fact this is
precisely what happens. Injection of LHRH agonist increases
the overall testosterone level in testicular IF in both
hypophysectomized (Sharpe et al., 1982a) and intact (Fig. 3)
rats. Moreover, when IF levels of testosterone are increased
3-fold by injection of intact rats with hCG, then both the
number of Leydig cell LHRH-receptors and the maximal testosterone response of these cells to LHRH agonist in vitro are
decreased, whereas the opposite changes accompany a reduction
in the concentration of testosterone in IF to grossly
subnormal levels as a result of hypophysectomy 3 days earlier

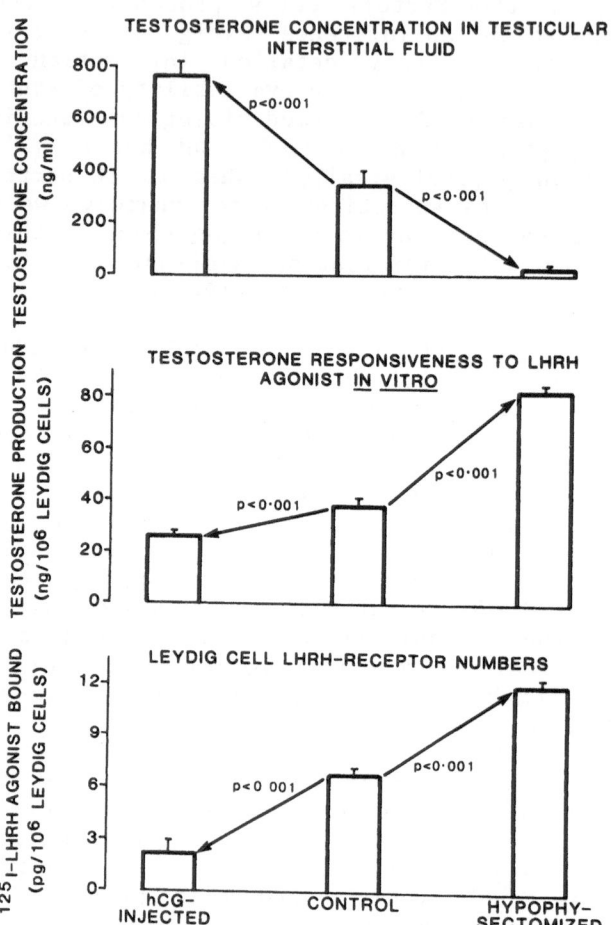

Figure 6. Inverse relationship between the levels of testosterone in testicular IF (top) and the in vitro responsiveness
of isolated Leydig cells to a maximally-stimulating concentration (2 ng/ml) of LHRH agonist (middle) and the number of
Leydig cell LHRH-receptors (bottom). Rats were 55 days old
and were either intact and treated with saline (control) or
treated with 50 IU hCG 3 days earlier (left) or had been
hypophysectomized 3 days earlier but left untreated (right).
All preparative procedures were as described elsewhere
(Sharpe and Fraser, 1980a,b; Sharpe et al. 1982a) and values
are the mean ± S.D. for either 4 rats (top) or triplicate
incubations (middle and bottom panels).

(Fig. 6). However, although the latter evidence appears convincing it should be noted that in the situations illustrated in Fig. 6, Leydig cell responsiveness to LH (hCG) decreased and increased in a somewhat similar manner to responsiveness to LHRH agonist, so that the apparent inverse relationship between IF levels of testosterone and steroidogenic responsiveness to LHRH agonist may simply be a fortuitous association. It should also be noted that Fig. 6 illustrates quite clearly that, in the absence of the pituitary, secretion of endogenous 'testicular LHRH' either did not occur or was in insufficient amounts to maintain normal IF levels of testosterone. This means that the suggested role for 'testicular LHRH' may be incorrect, or that physiologically it can only function as a modulator of LH action. This leads to the second possibility, namely that 'testicular LHRH' acts only within discrete areas of the testis where it locally modulates responsiveness to LH.

The basis for this possibility derives from the way in which spermatogenesis is organized as a wave along the seminiferous tubule, such that short sections of individual tubules are in different stages of spermatogenesis (Clermont, 1972). As the testosterone requirement changes according to the particular stage of spermatogenesis (Steinberger, 1971), it is evident that there is a potential need for some locally-produced and locally-acting factor that can modify testosterone output by the adjacent Leydig cells; presumably, the secretion of this factor would vary according to the stage of spermatogenesis. A factor such as 'testicular LHRH' has all the potential attributes for such a role, and although there is no direct evidence in support of this possibility, there are indications that such a system may function. Thus it is now well established that many aspects of Sertoli cell function change according to the stage of spermatogenesis with which they are associated (see Ritzen et al., 1981), and it has been shown recently that Leydig cells surrounding seminiferous tubules in stages VII to VIII are significantly larger than Leydig cells in association with other stages of spermatogenesis (Bergh, 1982). The fact that stages VII to VIII are probably the most androgen-dependent stages of spermatogenesis (Steinberger, 1971), and that at these stages the testosterone concentration within the seminiferous tubule is at its highest (Parvinen and Ruokonen, 1982), and the secretion of ABP is at its peak (Ritzen et al., 1982) also suggests that local factors may be at work. Further support for this interpretation is provided by the observation that localized interference with seminiferous tubule function by implantation of anti-androgens results in changes in Leydig cell size and number only in the immediate vicinity of the tubule damage (see Section 2.2).

Whilst the evidence presently available does not allow us to choose between the above possibilities concerning the physiology of Sertoli-Leydig cell communication, this review of the data can leave little doubt that local communication between the two principal compartments of the testis does occur and is likely to be of fundamental importance. The fact that this aspect of normal testicular physiology has only been regarded seriously in the last 3 to 4 years affords a further reminder of our general ignorance of the control of male reproduction, but offers hope for the future as any increase in our understanding of this important area cannot fail to have major reprecussions with respect to the regulation of male fertility.

ACKNOWLEDGMENTS: We are grateful to Dr. Jurgen Sandow and Hoescht, A. G. for the gift of LHRH and its agonist and antagonist.

REFERENCES

Aoki, A., and Fawcett, D. W., 1978, Is there a local feedback from the seminiferous tubules affecting activity of the Leydig cells? Biol. Reprod. 19:144.

Bambino, T. H., Schreiber, J. R., and Hsueh, A. J. W., 1980, Gonadotropin-releasing hormone and its agonist inhibit testicular luteinizing hormone receptor and steroidogenesis in immature and adult hypophysectomized rats, Endocrinology 107:908.

Bergh, A., 1982, Local differences in Leydig cell morphology in the adult rat testis: evidence for a local control of Leydig cells by adjacent seminiferous tubules, Int. J. Androl. 5:325.

Bourne, G. A., Regiani, S., Payne, A. H., and Marshall, J., 1980, Testicular GnRH receptors-characterization and localization on interstitial tissue, J. Clin. Endocrinol. Metab. 51:407.

Chen, Y. D. I., Kelch, R. P., and Payne, A. H., 1976, FSH stimulation of Leydig cell function in the hypophysectomized immature rat, Proc. Soc. Exp. Biol. Med. 153:473.

Clayton, R. N., Katikineni, M., Chan, V., Dufau, M. L., and
    Catt, K. J., 1980, Direct inhibition of testicular function
    by GnRH-mediation by specific GnRH receptors in inter-
    stitial cells, Proc. Natl. Acad. Sci. USA 77:4459.
Clermont, Y., 1972, Kinetics of spermatogenesis in mammals:
    seminiferous epithelium cycle and spermatogonial renewal,
    Physiol. Rev. 52:198.
Cooke, B. A., Magee-Brown, R., Golding, M., and Dix, C. J.,
    1981, The heterogeneity of Leydig cells from mouse and rat
    testes - evidence for a Leydig cell cycle? Int. J. Androl.
    7:355.
de Jong, F. H., Welschen, R., Hermans, W. P., Smith, S. D., and
    van der Molen, H. J., 1979, Effects of factors from ovarian
    follicular fluid and Sertoli cell culture medium on in vivo
    and in vitro release of pituitary gonadotropins in the rat:
    an evaluation of systems for the assay of inhibin, J.
    Reprod. Fert. Suppl. 26:47.
de Kretser, D. M., Sharpe, R. M., and Swanston, I. A., 1979,
    Alterations in steroidogenesis and hCG binding in the
    cryptorchid rat testis, Endocrinology 105:135.
DePhilip, R. M., Feldman, M., Spruill, W. A., French, F. S., and
    Kierszenbaum, A. L., 1982, The secretion of ABP and other
    proteins by rat Sertoli cells in culture: a structural and
    electrophoretic study, Ann. N. Y. Acad. Sci. 383:360.
Dorrington, J. J., and Armstrong, D. T., 1975, FSH stimulates
    estradiol-17β synthesis in cultured Sertoli cells, Proc.
    Natl. Acad. Sci. USA 72:2677.
Dutlow, C. M., and Millar, R. P., 1981, Rat testis immunore-
    active LHRH differs structurally from hypothalamic LHRH,
    Biochem. Biophys. Res. Commun. 101:489.
Grotjan, H. E. Jr., and Heindel, J. J., 1982, Effect of spent
    media from Sertoli cell cultures on in vitro testosterone
    production by rat testicular interstitial cells, Ann.
    N. Y. Acad. Sci. 383:456.
Hagenäs, L., and Ritzen, E. M., 1976, Impaired Sertoli cell
    function in experimental cryptorchidism, Mol. Cell.
    Endocrinol. 4:25.
Hansson, V., Purvis, K., Ritzen, E. M., and French, F. S., 1978,
    Hormonal regulation of Sertoli cell function in the rat,
    Ann. Biol. Anim. Biochem. Biophys. 18(2B):565.
Hsueh, A. J. W., and Erickson, G. F., 1979, Extra-pituitary
    inhibition of testicular function by LHRH, Nature 281:66.
Hsueh, A. J. W., and Jones, P. B. C., 1981, Extrapituitary
    actions of gonadotropin-releasing hormone, Endocrinol.
    Rev. 2:437.

Hsueh, A. J. W., Schreiber, J. R., and Erickson, G. F., 1981, Inhibitory effect of GnRH upon cultured testicular cells, Mol. Cell. Endocrinol. 21:43.

Hunter, M. G., Sullivan, M. H. F., Dix, C. J., Aldred, L. F., and Cooke, B. A., 1982, Stimulation and inhibition by LHRH analogues of cultured rat Leydig cell function and lack of effect on mouse Leydig cells, Mol. Cell. Endocrinol. 27:31.

Kerr, J. B., Rich, K. A., and de Kretser, D. M., 1979a, Effects of experimental cryptorchidism on the ultrastructure and function of the Sertoli cells and peritubular tissue of the rat testis, Biol. Reprod. 21:823.

Kerr, J. B., Rich, K. A., and de Kretser, D. M., 1979b, Alterations of the fine structure and androgen secretion of the interstitial cells in the experimentally cryptorchid rat testis, Biol. Reprod. 20:409.

Means, A. R., Fakunding, J. L., Huckins, C., Tindall, D. J., and Vitale, R., 1976, FSH, the Sertoli cell and spermatogenesis, Recent Prog. Horm. Res. 32:477.

Nozu, K., Dehejia, A., Zawistowich, L., Catt, K. J., and Dufau, M. L., 1982, Gonadotropin-induced desensitization of Leydig cells in vivo and in vitro: estrogen action in the testis, Ann. N. Y. Acad. Sci. 383:212.

Odell, W. D., Swerdloff, R. S., Jacobs, H. S., and Hescox, M. A., 1973, FSH induction of sensitivity to LH: one cause of sexual maturation in the male rat, Endocrinology 92:160.

Parvinen, M., and Ruokonen, A., 1982, Endogenous steroids in rat seminiferous tubules. Comparison of different spermatogenic stages isolated by transillumination-assisted microdissection, J. Androl. (in press).

Pomerantz, D. K., 1979, Effects of in vivo gonadotropin treatment on estrogen levels in the testis of the immature rat, Biol. Reprod. 21:1247.

Rich, K. A., Kerr, J. B., and de Kretser, D. M., 1979, Evidence for Leydig cell dysfunction in rats with seminiferous tubule damage, Mol. Cell. Endocrinol. 13:123.

Ritzen, E. M., Hansson, V., and French, F. S., 1981, The Sertoli cell, in: "The Testis", H. Burger and D. M. de Kretser, eds., p. 171, Raven Press, New York.

Ritzen, E. M., Boitani, C., Parvinen, M., French, F. S., and Feldman, M., 1982, Stage-dependent secretion of ABP by rat seminiferous tubules, Mol. Cell. Endocrinol. 25:25.

Risbridger, G. P., Kerr, J. B., Peake, R. A., Rich, K. A., and de Kretser, D. M., 1981a, Temporal changes in Leydig cell function after the induction of bilateral cryptorchidism, J. Reprod. Fert. 63:415.

Risbridger, G. P., Kerr, J. B., and de Kretser, D. M., 1981b,
    Evaluation of Leydig cell function and gonadotropin binding
    in unilateral and bilateral cryptorchidism: evidence for
    local control of Leydig cell function by the seminiferous
    tubule, Biol. Reprod. 24:534.
Risbridger, G. P., Kerr, J. B., Peake, R. A., and de Kretser,
    D. M., 1981c, An assessment of Leydig cell function after
    bilateral or unilateral efferent duct ligation: further
    evidence for local control of Leydig cell function,
    Endocrinology, 109:1234.
Rommerts, F. F. G., de Jong, F. H., Brinkman, A. O., and van der
    Molen, H. J., 1982, Development and cellular localization
    of rat testicular aromatase activity, J. Reprod. Fert.
    65:281.
Rommerts, F. F. G., Kruger-Sewnarain, B., Ch., van Woerkom-Blik,
    A., Grootegoed, J. A., and van der Molen, H. J., 1978,
    Secretion of proteins by Sertoli cell enriched cultures:
    effects of FSH, dibutyryl cyclic AMP and testosterone and
    correlation with secretion of oestradiol and ABP, Mol.
    Cell. Endocrinol. 10:39.
Setchell, B. P., and Sharpe, R. M., 1981, Effect of injected
    hCG on capillary permeability, extracellular fluid volume
    and the flow of lymph and blood in the testes of rats,
    J. Endocrinol. 91:245.
Sharpe, R. M., 1982a, The hormonal regulation of the Leydig cell,
    in: "Oxford Reviews in Reproductive Biology", C. A. Finn,
    ed., Oxford University Press, Oxford (in press).
Sharpe, R. M., 1982b, Cellular aspects of the inhibitory actions
    of LHRH on the ovary and testis, J. Reprod. Fert. 64:517.
Sharpe, R. M., and Cooper, I., 1982, Stimulatory effect of LHRH
    and its agonists on Leydig cell steroidogenesis in vitro,
    Mol. Cell. Endocrinol. 26:141.
Sharpe, R. M., and Fraser, H. M., 1980a, Leydig cell recep-
    tors for LHRH and its agonists and their modulation by
    administration or deprivation of the releasing hormone,
    Biochem. Biophys. Res. Commun. 95:256.
Sharpe, R. M., and Fraser, H. M., 1980b, hCG stimulation of
    testicular LHRH-like activity, Nature 287:642.
Sharpe, R. M., Fraser, H. M., Cooper, I., and Rommerts, F. F. G.
    1981, Sertoli-Leydig cell communication via an LHRH-like
    factor, Nature 290:785.
Sharpe, R. M., Doogan, D. G., and Cooper, I., 1982a, Stimula-
    tion of Leydig cell testosterone secretion in vitro and
    in vivo in hypophysectomized rats by an agonist of LHRH,
    Biochem. Biophys. Res. Commun. 106:1210.

Sharpe, R. M., Fraser, H. M., Cooper, I., and Rommerts, F. F. G.
    1982b, The secretion, measurement and function of a testic-
    ular LHRH-like factor, Ann. N. Y. Acad. Sci. 383:272.
Steinberger, E., 1971, Hormonal control of mammalian spermato-
    genesis, Physiol. Rev. 51:1.
van Beurden, W. M. O., Roodnat, B., de Jong, F. H., Mulder, E.,
    and van der Molen, H. J., 1976, Hormonal regulation of
    LH stimulation of testosterone production in isolated
    Leydig cells of immature rats: the effects of hypophysec-
    tomy, FSH and estradiol-17β, Steroids 28:847.

Gonadotropins and Target Cell Response

REGULATION OF STEROIDOGENESIS IN ISOLATED LEYDIG CELLS

F. F. G. Rommerts, G. H. Bakker, R. Molenaar and
H. J. van der Molen

Department of Biochemistry
Division of Chemical Endocrinology
Faculty of Medicine, Eramus University,
Rotterdam, The Netherlands

1.   Introduction

It is well-known that LH plays an important role in the
(acute) regulation of steroidogenesis in Leydig cells. In
the last years, it has become clear that in addition to LH,
hormones such as prolactin and oestradiol, as well as an
intratesticular LHRH-like factor, may also play an important
role in the (long-term) regulation of the responsiveness of
Leydig cells to LH. The ultimate regulation of the production
of biologically active steroids in Leydig cells is the result
of interactions of many stimulatory and inhibitory processes,
influenced by different hormones and/or factors. Investigation of isolated intact cells under defined conditions enables
a dissection of individual regulatory systems. It appears,
however, that the quality of isolated cells is not always
optimal and that different in vitro conditions may greatly
influence the steroid production by Leydig cells.

To define experimental conditions suited for studies on
hormonal control of steroidogenesis, the first part of this
chapter deals with effects of cell isolation and incubation
conditions on steroid production. In the second part, the
role of (phospho)proteins in the hormonal regulation of
cholesterol side-chain cleavage (CSCC) activity is described.
Details of methods used for isolation and incubation of
Leydig cells, as well as analytical methods, have been
described elsewhere (Bakker et al., 1981, 1982; Rommerts et
al., 1982a,b; Molenaar et al., 1982).

2.   Effects of Cell Isolation Technique and Incubation
      Condition on Steroid Production

        Freshly isolated Leydig cells have been used frequently
for investigations on the biochemical mechanism of acute
actions of trophic hormones (Dufau et al., 1978; Purvis et
al., 1978; Cooke et al., 1979a; Hall et al., 1979). However,
the use of freshly isolated cells has some disadvantages.
After collagenase dispersion techniques the number of the
cell surface receptors may be reduced and the cell membrane
may be damaged. Such artifacts of the cell preparation
technique may explain the large variation in steroidogenic
properties of isolated cells. LH-stimulated testosterone
production rates ranging from 3 to 100 ng/10^6 Leydig cells/hr
and stimulation factors ranging from 4- to 12-fold have been
reported (Janszen et al., 1976; Grotjan et al., 1978;
Cigorraga et al., 1980; Payne et al., 1980; Purvis et al.,
1980; Chen et al., 1981; Cooke et al., 1981; Sharpe and
Cooper, 1982). Subpopulations of Leydig cells, which differ
in LH-stimulated testosterone production (Janszen et al.,
1976; Schumacher et al., 1978; Payne et al., 1980; Chen et
al., 1981; Cooke et al., 1981) may also arise from various
degrees of cell damage during cell isolation. During preincubation in culture dishes, cells may recover from damages
obtained during the isolation procedure and viable cells can
be separated from dead cells by their attachment to the
coated plastic surface of the culture dish. This purification
technique has been applied to improve the quality of collagenase dispersed Leydig cells, isolated according to a standard
procedure (Janszen et al., 1976). The quality of the cells
was characterized by measuring the effect of LH (100 ng/ml)
and NADPH (1 mM) on steroid production (Table I). Damaged
cells were obtained using a crude method (shaking frequency
during incubation with collagenase 20-fold increased). They
showed no response to LH, but could be stimulated with NADPH.
Cells prepared by the standard procedure could be stimulated
with LH and also slightly with NADPH (Table I). Stimulation
of testosterone production by LH requires intact cells,
whereas NADPH can stimulate cells with damaged membranes
(Tsang and Stachenko, 1970; Goverde et al., 1980). The cell
preparations can therefore be characterized by the ratio of
the stimulation factor by LH, divided by the stimulation
factor by NADPH, providing a "quality factor". Intact cells
with a high stimulation factor by LH and a low NADPH response
show a high quality factor, whereas the factor for damaged
cells is low (Table II). The percentage of damaged cells can

Table I. Effect of LH and NADPH on Testosterone Production
by Different Leydig Cell Preparations from Mature Rats

| Cell preparation | Stimulation factor[a] | |
	LH	NADPH
Crude method	1.0 ± 0.0 (3)b	7.0 ± 0.5 (3)
Standard method		
I freshly isolated	8.6 ± 3.5 (4)	2.6 ± 0.4 (4)
II preincubated and attached to plastic surface	15.5 ± 4.0 (5)	2.1 ± 1.1 (5)

[a]Testosterone production with LH or NADPH/basal.

[b]Mean ± S.D. and number of cell preparations.

also be estimated histochemically, using an NADH-dependent
reduction of nitro blue tetrazolium (NBT). In cells with
damaged membranes NBT can be reduced by intracellular diaphorase activity, resulting in a blue staining. Cell preparations
with the highest quality factor show the lowest NBT-staining.
Using the quality factor and the diaphorase test as criteria
for cell viability, it appeared that the highest percentage
of intact cells can be selected from collagenase dispersed
cells by preincubation (2 hr) and attachment to plastic.
However, some damaged cells are still present in these preparations, as shown by the effect of NADPH. The maximal LH-
stimulated testosterone production by Leydig cells from
mature rats was 883 ± 465 (4) ng/1hr/10^6 cells with a
stimulation factor of 12 ± 3 (4) (mean ± S.D.). The steroid
production of these cells was at least 8-fold higher than
reported by other investigators (Molenaar et al., 1982).

Steroid production by Leydig cells isolated from
21-day-old rats preincubated and attached to culture dishes
could be stimulated by LH, but not by NADPH (Table III).

Table II. Effect of Cell Attachment to Plastic and Preincubation on the Quality Factor of Cell Preparations and the Percentage of Diaphorase Positive Cells

Criterion for quality	Crude cells	
	total	attached to plastic
Quality factor[a]	3.4 ± 1.0^b (3)	7.2 ± 2.2^b (3)
Percentage diaphorase positive cells	17.5 ± 6.5^c (4)	3.8 ± 4.8^c (4)

[a]Stimulation factor by LH/stimulation factor by NADPH.

[b]Significant increase after attachment: $P < 0.05$.

[c]Significant decrease after attachment: $P < 0.005$.

Means ± S.D.; number of cell preparations in parentheses.

These results indicate that damaged cells are virtually absent in cell preparations from immature rats. However, after a preincubation period of 24 hr, it was surprising to find that NADPH was as effective as LH in stimulating pregnenolone production (Table II). No cell damage was apparent from the diaphorase test indicating that the effect of NADPH cannot be attributed to damaged membranes. Experiments with structurally related compounds showed that $NADP^+$ was also active, that adenosine was most effective and that inosine was inactive. It has been described that adenosine can regulate adenylate cyclase in different tissues (brain tissue, artery strips) (Fain and Malbon, 1979) and in cultured adrenal and Leydig tumor cells (Wolff and Cook, 1977). Moreover, the stimulatory effects observed with NADPH, $NADP^+$, as well as the effects of other nucleotides and nucleosides, were shown to be caused by contamination of these compounds with adenosine and by adenosine-related compounds formed during the incubation (Fain and Malbon, 1979). The effect of NADPH on steroid production in Leydig cells from immature rats is therefore most likely an effect caused by adenosine or adenosine-related compounds, made from NADPH.

Adenosine is an important regulator in the cardiovascular system and the effects of adenosine on cultured Leydig cells suggest that this nucleoside may also play a role in physiological regulation of Leydig cells in the testis. No adenosine effects could be demonstrated with Leydig cells freshly isolated from testis tissue of immature and mature rats or from tumor tissue. However, all cell types responded to adenosine after a 24 hr incubation period. These results may be explained by removal of adenosine receptors during the cell isolation and resynthesis during the incubation period. It may also be possible that adenosine sensitivity, which is not present in normal Leydig cells, is obtained during culture. The latter possibility appears most likely, since Leydig cells in intact testis tissue from immature rats, not at all exposed to collagenase, do not respond to adenosine, whereas steroidogenesis can be stimulated with LH. The adenosine sensitivity which is developed during a 24 hr culture period of collagenase-dispersed Leydig cells, could be detected already after 2 hr incubation. These results show that the quality test for Leydig cells via measurement of the NADPH-stimulated steroid production can only be applied to 1 hr preincubated cells which do not respond to adenosine.

Table III. Effect of LH and NADPH on Pregnenolone Production by Leydig Cells from Immature Rats Attached to Plastic Dishes

Preincubation period	Stimulation factor[a]	
	LH	NADPH
1 hr	23.8 ± 2.8 (4)[b]	1.1 ± 0.6 (3)
24 hr	6.7 ± 2.5 (4)	7 ± 2.8 (4)

[a]Pregnenolone production with LH or NADPH/basal production.

[b]Means ± S.D. and number of cell preparations.

The development of new properties during culture has also been shown with mouse Leydig cells which become sensitive to catecholamines (Cooke et al., 1982). The development of responsiveness to adenosine and catecholamines in Leydig cells appears to be the only characteristic which increased during culture. Many other functional parameters related with steroidogenesis are decreased during culture: LH receptors (Hunter et al., 1982); cholesterol side-chain cleavage activity, 17α-hydroxylase (Rommerts et al., 198a); aromatase (Rommerts et al., 1982b). Changes in functional properties of Leydig cells in culture have been used (next part) to investigate the role of phosphoproteins in regulation of steroidogenesis. It is not known which culture conditions are required to maintain the original properties of isolated cells. A better understanding of the compounds or conditions which may influence the steroidogenic capacity and its regulation by hormones may help in the elucidation of the regulatory systems operating in Leydig cells.

In this respect it is also of interest to note that the LH-dependent cholesterol side-chain cleavage activity (CSCC) Leydig cells from immature rats incubated with a saturating dose of LH for 24 hr does not decline. The activity in perifused immature Leydig cells, however, declines within 60 min to approximately 50% of the original activity (Rommerts et al., 1982a). Similar results have been obtained by Segaloff et al. (1981) and Davies and Platzer (1981). Schumacher et al. (1982) showed that the LH-dependent steroid production, but not the LH-dependent cAMP production per 10^6 cells decreased when mouse Leydig cell suspensions were extremely diluted. At the present time these results cannot be explained. It may be possible, however, that the concentration of certain secretion products from Leydig cells is essential to maintain the LH-dependent CSCC activity. In addition to effects on CSCC activity, perifusion of cells also affects the rate of pregnenolone conversion to testosterone. In Leydig cells from mature rats this conversion was inhibited during perifusion and the initial activity was restored during subsequent static incubation (Table IV). These results are unexpected, because the conversion rate of pregnenolone is relatively low during perifusion, when product inhibition is minimal. The effects of medium flow on steroidogenic activities in isolated Leydig cells which cannot yet be understood, could be also physiologically important, because Leydig cells in vivo are continuously exposed to a flow of blood and/or interstitial fluid.

Table IV. Effect of Incubation Conditions on Conversion of
Pregnenolone (500 ng/ml) to Testosterone by Leydig Cells
from Mature Rat Testes Attached to Plastic Disks

Incubation condition	Rate of conversion (%) during each 30 min incubation period			
	1	2	3	4
period 1 - 4: static	100	-	84 ± 9 (4)	79 ± 8 (4)
period 1 and 4: static period 2 and 3: superfusion	100	-	36 ± 14 (6)	72 ± 38 (6)

Mean ± S.D. and number of cell preparations.

- = not determined.

3. Synthesis of (Phospho)Proteins and Regulation of Steroid
    Production

Increased phosphorylation of specific proteins after
activation of Leydig cells by LH probably is involved in
regulation of the mitochondrial CSCC activity (Cooke et al.,
1977; Bakker et al., 1981). The rapid stimulation of phosphorylation of these specific proteins did not permit a more
detailed kinetic analysis of the individual phosphoproteins,
to investigate which phosphorylated protein correlated best
with increased steroid production. A gradual decline in
the maximal LH-stimulated steroid production observed
during culture of isolated Leydig cells for 2 days, however,
enabled another comparison of the kinetics of LH-dependent
protein phosphorylation and steroid production.

The pattern of LH-independent protein phosphorylation
was not changed even after 5 days of culture. Hence, the
decrease in steroidogenesis appears to be induced by specific
alterations in enzymes involved in hormonal regulation of
steroid production. The concomitant decrease of LH-dependent
and dbcAMP-dependent pregnenolone production during the 2
days culture period suggests that these culture-induced
changes are not expressed at the level of the cell membrane.

Experiments with 25-hydroxycholesterol indicated that the decrease in LH-dependent pregnenolone production must have occurred at some step before the regulation of the CSCC activity. Pregnenolone production in the presence of 25-hydroxycholesterol is independent of LH action and protein synthesis and reflects the capacity of the CSCC activity and the endogenous generation of NADPH by intact mitochondria (Mason and Robidoux, 1978). The pregnenolone production in the presence of 25-hydroxycholesterol was more than 7 times higher than that stimulated by LH and this hydroxycholesterol-dependent steroid production also decreased during culture, although less rapidly than the LH-dependent pregnenolone production. It was inferred from these observations that the amounts of CSCC activity cannot be a limiting factor in steroid production. Apparently, alterations occur during culture in specific cellular activities involved in LH regulation of CSCC activity, which are localized between cAMP formation and stimulation of CSCC activity. Specific (phospho)proteins may play a role in this regulatory process. In cells incubated at 37°C instead of 32°C, pregnenolone production was initially stimulated, but steroid production was significantly more decreased after a 24 hr incubation period (Fig. 1). Cellular protein content and the rate of protein synthesis were increased after 24 hr incubation at 37°C to 115 $\pm$ 3% (3) and 147 $\pm$ 26% (3) of the respective values at the beginning of the culture. These results indicate that the specific changes which occur in stimulated steroidogenic activities of Leydig cells are time- and temperature-dependent.

During a 2 day culture of tumor Leydig cells, the effect of LH on protein phosphorylation decreased. Proteins with molecular masses of 170,000, 22,000, 2,400, 33,000 and 57,000 Da became less phosphorylated, whereas a protein of 20,000 Da, which was initially dephosphorylated under the influence of LH, could after two days of culture, be phosphorylated even in the presence of LH. The changes in LH-dependent protein phosphorylation were comparable for all proteins and occurred in parallel with changes in the LH-dependent pregnenolone production (Fig. 2). The 57,000 Da protein appears to be the regulatory subunit of the type II cyclic AMP-dependent protein kinase (Cooke et al., 1979b). Hence, this protein may constitute the common factor for activation of protein phosphorylation and the subsequent steroidogenesis. The observed decrease in phosphorylation of the 57,000 Da protein may therefore indicate reduced activity of the catalytic

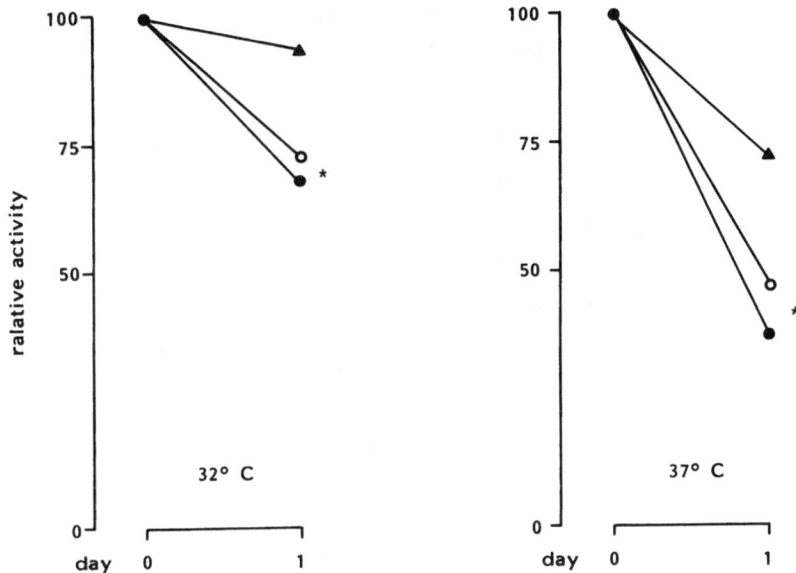

Figure 1. Effect of temperature and incubation time on the stimulated pregnenolone production (control production subtracted) by tumor Leydig cells. Pregnenolone production after 1 hr preincubation at 37°C was 137 ± 32% (12) of that at 32°C (p < 0.01). 25-hydroxycholesterol (closed triangles); dcAMP (open circles); LH/MIX (closed circles.

*significantly different from 25-hydroxycholesterol (p < 0.05).

subunit of protein kinase. This idea was tested by estimation of the enzymic activity of cAMP-independent and -dependent protein kinase in addition to phosphorylation of the 57,000 Da protein. The parallel decrease in phosphorylation and activity of protein kinase shown in Fig. 3 indicated that protein kinase activity had decreased during culture.

It is not clear which factors regulate the protein kinase activity. The decreased protein kinase activity is apparently not due to the absence of trophic hormones during the preincubation period of two days, since the presence of LH during the culture period could not prevent the decrease in steroid production. Moreover, tumor Leydig cells isolated from tumor-bearing mature rats, hypophysectomized 6 days

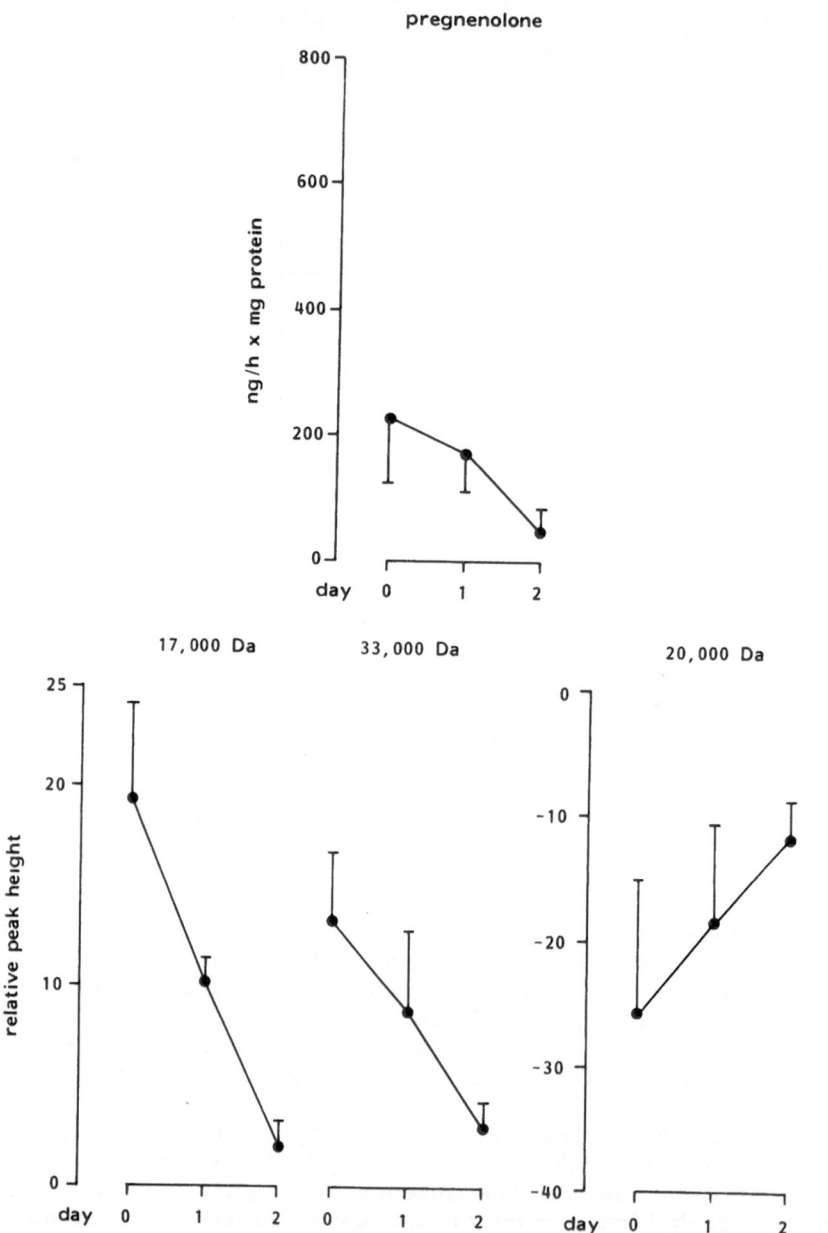

Figure 2. Effect of preincubation period on LH-stimulted pregnenolone production and phosphorylation of proteins in tumor Leydig cells. Phosphate-labeled proteins were separated

before the cell isolation, responded to LH stimulation in the same way as sham-operated animals.

Changes in hormone-dependent steroid production during culture have also been observed with Leydig cells isolated from testis tissue. Hsueh (1980) showed that after an initial decrease, LH-responsiveness was restored after culturing testicular cells for 10 days in the presence of LH, provided that the cells were obtained from hypophysectomized rats and cultured in the absence of foetal calf serum. These results indicate that in Leydig cells enzyme activities required for LH action, such as protein kinase, may be regulated by other factors than gonadotrophins.

The results of our long-term kinetic experiments have confirmed that protein kinase is important in regulation of steroidogenesis and that the kinase activity may be regulated by other factors than LH. It has not been possible, however, to indicate which LH-dependent phosphoprotein, in addition to cAMP-dependent protein kinase, may be important in the control of steroidogenesis.

The subcellular localization of phosphoproteins and its correlation with the function of the subcellular organelles may indicate how phosphoproteins are involved in LH action on steroidogenesis. Particular attention was paid to mitochondria, because the presence of LH-dependent phosphoproteins inside mitochondria could indicate a direct control of the CSCC activity.

Isolated (tumor) Leydig cells were fractionated in three different fractions: a nuclear fraction, a mitochondrial fraction, and a postmitochondrial supernatant fraction (Bakker et al., 1981). The fractions were characterized by determination of the CSCC activity as well as the DNA content and the

←——————————————————————————————————

on SDS-polyacrylamide gel electrophoresis. Peak height of proteins were measured from the densitograns and were expressed as a percentage of the peak height of a standard LH-independent phosphorprotein. The figure shows the decline in LH-dependent phosphorylation of the 17,000 Da and 33,000 Da proteins and the increase in phosphorylation of the protein of 20,000 Da initially dephosphorylated in the presence of LH.

activity of monoamine-oxidase and lactate dehydrogenase. The results showed that the nuclear fraction contained most of the DNA (55%) and that 96% of the lactate dehydrogenase activity was recovered in the postmitochondrial supernatant fraction. Most of the activities of the mitochondrial marker enzymes (70-80%) were present in the mitochondrial fraction, but significant nuclear contamination and some postmitochondrial supernatant activities were also present (Fig. 4a). The subcellular distribution of LH-independent phosphoproteins showed that most, if not all, of the phosphoproteins in the mitochondrial fraction may represent nuclear or cytoplasmic contamination.

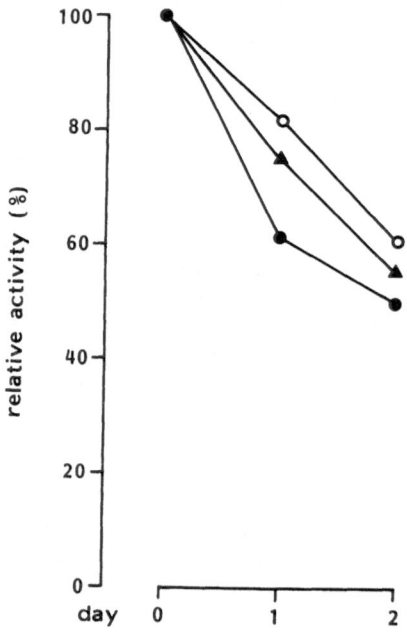

Figure 3. Effect of incubation period on LH-dependent phosphorylation of the 57,000 Da protein and protein kinase activity in tumor Leydig cells incubated at 32°C. Open circles = protein kinase activity with cyclic AMP; closed circles = protein kinase activity without cyclic AMP; closed triangles = stimulated phosphorylation of the 57,000 Da protein. The mean values from 3 different cell preparations shown for day 1 and day 2 are significantly different from day 0 (p < 0.05).

The distribution of the individual LH-dependent phosphoproteins is shown in Fig. 4b. The 17,000 Da protein could be
detected only in the nuclear fraction, whereas the 22,000,
24,000, 33,000 and 57,000 Da proteins were concentrated in
the postmitochondrial supernatant fraction. A small amount
of the 57,000 Da protein was present in the nuclear and
mitochondiral fraction. Contradictory to what has been
reported for adrenal cells treated with ACTH (Korocil and
Gallant, 1980), no LH-specific phosphoprotein could be
demonstrated in the purified mitochondrial fraction (Bakker
et al., 1981). Moreover, general protein phosphorylation
was low in mitochondria (cf. Fig. 4b). Stimulation of CSCC

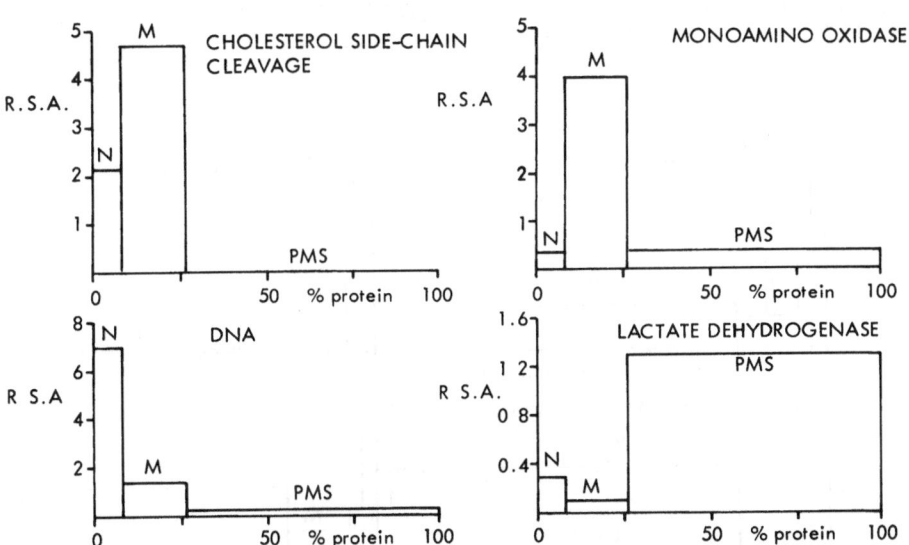

Figure 4a. Characterization of subcellular fractions isolated
from tumor Leydig cells. Subcellular distribution of choles-
terol-side-chain-cleavage activity, monoamine oxidate, DNA
and lactate dehydrogenase is shown. Abscissae: the percentage of the total protein content in each fraction is presented
as cumulative values. Ordinates: relative specific activity
(percentage of total enzyme activity or amount of DNA per
percentage of total protein content). Abbreviations used:
N, nuclear fraction; M, mitochondrial fraction; PMS, postmitochondrial supernatant fraction. Results shown are mean
values for three to five different cell preparations.

activity inside mitochondria via phosphoproteins may therefore occur indirectly by activation or synthesis of enzymes in other subcellular compartments.

The enrichment of the 17,000 Da protein in the nuclear fraction and the absence in other fractions clearly indicate a nuclear localization of this protein. Phosphorylation of the 17,000 Da protein may be involved in RNA synthesis or in transport of mRNA's out of the nucleus. LH could therefore possibly initiate activation of steroid production via phosphorylation of this protein and RNA synthesis.

This short-term activation of CSCC activity does not require RNA synthesis, since complete inhibition of RNA synthesis does not impair the LH stimulation of pregnenolone production for at least one hr (Table V). Direct inhibition of RNA synthesis only marginally influences LH-dependent

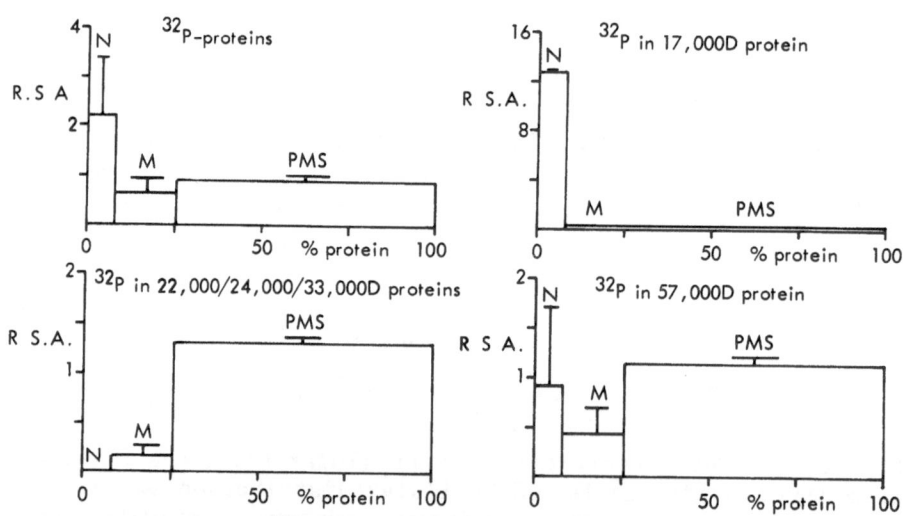

Figure 4b. Subcellular distribution of ^{32}P incorporation into phosphoproteins and lutropin-dependent phosphoproteins in fractions of tumor Leydig cells. Relative specific activities of the incorporation of (^{32}P)orthophosphate into proteins of subcellular fractions and relative-specific-activity values for the lutropin-dependent phosphoproteins. Results are means ± S.D. for twelve (^{32}P incorporation) are given and three (phosphoproteins) different cell preparations.

steroid production during the subsequent time period. This indicates that the mRNA(s) coding for protein(s) involved in stimulation of steroid production by LH are relatively stable. On the other hand, LH-stimulated steroid production is very rapidly decreased by inhibition of protein synthesis with cycloheximide (Cooke et al., 1979a; Bakker et al., 1982). This suggests the involvement of a rapidly-turning-over protein(s) in regulation of steroid production by LH. LH-induced changes in steroid production may thus occur via stimulation of translation of the stable mRNA(s) coding for the rapidly-turning-over protein(s) (through increased initiation or elongation). LH treatment could also cause phosphorylation of a protein with a high turn-over rate independent of LH action.

A stimulatory effect of LH on the synthesis of a 21,000 Da protein has previously been observed after a lag phase of approximately 2 hr (Janszen et al., 1978). However, this 21,000 Da protein is not a rapidly-turning-over protein. Phosphoproteins present in the postmitochondiral supernatant may directly regulate synthesis of the rapidly-turning-over protein, especially since phosphorylation and increased steroid production run in parallel (Bakker et al., 1981). The subcellular localization of the 33,000, 24,000, 22,000 and 20,000 Da proteins, mentioned above, has therefore been further investigated. In tumor Leydig cells the 33,000 Da phosphoprotein was present in 40S ribosomal subunits, whereas a phosphoprotein having the same molecular mass could also be demonstrated in Leydig cells from immature and mature rats (Bakker et al., 1982). The phosphorylation of this protein was stimulated by LH as well as by cycloheximide. The molecular mass, the subcellular localization and the sensitivity to phosphorylation in the presence of inhibitors of protein synthesis indicate that this 33,000 Da protein may be similar to the ribosomal protein S6, which has been observed in many different cell types (see reference Bakker et al., 1982). In these cell types increased phosphorylation of S6 as been correlated frequently with an increase in general protein synthesis. However, LH-stimulated phosphorylation of protein S6 in Leydig cells was not correlated with an increase in general protein synthesis. Theoretically, phosphorylation of protein S6 could participate in synthesis of the rapidly-turning-over protein discussed above, but it is not clear in what way this protein by itself could accomplish translation of specific mRNA(s).

Table V. Effect of Actinomycin D (10 µg/ml) on RNA Synthesis
and Steroidogenesis in Tumor Leydig Cells Preincubated for
2 hr at 37°C

	% Decrease
^{3}H-uridine incorporation	97 ± 3 (3)
LH-stimulated pregnenolone production	4 ± 5 (6)

Means ± S.D. and number of cell preparations; cells were
preincubated for 60 min.

The presence of 22,000 and 24,000 Da phosphoproteins in
microsomal fractions suggests that these phosphoproteins
could also be involved in protein synthesis. In this respect
the 24,000 Da protein may be the cap-binding protein which
participates in the initiation step of protein synthesis
(Thomas et al., 1981).

Synthesis of tryosine-aminotransferase in hepatocytes
can be specifically stimulated by dbcAMP, with no detectable
stimulation of general protein synthesis. It is unknown how
this specificity is achieved, but several results show that
control of initiation of translation is important (Snoek et
al., 1981). A similar situation may exist in the (tumor)
Leydig cells. The 33,000 Da protein, possibly in combination
with the 22,000 and 24,000 Da proteins, could be involved in
specific translation of a relatively stable mRNA, coding for
the protein with a short half-life. Cycloheximide inhibits
elongation of translation. Increasing concentrations of
cycloheximide progressively inhibit elongation. Inhibition
of protein synthesis occurs when the rate of elongation for a
particular messenger RNA becomes less than the rate of initiation. A stronger inhibition of synthesis of a specific
protein is observed when at the same low cycloheximide concentrations the rate of initiation is increased. Inhibition of
steroid production in tumor Leydig cells by low doses of
cycloheximide was significantly greater when cells were
stimulated with LH (Fig. 5). These results support the
hypothesis that control of initiation of translation by
LH-dependent phosphoproteins may constitute an important step
in regulation of steroidogenesis by LH.

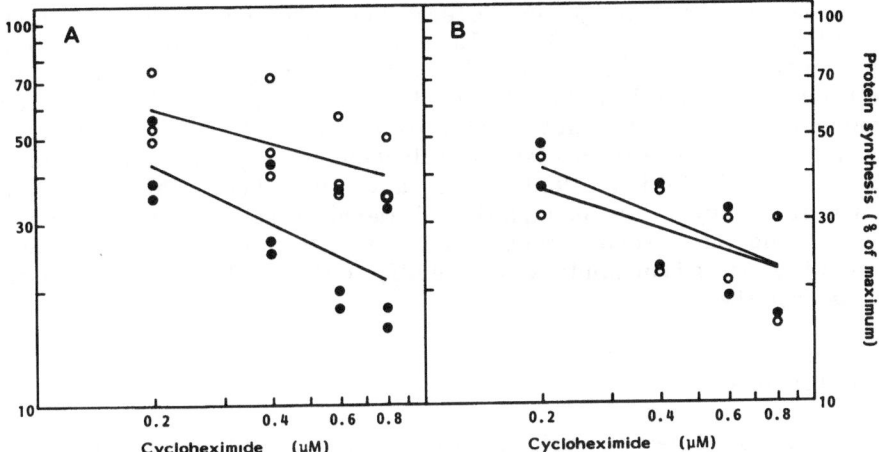

Figure 5. Effect of low concentrations of cycloheximide on pregnenolone production (A) and protein synthesis (B) in tumor Leydig cells. Controls, open circles; stimulated with LH, closed circles. Results shown were obtained in duplicate incubations with three (A) and two (B) different cell preparations. Inhibition of LH-stimulated pregnenolone production was significantly greater (p < 0.005) relative to control pregnenolone production, whereas no significant difference could be demonstrated between protein synthesis in the presence or absence of LH.

The 20,000 Da protein, dephosphorylated in the presence of LH, is localized in the cytosol and may be similar to myosin-light-chain present in microfilaments. Myosin-light-chain is dephosphorylated when its specific kinase is inhibited by phosphorylation (Bhalla et al., 1982). Phosphorylation of a protein of 76,000 Da has been observed in Leydig cells from immature and mature rat testes (Bakker et al., 1982), as well as in tumor Leydig cells. This 76,000 Da phosphorprotein may be identical to the myosin-light-chain kinase (cf. Bhalla et al., 1982). Phosphorylation of the 76,000 Da with ensueing dephosphorylation of the 20,000 Da protein may induce changes in the cytoskeleton, which is involved in regulation of intracellular activities, such as cholesterol transport (Crivello and Jeffcoate, 1978).

It is presently not clear how the putative rapidly-turning-over protein(s) could ultimately influence the CSCC activity in the mitochondria. Recent investigations of ACTH action on adrenal cells have shown that hormonally induced changes in metabolic activities of these cells include changes in phospholipid metabolism, which depend on protein synthesis (Farese and Sabir, 1980). We have not been able to show similar changes in phospholipid metabolism in tumor Leydig cells and the local mechanisms of activation of the CSCC activity in mitochondria of Leydig cells, therefore, remain to be resolved.

Conclusions

The quality of cell prepatations as well as incubation conditions (perincubation time, cell density, medium flow and temperature) greatly influence the responsiveness of Leydig cells to LH and other hormones. Therefore, isolated cells and incubation condition must be carefully characterized before results of different experiments can be compared and conclusions about hormone-dependent regulatory systems can be drawn. The phosphorylation of at least 5 proteins accompanies stimulation of steroidogenesis after addition of LH to isolated Leydig cells. Part of these phosphoproteins may regulate initiation of translation of a specific mRNA(s), resulting in synthesis of a rapidly-turning-over protein(s) involved in LH-dependent steroid production. This rapidly-turning-over protein(s) may increase steroid production by direct action at the level of the mitochondria, but the existence and the action of this rapidly-turning-over protein(s) have not yet been demonstrated.

REFERENCES

Bakker, G. H., Hoogerbrugge, J. W., Rommerts, F. F. G., and Van der Molen, H. J., 1981, Lutropin-dependent protein phosphorylation and steroidogenesis in rat tumor Leydig cells, Biochem. J., 198:339.
Bakker, G. H., Hoogerbrugge, J. W., Rommerts, F. F. G., and ban der Molen, H. J., 1982, Lutropin increases phosphorylation of a 33,000-Dalton ribosomal protein in rat tumor Leydig cells, Biochem. J. 204:809.

Bhalla, R. C., Sharma, R. V., and Gupta, R. C., 1982, Isolation of two myosin light-chain kinases from bovine carotid artery and their regulation by phosphorylation by cyclic AMP-dependent protein kinase, Biochem. J., 203:583.

Chen, G. C. C., Lin T., Murono, E., Osterman, J., Cole, B. T., and Nankin, H., 1981, The aging Leydig cell: two distinct populations of Leydig cells and the possible site of defective steroidogenesis, Steroids, 37:63.

Cigorraga, S. B., Sorrell, S., Bator, J., Catt, K. J., and Dufau, M. L., 1980, Estrogen dependence of a gonadotropin-induced steroidogenic lesion in rat testicular Leydig cells. J. Clin. Invest., 65:699.

Cooke, B. A., Golding, M., Dix, C. J., and Hunter, M. G., 1982, Catecholamine stimulation of testosterone production via cyclic AMP in mouse Leydig cels in monolayer culture, Molec. Cell. Endocrinol., 27:221.

Cooke, B. A., Lindh, L. M., and van der Molen, H. J., 1979a, The mechanism of action of lutropin on regulator protein(s) involved in Leydig-cell steroidogenesis, Biochem. J. 182:33.

Cooke, B. A., Lindh, L. M. and van der Molen, H. J., 1979b, Cyclic AMP-dependent phosphorylation of endogenous proteins in rat testis Leydig cells, J. Endocrinol., 83:32P.

Cooke, B. A., Magee-Brown, R., Golding, M., and Dix, C. J., 1981, The heterogeneity of Leydig cells from mouse and rat testes - evidence for a Leydig cell cycle? Int. J. Androl., 4:355.

Crivello, M., and Jeffcoate, C. R., 1978, Mechanism of corticotropin action in rat adrenal cells. I. The effects of inhibitors of protein synthesis and of microfilament formation on corticosterone synthesis, Biochim. Biophys. Acta, 542:315.

Davies, T. F., and Platzer, M., 1981, The perifused Leydig cell: system characterization and rapid gonadotropin-induced desensitization, Endocrinology, 108:1757.

Dufau, M. L., Horner, K. A., Hayashi, K., Tsuruhara, T., Conn, P. M., and Catt, K. J., 1978, Actions of choleragen and gonadotropin in isolated Leydig cells, J. Biol. Chem., 253:3721.

Fain, J. N., and Malbon, C. C., 1979, Regulation of adenylate cyclase by adenosine, Molec. Cell. Biochem., 25:143.

Farese, R. V., and Sabir, A. M., 1980, Polyphosphoinositides: Stimulator of mitochondrial SCC and possible identification as an ACTH-induced CX-sensitive, cytosolic, steroidogenic factor, Endocrinology, 106:1869.

Hall, P. F., Charponnier, C., Nakamura, M., and Gabbiani, G.,

1979, The role of microfilaments in the response of Leydig cells to luteinizing hormone, J. Steroid Biochem., 11:1361.

Hsueh, A. J. W., 1980, Gonadotropin stimulation of testosterone production in primary culture of adult rat testis cells, Biochem. Biophys. Res. Commun., 97:506.

Hunter, M. G., Magee-Brown, R., Dix, C. J., and Cooke, B. A., 1982, The functional activity of adult mouse Leydig cells in monolayer culture. Effect of lutropin and foetal calf serum. Molec. Cell. Endocrinol., 25:35.

Janszen, F. H. A., Cooke, B. A., van Driel, M. J. A., and van der Molen, H. J., 1976, Purification and characterization of Leydig cells from rat testes, J. Endocrinol., 70:345.

Janszen, F. H. A., Cooke, B. A., van Driel, M. J. A., and van der Molen, H. J., 1978, Regulation of the synthesis of lutropin-induced protein in rat testis Leydig cells, Biochem. J., 170:9.

Koroscil, T. M., and Gallant, S., 1980, On the mechanism of action of ACTH. The role of ACTH-stimulated phosphorylation and dephosphorylation of adrenal proteins, J. Biol. Chem., 255:6276.

Mason, J. I., and Robidoux, W. F., 1978, Pregnenolone biosynthesis in isolated cells of Shell rat adrenocortical carcinoma 494, Molec. Cell. Endocrinol., 12:299.

Molenaar, R., Rommerts, F. F. G., and van der Molen, H. J., 1983, Steroidogenic activities of isolated Leydig cells from mature rats depend on the isolation procedure. Int. J. Androl., in press.

Payne, A. H., Downing, J. R., and Wong, K. L., 1980, Luteinizing hormone receptors and testosterone synthesis in two distinct populations of Leydig cells, Endocrinology, 106:1424.

Purvis, K., Clausen, O. P. F., and Hansson, V., 1978, Age-related changes in responsiveness of rat Leydig cells to hCG, J. Reprod. Fert., 52:379.

Purvis, K., Clausen, O. P. F., and Hansson, V., 1980, Effect of age and hypophysectomy on responsiveness of rat Leydig cells to hCG, J. Reprod. Fert., 60:77.

Rommerts, F. F. G., de Jong, F. H., Brinkmann, A. O., and van der Molen, H. J., 1982b, Development and cellular localization of testicular aromatase activity, J. Reprod. Fert., 65:281.

Rommerts, F. F. G., van Roemburg, M. J. A., Lindh, L. M., Hegge, J. A. J., and van der Molen H. J., 1982a, The effects of short-term culture and perifusion on LH-dependent steroidogenesis in isolated rat Leydig cells, J. Reprod. Fert., 65:289.

Schumacher, M., Schäfer, G., Holstein, A. F., and Hilz, H., 1978, Rapid isolation of mouse Leydig cells by centrifugation in Percoll density gradients with complete retention of morphological and biochemical integrity, FEBS Lett. 91:333.

Schumacher, M., Schwarz, M., and Lichtenberg, V., 1981, Effect of cell concentration on the response of Leydig cells to hCG and dBcAMP, Acta Endocrinol., 96:suppl.240.

Segaloff, D. L., Puett, D., and Ascoli, M., 1981, The dynamics of the steroidogenic response of perifused Leydig tumor cells to human chorionic gonadotropin, ovine luteinizing hormone, cholera toxin and adenosine-3',5'-cyclic monophosphate, Endocrinology, 108:632.

Sharpe, R. M., and Cooper, I., 1982, Variations in the steroidogenic responsiveness of isolated rat Leydig cells, J. Reprod. Fert., 65:475.

Snoek, G. T., van der Poll, K. W., Voorma, H. O., and van Wijk, R., 1981, Studies on the post-transcriptional site of cyclic AMP action in the regulation of the synthesis of tryosine aminotransferase, Eur. J. Biochem., 114:27.

Thomas, A. A. M., Benne, R., and Voorma, H. O., 1981, Initiation of eukaryotic protein synthesis, FEBS Lett., 128:177.

Wolff, J., and Cook, G. H., 1977, Activation of steroidogenesis and adenylate cyclase by adenosine in adrenal and Leydig tumor cells, J. Biol. Chem., 252:687.

DISCUSSION

TAYLOR: Have you ever looked at adenosine production by the cultured Leydig cells? Might this in any way account for the differences you have observed between superfused cells and cells cultured under "static" conditions?

ROMMERTS: We have not measured adenosine production by Leydig cells. Superfused cells were frequently used after approximately 2 hr of preincubation and at this time adenosine effects can hardly be detected. So it appears unlikely that lack of adenosine can explain the decreased steroid production.

AAKVVAG: You used pregnenolone accumulation in the medium as a parameter of steroidogenic activity of the Leydig cells. Is it possible that variations in the activity of the subsequent reactions might influence the accumulation of pregnenolone?

ROMMERTS: We have used inhibitors of pregnenolone metabolism and changes in enzymes which metabolize pregnenolone are therefore irrelevant.

MEANS: The lack of parallelism in the cycloheximide experiment shown concerning pregnenolone production in the absence and presence of this compound suggests that the effect of LH does not primarily affect initiation of protein synthesis. Would you comment on this apparent discrepancy?

ROMMERTS: Our lines are indeed not parallel. This may indicate that LH regulates more than one protein. However, we have only a limited number of observations and we need more observations to test the significance of this apparent lack of parallelism.

HEDIN: I have some questions about your superfusion system. 1. Do you have the same recovery of steroids in the superfusion model as in the incubation system? 2. Have you used different media? 3. In one of your studies you showed steroid secretion in the superfusion model after a 25 min pulse of LH. Did you compare this output to the incubation results where LH was present for 24 hr?

ROMMERTS: The amount of pregnenolone produced under superfusion conditions is in the first hour similar to that when static incubations are employed. However, during the next hours superfused cells become less active.
We have not used other media but are planning to investigate the effect of Leydig cell conditioned media.
The presence of LH for 24 hr during static incubations did not affect the maximal steroid production during one hour in fresh medium.

GRIFFITHS: Does prolactin have a role in the control of steroidogenesis in the rat testis?

ROMMERTS: Several investigators have shown that prolactin in vivo may influence the number of LH receptors. We ourselves have not observed prolactin effects on isolated cells.

RAO: Can you speculate why one cannot maintain long-term cultures of Leydig cells in a functional state? Is it possible that Leydig cells have to be co-cultured with tubules?

ROMMERTS: It is obvious that Leydig cells lack something but we have not been able to prevent the decreased activities by addition of specific hormones like transferrin, EGF, insulin etc. We have not carried out enough co-culture studies with tubules. However, it appears that in the presence of tubules Leydig cells initially also show a decrease in steroidogenic activity.

PEPTIDE INHIBITORS OF INTRACELLULAR GONADOTROPIN ACTION

Kenneth W. McKerns

International Foundation for Biochemical
Endocrinology, Blue Hill Falls, Maine 04615

1.   Introduction

How is transcription regulated in trophic hormone-dependent tissues? What are the energy sources and the control mechanisms in the biosynthesis of nucleotides? Do hormones regulate DNA-dependent RNA synthesis? These are some questions to which I have given some answers and have proposed a general theory of regulation of the gonads by gonadotropins. Steroid hormone biosynthesis is also related to these mechanisms.

A chromatin preparation from nuclei isolated from ovarian corpus luteum tissues was found to respond to LH and hCG with an increase in RNA synthesis. This preparation was used in the initial evaluation of target specificity to gonadotropins, in the mechanism of the response, and in the initial search for possible inhibitors of LH or hCG action. If one could identify a peptide fragment of a linear sequence of LH or hCG, this might offer a rationale for the design of inhibitors. Enzymatic digests of LH were used initially. These were whole tryptic or chymotryptic digests. These mixtures of peptide fragments were found to be inhibitory in the chromatin preparation. It was planned to isolate individual peptides from the mixture and test these. However, in the meantime, ACTH analogues were used as a test for specificity. ACTH by itself did not influence transcription, but surprisingly, had a marked inhibitory effect on the stimulus to RNA synthesis by LH or hCG in the chromatin preparation. This at first seemed to be a disappointing lack of specificity.

However, this was pursued further and eventually led to the development of specific peptide inhibitors and to the identification of part of the active center of the gonadotropins. A number of similar amino acid sequences were identified in peptide hormones of widely differing functions.

2.   Energy Regulation in Steroid Hormone Biosynthesis

This is shown in Fig. 1 and has been described previously in detail (McKerns, 1978). In brief, the tropic hormone stimulates a unique species of glucose-6-phosphate dehydrogenase in its target tissue. This is the rate-limiting enzyme of the pentose phosphate pathway and its stimulation leads to an increase in reducing equivalents in the form of NADPH required in the rate-limiting steps of steroid biosynthesis from cholesterol in the mitochondria. One mechanism of coupling of NADPH to mitochondrial functions is through the formation of malate from NADPH plus pyruvate.

3.   Energy Regulation in Nucleotide Biosynthesis

Figure 2 shows how the tropic hormone activation of glucose-6-phosphate dehydrogenase leads to the generation of the rate-limiting ribose sugar, 5-phospho-D-ribosylpyrophosphate (5-PRP). The figures also demonstrate how the generation of 5-PRPP couples to the first enzymes of de novo pathways for pyrimidine and purine biosynthesis. This has also been explained in detail (McKerns, 1978).

4.   Gonadotropins and Transcription in Corpus Luteum
      Chromatin

Not only did the gonadotropins LH and hCG stimulate the de novo biosynthesis of pyrimidines and purines, they also stimulated polymerase activity in nuclei and chromatin. The methods used in the preparation of nuclei and chromatin and their use in the study of gonadotropin-stimulated RNA synthesis have been described previously (McKerns and Ryschkewitsch, 1976, 1977). The synthesis of all classes of RNA from [8-^{14}C]ATP was stimulated by the gonadotropins LH and hCG. There is an increase in both chain elongation and chain initiation. Some examples of these experiments are given in McKerns, 1982.

5. Gonadotropin Subunit Inhibition of Nucleotide
   Biosynthesis

Both the alpha and the beta subunits were found to
block the stimulatory effect of hCG on de novo pyrimidine
synthesis in nuclei prepared from corpus luteum.

6. Gonadotropin Peptide Inhibition of Chromatin Transcription In Vitro

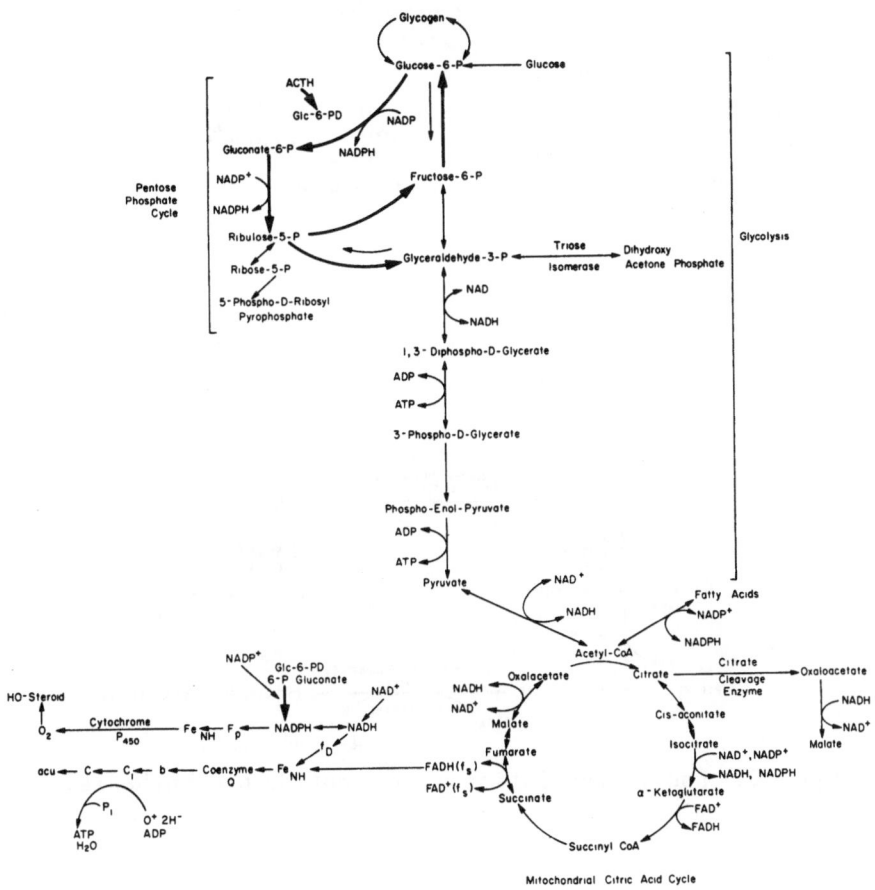

Figure. 1. Energy regulation in steroid hormone biosynthesis.

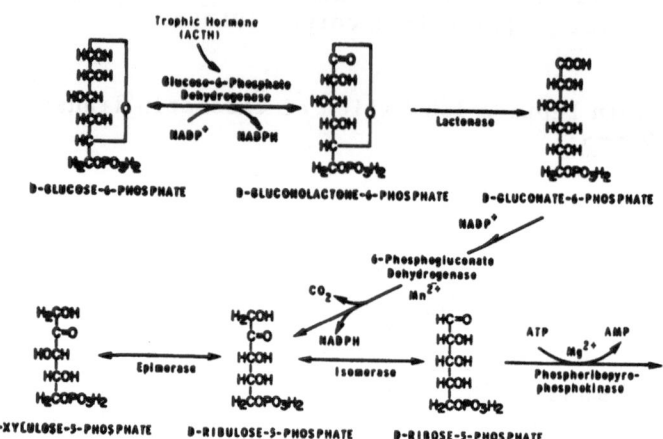

Figure 2.   Energy regulation of nucleotide biosynthesis.

It was interesting that the subunits of LH were inhibitory to the stimulatory action of the intact molecule. The possibility arose that a small peptide fragment, which may

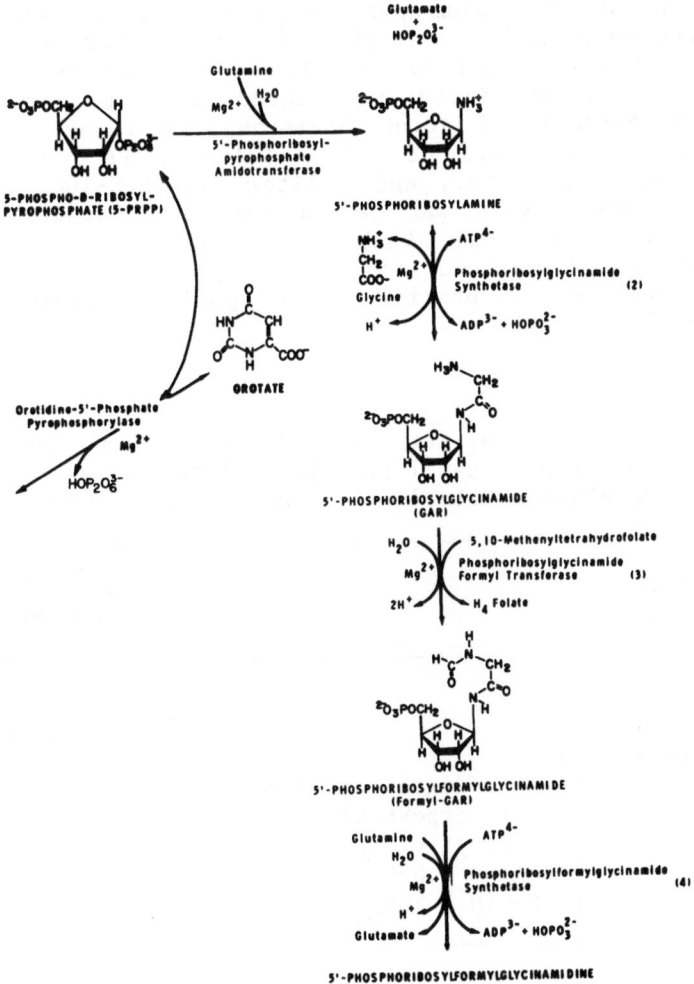

represent part of the active center of LH or hCG, might be an
inhibitor of gonadotropin action. A crude mixture of enzymatic digest of LH was tested in corpus luteum nuclei for
possible inhibitory effects. Typtic and chymotryptic digests
of lutropin (LH) were supplied by Dr. Darrell Ward, Houston,
Texas. An example of this experiment is given in Table I.
To the high strength buffer described in the text was added
0.5 µCi [6-^{14}C]orotate (spec.act. 8.15 Ci/mol), 4 µmol
glucose-6-P (except control), 0.006 µmol NADP (except control,
nuclei (6.32 µg DNA) and where indicated luteinizing hormone
(0.1 µg) and lutropin fractions (0.1 µg) in a total volume
of 0.5 ml. Incubation time was 10 min at 25°C. The reaction
was terminated by adding 5 ml of 5% trichloroacetic acid (TCA)
containing 0.2 M sodium pyrophosphate. The suspension was
collected on a millipore filter (1.2 micron pore) and washed
with a total of 15 ml of trichloracetic acid, 0.2 M sodium
pyrophosphate. The filter was placed in a 3 ml polyethylene
vial (INC Nuclear and Isotope Division) containing 3 ml Triton
X scintillation fluid (2 liters toluene; 11 g permablend,
Packard Instrument Co., and 1 liter Triton X-100, Rohm and
Hass). Radioactivity was determined in a Nuclear Chicago
scintillation counter. Each result is the mean of three
closely agreeing values expressed as µmol of [6-^{14}C]orotate
metabolized per incubation. 5.53 pmol is equivalent to
100 dpm.

Table I. Effect of Lutropin and its Fractions on the
Incorporation of Label from [6-^{14}C]orotate into Acid
Precipitable Material in Corpus Luteum Nuclei.

Gonadotropin compounds	pmol [6-^{14}C]orotate metabolized
Control	9.8
Glucose-6-P + NADP	18.4
+lutropin (LH)	70.0
+lutropin + tryptic digest of lutropin	44.4
+lutropin + tryptic digest of lutropin.SS0$_3$	38.3
+lutropin + chymotryptic digest of lutropin	69.0
+lutropin + lutropin α.SS0$_3$	46.3
+lutropin + lutropin β.SS0$_3$	6.7

The tryptic digestion products caused considerable inhibition. It was now apparent that the next step would be to isolate and test the individual peptides from the tryptic digests of LH. At about this point, a further check for specificity was carried out with the chromatin preparation using ACTH as a small peptide unrelated (or so we thought) to LH.

7.   ACTH Inhibition of Gonadotropin Stimulus to Transcription

A number of ACTH analogues were tested for their possible effect on the synthesis of RNA in the isolated chromatin preparation. Table II shows the effect of $^{1-39}$ACTH, $^{1-10}$ACTH and $^{11-24}$ACTH on the hCG stimulation to RNA synthesis in a chromatin preparation incubated in a low-ionic strength medium which favors polymerase I involved in rRNA synthesis. These ACTH peptides completely abolished the stimulatory effect of hCG. The ACTH peptides were also effective as inhibitors in a high-ionic strength buffer which favors mRNA

Table II.   Effect of ACTH Peptides on RNA Synthesis by Corpus Luteum Chromatin

Addition	$[8-^{14}C]$ - ATP incorporated (pmol)
Control	200
hCG + ACTH$^{1-39}$	640
hCG + ACTH$^{1-10}$	200
hCG + ACTH$^{11-24}$	230

Chromatin (1.0 µg DNA) was incubated in a Mg^{2+} - low salt buffer containing albumin and 1 µmol $[8-^{14}C]ATP$, 1 µmol each CTP, GTP, and UTP; hCG and ACTH peptides at $10^{-9}M$ in a total volume of 0.25 ml. Incubation was for 10 min at 25°C. Each value is the mean of 3 closely agreeing values.

synthesis. The $^{1-24}$ACTH analogues were also studied as
ovulation inhibitors in cycling rats given nembutol in the
early afternoon of proestrus.   The rats were given either LH
or LH plus peptide into the jugular vein at 15 and 30 min.
When used at a total dose of 300 µg per rat in three doses,
the peptides suppressed ovulation.

Other peptides that contained the ACTH sequence or part
of the sequence were also tested.   Table III shows the effect
of alpha MSH and beta LPH in inhibiting RNA synthesis in the
chromatin preparation.   They were somewhat less effective as
inhibitors.

Because of these interesting findings, it was decided to
synthesize a peptide overlapping the two halves of ACTH,
beginning with Arg^8 and ending with Lys^{16}, with the addition
of D-Ser at the amino end and Val-amide at the carboxy end.
This would be the peptide D-Ser-Arg-Tyr-Gly-Lys-Pro-Val-Gly-
Lys-Lys-Val-NH$_2$, the synthesis of which has been described
(McKerns, 1982).

When this peptide was given intravenously via the jugular
vein in doses of 50 µg, each, at 0, 15 and 30 min with 10 µg
of LH at 0 on the afternoon of proestrus, it blocked ovulation

Table III.   Effect of MSH and β LPH on RNA Synthesis by
Corpus Luteum Chromatin

Addition	$[8-^{14}C]$-ATP incorporated (pmol)
Control	280
hCG	490
hCG + MSH	300
hCG + β LPH	340

Chromatin (2.0 µg DNA) was incubated as described in Table
II, with peptides at 10^{-9}M.

in the rat. However, amino acid analysis showed no Lys and it was realized that the Lys used was the BOC-Lys (CL-Z). The chlorocarbobenzoxy was removed and the synthesis was repeated. This peptide was much less active. It would seem that the active inhibitor peptide was D-Ser-Arg-Tyr-Gly-Pro-Val-Gly-Val-NH$_2$.

The effects of this peptide and two other lysine containing peptides which are less active are given in Table IV. The effects of peptide inhibition of corpora lutea chromatin and ovulation have been given in detail previously (McKerns, 1982).

The peptide was compared with the linear sequences of the alpha and beta subunits of hCG and LH to see if there were similar sequences. The similarities are:
   residues 43-48 in hCG beta: Arg-Val-Leu-Gln-Gly-Val
   residues 132-138 in hCG beta: Ser-Arg-Leu-Pro-Gly-Pro-Ser
   residues 43-50 in hCG beta: Arg-Val-Leu-Gln-Gly-Val-Leu-Pro
   residues 38-43 in LH alpha: Ser-Arg-Ala-Tyr-Pro-Thr
   residues 34-38 in hCG alpha: Ser-Arg-Ala-Tyr-Pro

The peptides also show a striking similarity to the enkephalins Arg-Thr-Gly-Gly-Phe-Leu. The peptide D-Syr-Arg-Tyr-Gly-Pro-Val-Gly-Val-NH$_2$ has been synthesized on two occasions by Beckman Bioproducts according to my protocols and to FDA specifications. It was tested fairly extensively in Rheus monkeys in the late luteal phase, which were stimulated with an infusion of hCG to increase the synthesis of progesterone. When the peptide was infused in the range 20-100 μg per hr, there was suppression of the hCG response. At 200 μg per hr there was a total suppression of stimulus to progesterone by hCG. A small number of baboons in the early to mid-luteal phase were given the peptide intravenously in multiple doses. These experiments were carried out by others. The experimental design was restricted to the early stages of the luteal cycle and without the administration of exogenous gonadotropin and thus they may not have been very sensitive to suppression. Nevertheless, if each baboon served as its own control, there was a drop in the progesterone level due to the peptide.

8.   Projections for the Future

A number of analogue peptides that may be more stable to enzymatic degradation have been synthesized and they will be

Table IV. Effect of Inhibitor Peptides on Lutropin-Induced
Ovulation in the Nembutal-Blocked Rat

Compound	Dose(μg)	# of animals		Average # of eggs	
		LH	LH + compound	LH	LH + compound
[a]E$_2$	200	6	8	10	0
[a]E$_2$	100	3	8	11	0
[a]E$_2$	50	1	2	10	0
[b]I	100	4	4	11	8
[b]I	50	2	2	10	6
[b]I	20	2	3	12	10
[c]III	300	1	3	12	5
[c]III	200	1	3	12	10
[c]III	100	1	3	12	10
[d]E$_1$	100	3	2	12	8

[a]E$_2$:   D-Ser-Arg-Tyr-Gly-Pro-Val-Gly-Val-NH$_2$.
[b]I: D-Ser-Arg-Ala-Tyr-Pro-Thr-Pro-Ala-Arg-Ser-Lys-Lys-NH$_2$.
[c]III: D-Ser-Arg-Tyr-Gly-Lys-Pro-Val-Gly-Lys-Lys-NH$_2$.
[d]E$_1$:   D-Ser-Pro-Val-Gly-Val-NH$_2$.

tested in various systems including Leydig cell suspension,
corpus luteum cell suspension, chromatin prepared from corpus
luteum tissue, and as inhibitors of ovulation in cycling
rats. The compounds will also be tested for any enkephalin-
like activity and for possible effects on the release of
LH-RH.

The model peptide has been designated E2. After discus-
sions with a number of collagues, the following peptides have

been synthesized by Dr. John M. Stewart's group in Denver, Colorado: E2-HOAc; E2-TFA; DAla4,7-E2-TFA; Ac-DAla4,7-E2-TFA; pClPhe3-E2-TFA; OMeTyr3-E2-TFA; Ile3-E2-TFA; Phe3-E2-TFA; Acetyl-E2-HOAc; Stearoyl-E2; Benzoyl-E2-HOAc; Pro4,7-E2-TFA; D-TYR-3-E2; HCG(34-38)-amide.

REFERENCES

McKerns, K. W., 1969, Studies on the regulation of ovarian function by gonadotropin, in: "The Gonads", K. W. McKerns, ed., pp. 137-173, Appleton-Century-Crofts, New York.

McKerns, K. W., 1973a, ACTH stimulation of purine nucleotide biosynthesis in the adrenal cortex, Arch. Biochem. Biophys. 154:341.

McKerns, K. W., 1973b, Gonadotropin regulation of nucleotide biosynthesis in corpus luteum, Biochemistry, 12:5206.

McKerns, K. W., and Ryschkewitsch, W., 1974, Interaction of luteinizing hormone and its subunits in corpus luteum supernatant, Endocrinology, 95:847.

McKerns, K. W., and Ryschkewitsch, W., 1976, Regulation of RNA synthesis in corpora lutea by luteinizing hormone and derivatives, Biochim. Biophys. Acta, 454:51.

McKerns, K. W., and Ryschkewitsch, W., 1977, Lutropin stimulation of RNA synthesis in corpus luteum chromatin, Biochim. Biophys. Acta, 478:68.

McKerns, K. W., 1978, Regulation of gene expression in the nucleus by gonadotropins, in: "Structure and Function of the Gonadotropins", K. W. McKerns, ed., pp. 315-338, Plenum Press, New York.

McKerns, K. W., 1982, The search for the active center of the gonadotropins, in: "Hormonally Active Brain Peptides: Structure and Function", K. W. McKerns and V. Pantić, eds., pp. 71-84, Plenum Press, New York.

DISCUSSION

ROMMERTS: I am a little bit confused by your experimental data. What could be the mechanism of the stimulation of the different enzymes? Have you investigated effects of hormones on purified enzymes?

McKERNS: We have prepared purified glucose-6-P dehydrogenase from cow adrenal cortex and from cow corpus luteum of the mid-luteal phase. These and other glucose-6-P dehydrogenases are separate molecular species with different amino acid compositions. The corpus luteum enzyme is stimulated in an allosteric fashion by LH or hCG and the adrenal enzyme by ACTH only. In the other site of action, the polymerase-chromatin interaction is modified such that both RNA chain initiation and elongation is activated. The mechanism of this stimulation is unknown.

MEANS: Do you ascribe any physiological significance to your studies suggesting direct stimulation of RNA synthesis upon addition of the hCG molecule to isolated chromatin? This would require that the α/β dimer be internalized intact in order to function.

McKERNS: Yes, we propose that hCG and LH directly regulate cytoplasmic and nuclear function as part of their physiological function. The whole molecule seems to be internalized intact and is found in the cytoplasm and nucleus. Processing also occurs and it is possible that a small biologically active fragment could be formed.

ROSBERG: How fast is the inhibitory effect on progesterone formation? If the peptide blocks hCG-binding, you would expect a rapid effect. If the effect is on internalized hCG-molecules, you would expect a time-lag before inhibition.

McKERNS: The inhibitory effect is in the corpus luteum cell, in the cytoplasm and nucleus. The in vitro experiments were done with chromatin prepared from corpus luteum nuclei and the effect is almost immediate. The in vivo experiments with rats, for example, were done by injection of several doses over a one hr period. Studies, done by others, show internalization to be quite rapid.

ROLE OF TROPHIC HORMONES IN REGULATION OF GROWTH AND FUNCTION OF RESPONSIVE CELLS

A. Jagannadha Rao[a], J. A. Long[b], B. D. Gondos[c],
J. G. Lehoux[d], and J. Ramachandran[e]

[a]Department of Biochemistry, Indian Institute of
Science, Bangalore-560 012, India
[b]Department of Anatomy, University of California,
San Francisco, CA 04143 USA
[c]Department of Pathology, University of Conneticuit
Health Centre, Farmington, CT 060032, USA
[d]Faculty of Medicine, University of Sherbrooke,
Sherbrooke, Quebec J1H 5N4, Canada
[e]Hormone Research Laboratory, University of
California, San Francisco, CA 04143 USA

The role of the trophic hormones, Adrenocorticotropic
hormone (ACTH) and Luteinizing hormone (LH) in regulating
growth and function of adrenocortical cells and Leydig cells
respectively, has been investigated using an immunological
approach. Antisera to porcine ACTH and ovine LH were raised
in rabbits and characterized for specificity, ability to
neutralize rat ACTH and LH respectively. Administration of
ACTH antiserum to rats for 6 to 10 days did not cause any
decrease in the weight of the adrenals, but resulted in a
significant decrease in serum corticosterone. Also when the
adrenocortical cells isolated from normal rabbit serum (NRS)
or ACTH antiserum treated rats were examined for their ability
to respond to exogenous ACTH, there was a drastic decrease in
the response of the latter as judged by corticosterone production. It is known that in an unilaterally adrenalectomized
rat there is compensatory hypertrophy of the remaining adrenal
and this growth has been shown to be due to actual increase
in cell number. Administration of ACTH antiserum to unilaterally adrenalectomized rats did not in any way prevent the
compensatory hypertrophy response of the remaining adrenal as
judged by weight, DNA, protein or yield of adrenocortical
cells. However, once again there was a drastic decrease in

the response of the adrenocortical cells isolated from ACTH
antiserum treated rats as compared to cells from NRS treated
rats. Studies on chronic treatment of rats with ACTH showed
that there was a significant decrease in ^{125}I labelled Angio-
stensin II binding to the zona glomerulosa cells indicating
that functional differentiation induced by ACTH includes
changes at the receptor level also. Using the system of LH
and rat Leydig cells, it was found that deprivation of endogenous LH by use of antiserum to ovine LH did not affect the
yield of Leydig cells that could be isolated from the antiserum treated animals. However, a significant decrease in
serum testosterone and the in vitro response of the Leydig
cells to exogenous LH was noticed. Light and electron microscopic study of testes from NRS and LH antiserum treated
animals revealed that in the antiserum treated group, there
was a highly significant increase in the number of undifferen-
tiated cells.

Based on these results it is proposed that the trophic
hormones mainly regulate functional differentiation of
responsive cells and may not have a major role in stimulating
growth.

1.   Introduction

It is now a well accepted fact that the main role of
tropic hormones is regulation of growth and function of
target tissues. Regulation of function involves maintenance
and stimulation of both acute and long-term responsiveness.
Growth as considered in a classical sense involves increase
in size and weight. This is generally supposed to be due to
increase in cell number i.e., hyperplasia. During the early
investigations the presence of pituitary tropic hormones
[Somatotropic hormone (STH), Adrenocorticotropic hormone
(ACTH), Thyroid stimulating hormone (TSH), Follicle stimulating hormone (FSH), Luteinizing hormone (LH)] were demonstrated
by employing the technique of hypophysectomy (Greep, 1974).
Thus, removal of the pituitary in rats resulted in decrease
in size, weight and also impairment in the function of
thyroid, adrenals, gonads and several other tissues. Conclusions on the regulation of function of these glands by tropic
hormones was based on metabolic disturbances observed in
the body due to atrophy of a target gland following hypophysectomy. However, involvement in regulation of growth was
mostly based on gross changes in size and weight and, some-
times on histological data. These effects of hypophysectomy

could be reversed by supplementation with crude pituitary extracts or partially purified hormones. Based on these studies involving changes in weight and function, it was generally agreed that the tropic hormones regulate the growth and function of the target tissues. However, now it is known that changes in size and weight are not true indicators of growth and that increase in size of a tissue can occur not only due to hypertrophy, but also due to absorption of fluids without involving actual increase in cell number. Also in some cases like testes, the Leydig cells which are responsive to LH comprise only 10% of the total cell population (Bascom and Osterud, 1925) and the bulk of the weight is due to seminiferous tubules. Thus changes in weight of testes due to removal or supplementation of gonadotrophic support do not reflect actual changes in Leydig cell growth. During the recent years, attempts have been made to provide biochemical evidence for growth promotion by trophic hormones particularly in the case of ACTH. However, the evidence seems to be inconclusive as reports have appeared both for and against ACTH as a growth promotor (Farese and Reddy, 1971; Masui and Garren, 1971; Ramachandran and Suyama, 1975; Garren et al., 1971; Gill, 1972). It is known that removal of the pituitary involves trauma to the animal as well as deprival of an entire array of known pituitary hormones and possibly other unknown factors present in the pituitary. In view of this it is desirable to examine the role of tropic hormones in regulation of growth and function of target tissues by selective deprival of endogenous hormones in an animal. This can be achieved by use of specific antisera to the tropic hormones. The use of spefific antisera not only eliminates the trauma associated with hypophysectomy but also permits selective deprival of one or more endogenous hormones at will for the duration of the experiment. This technique in recent years has been extensively used to delineate the role of gonadotrophins in the reproductive physiology of rat, hamster and other mammals (Jagannadha Rao, et al., 1972, 1974; Sairam et al., 1974, 1975; Moudgal et al., 1974; Nieschlag, 1975; Jagannadha Rao, 1982). The studies reported herein are restricted to only two tropic hormone systems, namely, ACTH and LH. Selective deprival has been achieved by neutralizing endogenous hormones in rats by the use of antisera to either ACTH or LH. In the present paper the results obtained by the use of the immunological approach as well as by administering tropic hormone to intact rats, on the growth and function of adrenal and testis are reviewed.

2.   Role of ACTH in Regulation of Growth and Function of
      Adrenal Cortex

      A.   Effect of ACTH antiserum administration to male
rats on adrenal weight and responsiveness of adrenocortical
cells to ACTH. The effect of deprivation of endogenous ACTH
on the weight of the adrenal and function of adrenocortical
cells in the rats was examined by injecting a highly specific
and potent antiserum to porcine ACTH, raised in rabbits. The
details of production and characterization of antiserum have
been described in earlier papers (Jagannadha Rao, et al.,
1978, 1980).   Antiserum to ACTH was injected into male rats
ranging in age from 3 to 12 weeks by the subcutaneous route.
Animals which received equal quantity of normal rabbit serum
(NRS) served as controls. At the end of the treatment which
ranged from 6 to 10 days, changes in adrenal weight, serum
corticosterone concentration and responsiveness of isolated
adrenocortical cells from control and antiserum treated
animals to exogenous ACTH was evaluated. The details of
isolation of adrenocortical cells, radioimmunoassay of corticosterone have also been described in an earlier paper
(Jagannadha Rao, et al., 1978).

      It can be seen from the data presented in Table I that
selective deprival of endogenous ACTH had no effect on the
adrenal weight in any age group of animals. It should be
pointed out that the ability of the antiserum to neutralize
endogenous ACTH was established earlier and the quantity of
the antiserum administered was more than sufficient to neutralize the quantity of ACTH present in circulation.

      It is also evident from Table II that administration of
ACTH antiserum caused a significant decrease in the serum
corticosterone levels indicating the efficacy of ACTH antiserum in neutralizing endogenous ACTH.

      Experiments were also conducted to examine the responsive-
ness of the adrenocortical cells isolated from the control and
antiserum treated animals to exogenous ACTH in vitro in all
the five experiments listed in Table I. The results obtained
in one such experiment are presented in Table III, though,
essentially similar results were obtained in all the experiments. It can be seen that whereas in cells from the control
group a 94-fold stimulation was induced by 0.7 nM ACTH, this
concentration of hormone caused only a 4-fold stimulation in
the cells from antisera treated animals indicating a significantly lowered response following anti-serum treatment.

Table I. Effect of ACTH Antiserum Administration of Paired
Adrenal Weight in Growing Male Rats

Exp. no.	Age of rats (weeks)	No. of animals	Adrenal wt (mg) ± SE	
			NRS-treated	ACTH A/S-treated
1	3	6	19.7 ± 0.7	21.5 ± 1.2
2	3	6	18.8 ± 1.1	23.3 ± 2.4
3	3	8	17.1 ± 1.1	16.7 ± 0.7
4	6	6	27.3 ± 1.9	29.6 ± 1.4
5	12	8	37.9 ± 3.7	39.7 ± 3.0

NRS or ACTH antiserum (A/S) was administered once daily ip
for a minimum of 6 and a maximum of 10 days before autopsy
(from Jagannadha Rao, et al., 1978).

Table II. Effect of ACTH Antiserum Treatment on Serum
Corticosterone Levels

	Corticosterone μg/dl	P
NRS treated	30.1 ± 1.0 (8)[a]	
ACTH antiserum-treated	22.9 ± 1.4 (8)	< 0.001

[a]Mean ± S E; number of animals shown in parenthesis.
Number in parenthesis indicate number of animals per group
and corticosterone was determined by radioimmunoassay.
From Jagannadha Rao et al., 1978.

Table III.   Responsiveness of the Isolated Adrencortical
              Cells to Exogenous ACTH

	Corticosterone[a] Production in Adrenal Cells		
Additions	NRS treated rats	ACTH A/S-treated rats	P
None	1.7 ± 0.1	1.0 ± 0.1	
ACTH (0.7 nM)	160 ± 20	7.3 ± 5	< 0.001
ACTH (2 nM)	312 ± 8	208 ± 28	< 0.05

The results from experiment 3 of Table I.
[a]Nanograms per 10^5 cells per h. Mean ± S E of triplicate
incubations.
From Jagannadha Rao et al., 1978.

B.   Effect of ACTH antisera on the compensatory adrenal
hypertrophy response.   It is well known that removal of one
adrenal gland results in the enlargement of the remaining
adrenal, (Tepperman et al., 1943; Ingle, 1951; Carr, 1959;
Bransome and Reddy, 1961), and this enlargement has been
shown to be due to an increase in the number of cells.   This
hypertrophy is considered to result from the increase in ACTH
secretion caused by the low circulating levels of corticosterone.   Thus the unilaterally adrenalectomized animal
appeared to be a good experimental model to examine the role
of ACTH in adrenal growth.   The results of injecting normal
rabbit serum or ACTH antiserum into unilaterally adrenalectomized animals are presented in Table IV.   It can be seen
that in group B there is a significant increase in the adrenal
weight and the administration of ACTH antiserum to animals in
group C did not in any way prevent this increase.   The fact
that the increased weight indeed represents actual growth is
reflected in the increased number of cortical cells that
could be isolated, as well as the increase in DNA and protein
and this is also not prevented by ACTH antiserum treatment.
Thus by all the three criteria growth seems to be unaffected.

However, there is a significant decrease in the serum corticosterone level indicating, once again the efficacy of the injected ACTH antiserum. This becomes all the more evident when we examine the response of the adreno-cortical cells from the control and antiserum treated animals.

It can be seen from the data presented in Fig. 1 that the steroidogenic response of the cells from group B is significantly increased over Group A, while in group C the response was less than that of the controls indicating a drastic impairment in functional response. In order to rule out the possibility that the observed effects are not due to insufficient antibody administered, the serum of the antisera treated rats was checked for its ability to bind tritiated ACTH. It was found that each ml of the serum in these animals was capable of binding 3.3 ng ACTH, indicating the presence of excess antibody.

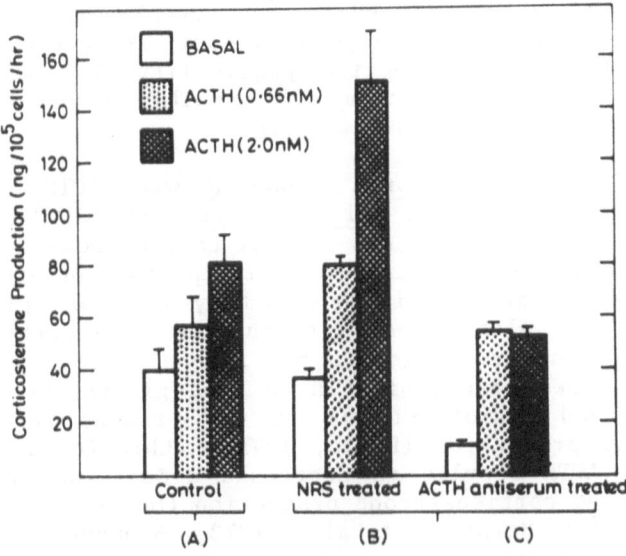

Figure 1. Effects of unilateral adrenalectomy and ACTH antiserum on the responsiveness of adrenocortical cells to exogenous ACTH. Cells were isolated from the right adrenals of the three experimental groups and incubated with ACTH. Corticosterone production was measured by radioimmunoassay. From Jagannadha Rao et al., 1978.

C. A comparative ultrastructural study of hypophysectomized or ACTH antiserum treated rat adrenal. It is known
that there are dramatic changes in the ultrastructure of the
cells of zona fasciculata of the adrenal cortex following
hypophysectomy (Idelmen, 1970). The reorganization of the
tubulolamellar cristae of the mitochondria to vescicular
cristae and the increase in smooth surfaced endoplasmic
reticulum are well established changes caused by ACTH (Kahri,
1966; Idleman, 1970; O'Hare and Neville, 1973; Manuelidis
and Mulrow, 1974; Nussdorfer et al., 1977; Suyama et al.,
1977). The use of antiserum facilitates specific deprivation
of only ACTH in contrast to hypophysectomy which removes a
whole array of hormones. So it was felt that a comparison
of the effects at the ultrastructural level should reveal
differences and these are summarized in Table V. While
there was a large reduction in cell volume within 7 days
after hypophysectomy, antiserum treatment did not affect the
cell volume significantly. However, neutralization of
endogenous ACTH did result in significant decreases in the
absolute volume of mitochondria, cytoplasmic matrix and
nuclei although the changes were not as large as after
hypophysectomy suggesting the possibility that the effects
observed after hypophysectomy may possibly be due to removal
of other factors in addition to ACTH.

D. Effects of chronic treatment with ACTH on the rat
adrenal zona glomerulosa cell function. It is a well established fact that in the rat adrenal cortex, zona fasciculata
and zona reticularis contribute to the production of corticosterone and aldosterone is produced by the zona glomerulosa
(Long, 1975). Although ACTH stimulated both corticosterone
and aldosterone production in the adrenal cortex, it is now
known that the effects of ACTH on zona glomerulosa are only
transient and Angiotensin II is the primary regulator of
aldosterone production (Dabis, 1975). Chronic treatment of
rats with ACTH results in decreased aldosterone production
and increased corticosterone production (Muller et al., 1956;
Muller, 1970; Hornsby et al., 1973; Baumann and Muller,
1974). This experimental observation has been elegantly made
use of both in vivo and in vitro (Muller, 1970; Hornsby et
al., 1974; Kahri et al., 1976) to investigate the role of
ACTH as a differentiating hormone. In vitro studies (Kahri,
1966; Kahri et al., 1976) revealed that the foetal rat
adrenals in culture appeared like glomerulosa cells in the
absence of ACTH and were transformed into zona fasciculata
type with characteristic morphology when treated with

ACTH. Hornsby et al. (1974) observed that treatment of glomerulosa cells isolated from rat adrenals and maintained in monolayer culture with ACTH not only caused the mitochondrial cristae of the cells to change from a tubule to a vescicular form but also induced the secretion of corticosterone instead of aldosterone. These results suggest that ACTH in addition to acutely stimulating steroidogenesis can also induce differentiation in the adrenocortical cells. Our studies (Jagannadha Rao and Lehoux, 1979) on the effects of chronic treatment of adult male rats with ACTH on Angiotensin II receptors in adrenal zona glomerulosa cells has provided additional support for this concept. It is well known now that Angiotensin II is a potent stimulator of aldosterone production in a number of experimental animals (Blair West et al., 1963; Haning et al., 1970; Peytremann et al., 1973; Fredlund et al., 1975; Douglas et al., 1978). Studies using ^{125}I labelled Antiotensin II have shown that specific Angiotensin II receptors are localized mainly in the glomerulosa cells (Glossmann et al., 1974; Fredlund et al., 1975; Douglas and Catt, 1976; Douglas et al., 1978; Aguilera et al., 1980a,b). In view of the significant morphological and functional changes induced by ACTH resulting in differentiation of glomerulosa cells into fasciculata type it was of interest to examine whether ACTH also induces changes at the Angiotensin II receptor levels, as the fasciculata type cells are not responsive to Angiotensin II. The details of treatment with ACTH, isolation of glomerulosa cells, radioimmunoassay of cortical steroids have been described earlier (Jagannadha Rao and Lehoux, 1979). The data presented in Table VI indicates that administration of ACTH to male rats for 4 to 8 days caused a significant decrease in the quantity of ^{125}I labelled Angiotensin II bound by the glomerulosa cells compared to cells from control group, suggesting partial loss of one of the features characteristic of glomerulosa cells. The decrease which was observed in all the three experiments ranged from 19 to 54% and seems to be influenced by duration and/or dose of ACTH treatment. The data from Table VII indicates that there is a significant decrease in serum aldosterone concentration indicating that not only a decrease in binding but also a functional change has been induced. The results of the in vivo ACTH treatment on the in vitro response of the glomerulosa cells to Angiotensin II and ACTH are presented in Table VIII. It can be seen that while the cells from the control group exhibited the expected response to both hormones, the response of the cells from ACTH treated groups is greatly diminished. These observations

Table IV. Effect of ACTH Antiserum on Compensatory Hypertrophy of Right Adrenal

Group	Treatment	Right adrenal wt (mg)	Cell Yield $(X10^{-5})$	Protein/adrenal (mg)	g DNA/mg protein	Serum Corti- sterone $(\mu g/dl)$
A	Unoperated controls	25.4 ± 2.9 (8)[a]	7.2[b]	1.05 ± 0.09 (4)[a]	46.6 ± 3.1 (4)[a]	5.88 ± 0.75 (8)[a,c]
B	Unilaterally adrena- lectomized and NRS treated	35.4 ± 1.8 (8)	9.3	1.53 ± 0.12 (4)	65.4 ± 4.4 (4)	9.75 ± 1.45 (8)
C	Unilaterally adrena- lectomized and ACTH antiserum treated	34.9 ± 2.4 (8)	10.6	1.48 ± 0.10 (4)	73.7 ± 4.1 (4)	5.70 ± 0.63 (8)

Unilaterally adrenalectomized animals were administered 0.5 ml ACTH antiserum dialy for 8 days ip. The animals were killed on the nineth day.

[a] Mean ± SE; number of replicates is shown in parenthesis.

[b] Cells were isolated from four adrenals in each group.

[c] Values: 9.75: 5.88, $P<0.05$; 9.95: 5.70, $P<0.02$.

From Jagannadha Rao, et al., 1978.

Table V. Effects of ACTH Antiserum Treatment on Absolute Volumes of Fasciculate Cells and Subcellular Organelles

Volume	NRS-treated controls	Hypophysectomized	ACTH antiserum-treated
Cell	1481.3±88.1	615.3±23.1	1305.0±37.3
Δ%		-58.5	-11.9
P		< 0.001	NS
Nucleus	180.9± 4.0	121.3±10.2	154.0±11.3
Δ%		-32.9	-14.9
P		< 0.005	< 0.05
Cytoplasmic matrix	655.6±21.7	297.2± 8.4	569.2±13.8
Δ%		-54.7	-13.2
P		< 0.001	< 0.005
Lipid	117.1±17.2	15.9± 6.3	129.3±21.4
Δ%		-86.4	+10.4
P		< 0.005	NS

Three week old rats were hypophysectomized and adrenals removed 7 days later for ultrastructural studies. P values refer to a comparison with controls.

[a] Mean ± SE.

From Jagannadha Rao, et al., 1978.

have been recently confirmed by studies of Aguilera et al. (1981). Thus, although Angiotensin plays a significant role in regulation of aldosterone production by glomerulosa cells ACTH appears to have a dominating influence over the morphological and functional differentiation of these cells.

3. Role of LH in Regulation of Growth and Function of Testes

A. <u>Effect of LH antiserum injection to rats on testes weight and responsiveness of Leydig cells to LH</u>. The dependance of the testis on gonadotrophic stimulation for normal growth and function was established almost five decades ago. As mentioned in the introduction all the earlier studies on the role of gonadotrophins were carried out using the technique of hypophysectomy which resulted in atrophy of the gonads. Interestingly the neutralization of endogenous LH in male and female mammals by adminis-tration of LH antiserum not only interferes with function but also results in a drastic decrease in a gonadal weight (Contropulous and Hayashida, 1963; Bourdel and Li, 1963; Qudri and Spies, 1966; Madhwa Raj and Moudgal, 1970; Jagannadha Rao et al., 1972; Moudgal et. al., 1974; Jagannadha Rao, 1982). However, in contrast to the adrenals, cellular organization of testes and their hormonal dependence is a complex one. The testes is composed of seminiferous tubules, Sertoli cells and Leydig cells. Although it is well accepted now that FSH acts primarily on Sertoli cells, LH on Leydig cells and testosterone on germ cells, it is also known that the growth and function of these cells are interre-lated. The increase in weight of testes has been shown to be proportional to the increase in the level of gonado-tropins (Steinberger and Steinberger, 1972). However, the relative roles of gonadotropins is still not clear since, to a great extent, testosterone can replace the need for gonadotropins in spermatogenesis and also cause an increase in the weight of testes in the absense of gonadotropin. Thus the use of weight and size as parameters of growth stimulation by LH is all the more questionable in the case of testes. Also the results obtained with the adrenal cell system and ACTH as well as the fact that Leydig cells contribute negligibly to the bulk of testes

Table VI. Effect of In Vivo ACTH Treatment on ^{125} Labeled
Ag II Binding by Rat Adrenal Glomerulosa Cells

| | fg Ag II bound/10^5 cells | | |
	Expt 1	Expt 2	Expt 3
Control	1004 ± 58	1648 ± 26	946 ± 42
ACTH treated	812 ± 33[a]	1010 ± 111[b]	444 ± 17[b]
Decrease (%)	19	39	54

[a] $P = 0.05 - 0.025$.
[b] $P < 0.001$.
Expt. 1, 50 μg ACTH.rat^{-1}day^{-1} for 4 days, N = 5;
Expt. 2, 100 μg ACTH.rat^{-1}.day^{-1} for 8 days, N = 9;
Expt. 3, 150 μg ACTH.rat^{-1} day^{-1} for 8 days, N = 8.
All values mean ± S E. N = number of determinations.
From Jagannadha Rao and Lehoux, 1979.

Table VII. Effect of ACTH Treatment on Plasma Aldosterone
and Corticosterone Concentrations

	Aldosterone (ng/dl)	Corticosterone (μg/dl)
Control	14.6 ± 1.66	1.08 ± 0.45
ACTH-treated	8.2 ± 1.07[a]	0.66 ± 0.19[b]

[a] $P < 0.001$.
[b] P, not significant.
Data from expt. 3 of Table VI. Values represent mean ± S E
of 8 determinations.
From Jagannadha Rao and Lehoux, 1979.

Table VIII.   Effect of <u>In Vivo</u> ACTH Treatment on <u>In Vitro</u>
Response of Rat Glomerulosa Cells to Ag II and ACTH

	ng Aldosterone/10^5 cells	
Group	Control	Treated
No hormone	2.03 ± 0.06	0.80 ± 0.14
Ag II 1 × 10^{-9}M	4.34 ± 0.09	0.71 ± 0.07
Ag II 1 × 10^{-8}M	9.00 ± 0.61	0.89 ± 0.05
Ag II 1 × 10^{-7}M	5.00 ± 0.03	0.71 ± 0.14
ACTH 0.3 × 10^{-12}M	2.38 ± 0.12	0.42 ± 0.10
ACTH 0.3 × 10^{-11}M	7.19 ± 0.90	0.76 ± 0.15
ACTH 3.0 × 10^{-10}M	12.30 ± 1.32	1.33 ± 0.15

Approximately 5×10^4 cell/tube were incubated with or with-
out hormone for 2 hr at 37°C under 95% O_2 and 5% O_2.
Aldosterone were determined by radioimmunoassay after extrac-
tion of cell suspension with dichloromethane.   Values are mean
± S E of triplicate determinations.
From Jagannadha Rao and Lehoux, 1979.

weight prompted us to re-examine the role of LH in regulation
of growth and function of Leydig cells using the immunological
approach.

The details of production of antiserum to ovine LH, its
characterization ability to neutralize rat LH, radioimmunoassay of testosterone, isolation of leydig cells and electron
microscopy of testes have been described in earlier communica-
tions (Jagannadha Rao et al., 1974; Gondos et al., 1981).
The study was carried out using adult male rats which received
0.5 ml of normal rabbit serum (NRS) or 0.5 ml of antiserum to
ovine LH raised in rabbits, by the subcutaneous route daily

ovine LH raised in rabbits, by the subcutaneous route daily
for 8 days. After the treatment the effects on the weight of
testes, serum testosterone and the responsiveness of the
isolated leydig cells to exogenous LH were examined. In one
batch the testicular tissue was processed for light and
electron microscopic study. Neutralization of endogenous LH
for 8 days resulted in the marginal but significant decrease in
the testes weight (Table IX) and there was also a significant
decrease in serum testosterone levels indicating the efficacy
of the antiserum. However, there was no difference in the
number of Leydig cells that could be isolated in the control
and antiserum treated group. If LH were needed for proliferation of Leydig cells in the present experiment, deprivation
of LH must have resulted in decreased yield of cells. The
possibility that the lack of effect on cell yield is due to
incomplete neutralization of LH can be ruled out as there is
a significant decrease in serum testosterone levels which has
resulted in a decrease in the testes weight. Since it is
known that testosterone maintains seminiferous tubule growth,
the decrease in testes weight must have been due to a decrease
in the weight of the seminiferous tubule compartment. The
data presented in Table X clearly indicates that there is a
decrease in the basal rate of testosterone production as well
as response to LH.

B. Light and electron microscope study of Leydig cells
from NRS and antisera treated rats. In the normal rabbit
serum treated group, the interstitial regions showed predom-
inantely Leydig cells and partially differentiated cells with
occasional scattered undifferentiated mesenchymal cells.
The Leydig cells were characteristically arranged in clusters
around blood vessels. In the group treated with antiserum to
LH, fully differentiated Leydig cells were found only as rare
isolated cells and the predominant cell type was the mesenchymal cell. The amount of space occupied by the interstitial
regions was significantly reduced in comparison to the control
group. The relative percentage of different cell types
is presented in Table XI. There was a clear shift to less
differentiated forms in the experimental group with almost
a complete absence of fully differentiated cells. Electron
microscopic study revealed that antiserum treatment resulted
in disruption of the endoplasmic reticulum and accumulation
of dense bodies resembling lysosomes in the Leydig cells
and such changes were not seen in Leydig cells from the
normal rabbit serum treated group.

4.   Role of Trophic Hormones in Promoting the Growth of
      Target Tissues

        Since the classic demonstration of the presence of
trophic hormones in the pituitary (Smith, 1927, 1930), it is
widely accepted that the trophic hormones in addition to
regulating the function also regulate the growth of the target
tissue. While the earlier studies were based on gross changes
in target glands, recently attempts have been made to provide
biochemical evidence to support this conclusion. Several
studies with ACTH and the adrenocortical cell system (Farese
and Reddy, 1963; Imrie et al., 1965; Masui and Garren, 1970)
indicated that ACTH promoted cell proliferation which was
based on increased ^{3}H thymidine uptake. However, reports also
exist (Bransom and Reddy, 1961; Masui and Garren, 1971; Gill,
1972; Ramachandran and Suyama, 1975; Dallman et al., 1980)
which show that ACTH did not promote DNA synthesis, but infact
inhibited DNA synthesis. In vivo studies using anti-serum to
ACTH clearly suggest that neutralization of ACTH did not
interfere with growth of adrenal. This is evident from both
intact and unilaterally adrenalectomized rat models. Several
studies have clearly established that the increase in weight
during adrenal hypertrophy in unilaterally adrenalectomized

Table IX. Effects of Antiserum to LH and Normal Rabbit Serum
Given to Ten Rats/Group on the Weight and Number of Interstitial
Cells in Adult Rat Testes and on Levels of Testosterone in Serum
            (Values are means ± S. E. M.)

Treatment	Paired testes weight (g)	Interstitial cells/testis ($\times 10^{-6}$)	Serum testoserone (ng/ml)
Normal rabbit serum	3.10 ± 0.07	13.7 ± 1.01	2.19 ± 0.19
LH antiserum	2.61 ± 0.06[a]	13.1 ± 2.50	1.03 ± 0.13[a]

[a]P < 0.001: compared with control group (Student's t-test).
From Gondos et al., 1980.

Table X. Effects of Administration of Antiserum to LH or Normal Rabbit Serum (NRS) or In Vitro Responsiveness of Rat Interstitial Cells. Values are means ± S. E. M. of Triplicate Incubations

LH Concentration (nmol/l)	Testosterone (ng/10^5 cells in 2 hr)	
	NRS-treated	LH antiserum-treated
0.025	1.69 ± 0.15	0.29 ± 0.10
0.10	3.90 ± 0.04	2.79 ± 0.06
0.40	5.38 ± 0.14	3.67 ± 0.15
4.00	4.10 ± 0.26	2.87 ± 0.11

From Gondos et al., 1980.

Table XI. Mean (± S. E. M.) Percentage Distribution of Cell Types in the Testicular Interstitial Tissue of Rats Treated with Antiserum to LH or Normal Serum (NRS)

	Mesenchymal (undifferentiated cells	Partially differen- Leydig cells	Fully differen- Leydig cells
NRS treated	14.7 ± 1.3	41.4 ± 1.7	43.9 ± 1.5
LH antiserum-treated	79.5 ± 1.0	20.2 ± 0.9	0.3 ± 0.0

From Gondos et al., 1980.

rat is indeed due to cell division (Tepperman et al., 1943; Dallman et al., 1976, 1977; Dallman et al., 1980). Recently (Dallman et al., 1980) using an unilaterally adrenalectomized animal model, it has been shown that ACTH is not involved in the regulation of growth of adrenal. These studies revealed that treatment of rats with ACTH inhibited the proliferative response of the remaining adrenal after unilateral adrenal-ectomy. It was also found that the initial effects of ACTH treatment was the increase in adrenal RNA content without a concurrent increase in DNA. They also observed that the use of synthetic ACTH did not cause increase in adrenal weight and increase in weight could be demonstrated only with pharma-cological doses. Based on these studies they concluded that ACTH is not the agent involved in the proliferative process involved in the adrenal compensatory hypertrophy. Our studies using Leydig cells and LH also lend support to this concept that trophic hormone may not be a mitogenic factor. Deprival of endogenous LH did not result in decreased yield of cells and instead there was an increase in the number of undifferen-tiated cells. However, it has been reported that there is an increase in Leydig cell number following hCG treatment in rats (Christensen and Peacock, 1980). These studies were based on histological parameters and morphometry. Interest-ingly, the same authors have also commented that no dividing Leydig cells could be noticed during their extensive counting process. In contrast, Schafer et al. (1982) have reported only an increase in cell volume and not in cell number with advancing age in rats. Huhtaniemi (1981) also has reported no changes in Leydig cell number when neonatal rats were treated with hCG. It is known from several histological studies (Christensen, 1975) that mature Leydig cells in the adult testes are never seen in cell division and yet their number based on histological criteria increases under LH stimulation. This suggests the possibility that LH may be stimulating the process of differentiation of some precursor cells into Leydig cells. It may be pertinent to point out that in most mammals studied Leydig cells undergo two distinct periods of development, the first occuring during foetal stage and second at the time of puberty. Recently, Payne et al. (1980) have reported that even in adult testes two types of Leydig cells exist and these differ only in the responsive-ness to hCG. They suggest that the cells with decreased responsiveness to hCG may represent immature Leydig cells. Using entirely different parameters Purvis et al. (1978) also have reported that the rat Leydig cells, within the same testes, exhibit various degrees of maturation and Leydig cell population is not functionally synchronized. These observa-tions suggest that the increase in Leydig cells may be a continuous process and may include differentiation of some precursor cell into a functional Leydig cell and this process may be under the control of LH and/or other factors. The suggestion that the trophic hormones may not be the growth promoter in target tissue obviously raises the question of what regulates the growth of these tissues. While there is no definite answer, several earlier studies lend evidence to the existence of distinct pituitary growth promoting factors. In fact it was observed that during the course of the isolation and characterization of ACTH, the partially purified pituitary extracts which were weak in corticotrophic activity as measured by adrenal ascorbic acid depletion caused changes in weight and structure of the adrenal cortex (Astwood, 1955). Dixon et al. (1951) also reported that the adrenal ascorbic acid depleting factor could be separated from an adrenal weight increasing activity. Clinical studies (Liddle et al., 1954) revealed that the increased adrenal responsiveness could be observed in patients treated with a pituitary fraction devoid of the immediate steroid discharging property of ACTH. Interestingly adrenal weight maintenance activity was detected in plasma of patients with Cushing's syndrome due to bilateral adrenal hyperplasia but not in the plasma of patients with Cushing's syndrome due to adrenal tumor or in normal subjects (Jailer et al., 1957). It was also demonstrated (Carter and Stack Dunne, 1953; Cater and Stack Dunne, 1955) that although ACTH induced the secretion of steroids and maintained adrenal responsiveness, it was relatively ineffective in stimulating mitotic activity in the adrenals of hypophysectomized rats. In contrast, they found that the pituitary growth hormone preparations induced a marked stimulation of cell division with relatively little effects on adrenal weight. But when ACTH and GH were injected together there was a synergistic increase in adrenal weight. Similar observations have also been made by Lostroh and Li (1957). Thus while earlier studies suggest that other pituitary hormones may have synergistic roles in adrenal growth regulation, recent studies show that hormones like insulin or factors like FGF may be involved in this growth regulating process. In these studies (Ramachandran and Suyama, 1975) it was found that insulin caused a significant increase in adrenocortical cell proliferation in primary monolayer cultures. The fibroblast growth factor (FGF) isolated from bovine pituitaries was also found to stimulate the replication of Y-1 mouse adrenal tumor cells in culture (Gospadorowicz and Handley, 1975). Gill et al. (1977) have also reported that Angiotensin II stimulated cell proliferation and ^{3}H thymidine incorporation into DNA in monolayer cultures of bovine adrenocortical cells. Payet and Isler (1976) have also reported that Oxytocin is a potent mitogenic factor for zona glomerulosa cells. It may be pertinent to mention here that the isolation of ovarian growth factor distinct from pituitary FSH and LH has also been reported (Gospadorowicz et al., 1974).

Though no specific studies are available with FSH or TSH it is possible to draw some supportive evidence from the available data. It is known that specific FSH receptors exist in Sertoli cells only and Sertoli cells stop dividing very early in age in rat and no receptors for FSH have been demonstrated in germ cells (Means, 1980). It is clear that the stimulation of DNA synthesis observed in the seminiferous tubules following FSH treatment is not a direct effect of FSH and must be mediated through some Sertoli cell factor.

5.   Role of Trophic Hormones in Functional Differentiation

The ability of trophic hormones to maintain and stimulate the function of the responsive tissue is a well established fact. While in the case of somatotropin and prolactin, no specific parameter is used, the response to ACTH, Gonadotropins and Thyroid stimulating hormone is evaluated by quantitating the hormones produced by the responsive tissues or cells in response to trophic stimulus. Our studies using an immunological approach clearly show that deprivation of trophic support for the adrenal and testes results in a decrease in basal rate of hormone secretion as well as response to exogenous hormonal stimulus. In addition, significant changes in the ultrastructure of the adrenocortical and Leydig cell was also noticeable. The ability of ACTH to induce changes in the ulstructure of adrenocortical cells have been extensively studied (Nussdorfer et al., 1977; Kahri, 1976, 1966; Hornsby et al., 1973, 1974; Haning, 1970; Ramachandran et al., 1977). Studies of Kahri et al. (1976) has clearly indicated that ACTH also acts as a differentiating hormone, particularly in the case of human foetal adrenals. It is known that human adrenal cortex consists, during foetal life mainly of two different zones, namely foetal zone and definitive zone. It is reported that ACTH induces a very dramatic increase in the secretion of steroids of the adult type i.e., cortisol. Thus a change in functional capacity was also reflected in the changes in ultrastructure of cortical cells. Studies using rat adrenals both under in vivo and in vitro condition have also shown that the changes are induced at the receptor level also in the zona glomerulosa cells by ACTH. The studies reported here with Leydig cells also show a drastic change in ultrastructure following LH deprival and there is a sharp decrease in the proportion of fully differentiated Leydig cells. The relative increase in partially differentiated Leydig cells implies a regression to less differentiated forms. The present studies reported here show degenerative changes in the cytoplasma of Leydig cells which may be responsible for the decreased steroidogenic capacity. Thus our studies confirm the earlier observations of Dym et al. (1977) and essentially point out that LH may also act as a differentiating hormone, in addition to maintaining both acute and long-term steroidogenesis. The fact that the Leydig cells undergo two distinct periods of development, one during foetal stage and the other during puberty (Christensen, 1975) suggest that this latter period may correspond to the period at which Leydig cells may undergo differentiation into the adult type of Leydig cells. Studies have shown that in the immature rat testis the major products of Leydig cells are 5 reduced steroids and these secrete very little testosterone (Purvis et al., 1981). However, with the development of adult type of Leydig cell population between 20 and 30 days of age, there is parallel increase in the activity of three enzymes, which in the adult are primarily concerned with testosterone production. Along with this there is a decrease in the steroidogenic enzyme characteristic of foetal leydig cells. It may be pertinent to point out that the immature rat is more sensitive to the effects of hypophysectomy than the adult rat (Purvis et al., 1980). All these facts together suggest that gonadotropins may have an important role during this period of differentiation of foetal Leydig cells into the adult type of Leydig cells. Very little information is available on the actual process of differentiation itself. It may involve synthesis of new enzymes or specific proteins or both. It is also known that both ACTH and LH as well as prolactin induce changes in several steroidogenic enzymes and other functional features in adrenocortical cells and Leydig cells, respectively (Garren, 1968; Kimura, 1969; Eiknes, 1970; Hall, 1970; Kowal, 1970; Purvis et al., 1973; Steinberger and Steinberger, 1975; Hansson et al., 1978, Kortiz, 1977; Purvis et al., 1981). However the relationship of these changes following hormone exposure to differentiation is yet to be studied. Recently studies of Liles and Ramachandran (1977) and Rybak and Ramachandran (1982) have shown that when rat primary culture of normal rat adrenocortical cells were maintained in the absence of ACTH, there was a rapid decay of the enzyme Δ^5 3βhydroxy steroid dehydrogenase as judged by histochemical staining as well as by progesterone formation. They also demonstrated that addition of ACTH to cultures kept in the absence of the hormones for two weeks resulted in the induction of Δ^5 3βhydroxy steroid dehydrogenase within about 4 hr. Clear difference in the pattern of proteins in cells maintained in the presence and absence of ACTH was also discernable in sodium dodecyl sulphate polyacrylamide gel electrophoresis. Thus it is apparent that one of the functions of ACTH is maintenance of the steroidogenic enzymes and it is to be expected that this maintenance function may not be restricted to one enzyme only but may also include several other enzymes, proteins or factors.

Studies with leydig cells have shown that there is rapid protein synthesis following exposure to LH (Cook et al., 1975) and this is a prerequisite for a normal steroid response, since inhibitors of protein synthesis will block testosterone production, within a short time of exposure to LH. As these changes are in response to acute stimulus it is difficult to relate to them to the process of differentiation. However, Janszen et al. (1977) have described several proteins which are induced by LH stimulation in normal and tumor Leydig cells and these appear only two hours after exposure to LH. Recently, we have observed (Jagannadha Rao, unpublished studies) that there is a distinct difference in proteins on sodium dodecyl sulphate polyacrylamide gel electrophoresis between cytosolic proteins of the Leydig cells isolated from NRS and LH antiserum treated new born rats and some proteins were completely absent in the antisera treated group. It is possible that these changes may be related to the differentiation process.

6.   Concluding Remarks

The action of trophic hormone is a complex one involving both acute stimulation as well as long-term maintenance of functional status of target cell and this latter function can be interpreted to include the process of "growth" though not in the classical sense. It is difficult to make a clear distinction between the two processes, namely growth and function as these two are interrelated. As mentioned earlier, pituitary or non pituitary factors may be involved along with the trophic hromones in regulating the growth of responsive cells. The trophic hormones mainly induce functional differentiation, which consists of changes at the ultrastructural level as well as in the various enzymes and proteins. It is possible that the processes of growth and differentiation may take place sequentially or simultaneously depending upon the type of responsive cell.

ACKNOWLEDGEMENT. The work reviewed above was supported by NIH (USA) grants, CA 16417 and GM 2907 (to J. R.), Medical Research Council, Canada (to J. G. L.) and Indian Institute of Science, Bangalore, Family Planning Foundation, India (to A. J. R.). The permission to reproduce tables from journals, Endocrinology, Journal of Endocrinology and FEBS Letters is gratefully acknowledged. One of the authors (A. J. R.) is grateful to Prof. N. R. Moudgal, Department of Biochemistry, Indian Institute of Science, Bangalore for his encouragement and to Mr. M. Vadeendra for typing the manuscript.

REFERENCES

Aguilera, G., Menard, R. H., and Catt, K. J., 1980a, Regulatory actions of angiotensin II on receptors and steroidogenic enzymes in adrenal glomerulosa cells, Endocrinology 107:55.

Aguilera, G., Schirar, A., Baukal, A., Catt, K. J., 1980b, Angiotensin II receptors: Properties and regulation in adrenal glomerulosa cells, Circ. Res. Suppl. 46:118.

Aguilera, G., Fujita, K., and Catt, K. J., 1981, Mechanism of inhibition of aldosterone secretion by adrenocorticotrophin, Endocrinology 108:522.

Astwood, E. B., 1955, Growth hormone and adrenocorticotrophin, in: "The Hormones" Volume 3, p. 235, G. Pincus and K. V. Thimann, eds., Academic Press, New York.

Bascom, K. F., and Osterud, H. L., 1925, Quantitative studies of the testicle. II Pattern and total tubule length in the testicles of certain mammals, Anat. Rec. 31:159.

Baumann, K., and Muller, 1974, Effects of hypophysectomy with or without ACTH maintenance therapy on the final steps of aldosterone biosynthesis in the rat, Acta Endocrinol. (kbh) 76:102.

Blairwest, J. R., Coghlan, J. P., Denton, D. A., Goding, J. R., Wintour, M., and Wright, R. D., 1963, The control of aldosterone secretion, Rec. Prog. Horm. Res. 19:311.

Bourdel, G., and Li, C. H., 1963, Effect of rabbit antiserum to sheep pituitary interstitial stimulating hormone in adult female rats, Acta Endocrinol.(kbh) 42:473.

Bransome, E. D., and Reddy, W. J., 1961, Studies of adrenal nuclei acids: The influence of ACTH, unilateral adrenalectomy and growth hormone upon adrenal RNA and DNA in the dog, Endocrinology 69:997.

Carr, I., 1959, The human adrenal gland at the time of death, J. Path. Bacteriol. 78:533.

Cater, D. B., and Stack-Dunne, M. P., 1953, Histological changes in the adrenal of the hypophysectomized rat after treatment with pituitary preparations, J. Path. Bacteriol. 66:119.

Cater, D. B., and Stack-Dunne, M. P., 1955, The effects of growth hormone and corticotrophin upon the adrenal weight and adrenocortical mitotic activity, J. Endocrinol. 12:174.

Christensen, A. K., 1975, Leydig cells in: "Handbook of Physiology", Section 7, Volume 5, p. 57, R. O. Greep, E. B. Astwood, eds., Williams and Wilkins, Baltimore, MD.

Christensen, A., and Peacock, K., 1980, Increase in leydig cell number in testes of adult rats treated chronically with an excess of human chorionic gonadotrophin, Biol. Reprod. 22:383.

Cooke, B. A., Manszen, F. H. A., Clotscher, W. F., and Van Der Molen, H. J., 1975, Effect of protein synthesis inhibitors on testosterone production in rat testes interstitial tissue and leydig cell preparations, Biochem. J. 150:413.

Contopoulous, A. N., and Hayashida, T., 1963, Neutralization of activity of circulating gonadotrophic hormones by antiserum to rat pituitary, J. Endocrinol. 25:451.

Dallman, M. F., Engeland, W. C., Schinsako, J., 1976, Compensatory adrenal growth: a neorally mediated reflex, Am. J. Physiol. 231:408.

Dallman, M. F., Engeland, W. C., McBride, M. H., 1977, The neural regulation of compensatory hypertrophy, Ann. New York Acad. Sci. 297:373.

Dallman, M. F., Engeland, W. C., Holzwarth, M. A., Scholz, P. M., 1980, Adrenocorticotropin inhibits compensatory adrenal growth after unilateral adrenalectomy, Endocrinology 107:1397.

Davis, J. O., 1975, Regulation of aldosterone secretion in: "Handbook of Physiology", Section 7, Volume 4, p. 77, R. O. Greep and E. B. Astwood, eds., Williams and Wilkins, Baltimore, MD.

Dixon, H. B. F., Stack-Dunne, M. P., Young, F. G., and Carter, D. B., 1951, Influence of adrenotrophic hormone fractions on adrenal repair and on adrenal ascorbic acid, Nature 168:1084.

Douglas, J., Catt, 1976, Regulation of Angiotensin II receptors in rat adrenal cortex by dietary electrolytes, J. Clin. Invest. 58:834.

Douglas, J., Aguilera, G., Kondo, T., Catt, K. J., 1978, Angiotensin II receptors and aldosterone production in rat adrenal glomerulosa cells, Endocrinology 102:685.

Dym, M., Madhwaraj, H. G., and Chemes, H. E., 1977, Response of the testes to selective withdrawl of LH or FSH using anti-gonadotropic sera in: "The Testes in Normal and Infertile Man", p. 97, P. Troen and H. R. Nankin, ed., Raven Press, New York.

Eik-Nes, K. B., 1970, Synthesis and secretion of andostenedione and testosterone, in: "The Androgens of the Testis", p. 1, K. B. Eik-Nes, ed., Marrel and Dekker, New York.

Farese, R. V., and Reddy, W. J., 1963, Observations on the interactions between adrenal protein RNA and DNA during prolonged ACTH administration, Biochem. Biophys. Acta 76:145.

Fredlund, P., Saltman, S., and Catt, K. J., 1975, Aldosterone production by isolated adrenal glomerulosa cells: stimulation by physiological concentrations of Angiotensin II, Endocrinology 97:1577.

Garren, L. D., 1968, The mechanism of action of adrenocorticotropic hormone, Vit and Horm. 26:119.

Garren, L. D., Gill, G. N., Masui, H., and Walton, G. M., 1971, On the mechanism of action of ACTH, Rec. Prog. Horm. Res. 27:433.

Gill, G. N., 1972, Mechanism of ACTH action, Metabolism, 21:571.

Gill, G. N., III, C. R., Simonian, M. H., 1977, Angiotensin stimulation of bovine adrenocortical cell, Proc. Natl. Acad. Sci. USA 74:5569.

Glossmann, H., Baukal, A., and Catt, K. J., 1974, Properties of angiotensin receptors in the bovine and rat adrenal cortex, J. Biol. Chem. 249:825.

Gondos, B., Jagannadha Rao, A., and Ramachandran, J., 1980, Effects of antiserum to luteinizing hormone on the structure and function of rat leydig cells, J. Endocrinol. 87:265.

Gospadorowicz, D., Jones, K., Sato, G., 1974, Purification of a growth factor for ovarian cells from bovine pituitary gland, Proc. Natl. Acad. Sci. USA 71:2295.

Gospadorowicz, D., and Handley, H. H., 1975, Stimulation of
    division of Y-1 adrenal cells by a growth factor isolated
    from bovine pituitary glands, Endocrinology 97:102.
Greep, R. O., 1974, History of research on anterior typophysical
    hormones, in: "Handbook of Physiology", Section 7, Volume
    4, p. 1, R. O. Greep, E. B. Astwood, eds., Williams and
    Wilkins, Baltimore, MD.
Hall, P. F., 1970, Gonadotrophic regulation of testicular
    function, in: "The Androgens of the Testis", p. 73,
    K. B. Eik-Nes, ed., Mercel Dekker Inc., New York.
Haning, R., Tait, S. A., and Tait, J. F., 1970, In vitro effects
    of ACTH, Angiotensin, Serotonin and Potassium on steroid
    output and conversion of corticosterone to aldosterone by
    isolated adrenal cells, Endocrinology 87:1147.
Hornsby, P. J., O'Hare, M. J., and Neville, A. M., 1973, Effect
    of ACTH on biosynthesis of aldosterone and corticosterone
    by monolayer culture of rat adrenal zona glomerulosa cells,
    Biochem. Biophys. Res. Comm. 54:1554.
Hornsby, P. J., O'Hare, M. J., and Neville, A. M., 1974,
    Functional and morphological observations on rat adrenal
    zona glomerulosa cells in monolayer culture, Endocrinology
    95:1240.
Huhtaniemi, I. T., Mohan, K., and Catt, K. J., 1981, Regulation
    of LH receptors and steroidogenesis in the neonatal rat
    testes, Endocrinology 109:588.
Hansson, V., Ritzen, M., Purvis, K., French, F. S., 1978,
    Endocrine approaches to male contraception, Scriptor,
    Copenhagen.
Idleman, S., 1970, Ultrastructure of the mammalian adrenal
    cortex, Int. Rev. Cytol. 27:181.
Imrie, R. C., Ramaiah, T. R., Antoni, F., Hutchinson, W. C.,
    1965, The effect of ACTH on the nuclei acid metabolism of
    the rat adrenal gland, J. Endocrinol. 32:302.
Ingle, D. J., 1951, The functional interrelationship of the
    anterior pituitary and adrenal cortex, Ann. Inter. Med.
    35:652.
Jagannadha Rao, A., Madhwa Raj, H. G., and Moudgal, N. R., 1972,
    Effect of LH, FSH and their antisera on gestation in the
    hamster, (Mesocricetus auratus), J. Reprod. Fert. 29:239.
Jagannadha Rao, A., Moudgal, N. R., Madhwa Raj, H. G., Lipner,
    H., Greep, R. P., 1974, The role of FSH and LH in the
    initiation of ovulation in rats and hamsters; a study using
    rabbit antisera to ovine FSH and LH, J. Reprod. Fert.
    37:323.
Jagannadha Rao, A., Long, J. A., and Ramachandran, J., 1978,
    Effects of antiserum to adrenocorticotropin on adrenal
    growth and function, Endocrinology 102:371.

Jagannadha Rao, A., and Lehoux, J. G., 1979, Effect of ACTH on ^{125}I labelled angiotensin II binding and response by rat adrenal glomerulosa cells, FEBS Letters 105:325.

Jagannadha Rao, A., Behrens, C., and Ramachandran, J., 1980, Immunochemical studies of adrenocorticotropin using tritium labelled hormone, Int. J. Peptide Protein Res. 15:480.

Jagannadha Rao, A., 1982, Effect of rabbit antiserum to ovine LH on reproductive organs in male hamsters and guinea pigs, Experientia, 38:279.

Jailer, J. W., Longson, D., Christy, N. D., 1957, Cushing's Syndrome II. Adrenal weight maintaining activity in the plasma of patients with cushing's syndrome, J. Clin. Endocrinol. Metab. 36:1608.

Janszen, F. H. A., Cooke, B. A., Van Der Molen, H. J., 1977, Specific protein synthesis in isolated rat leydig cells, Biochem. J. 162:341.

Kahri, A. J., 1966, Histochemical and electron microscopic studies on the cells of rat adrenal cortex in tissue culture, Acta Endocrinol. 52: Suppl. (108) 1.

Kahri, A. I., Huhtaniemi, I., and Salmenpera, M., 1976, Steroid formation and differentiation of cortical cells in tissue culture of human foetal adrenals in the presence and absence of ACTH, Endocrinology 98:33.

Kimura, T., 1969, Effect of hypophysectomy and ACTH administration on the level of adrenal cholesterol side chain desmolase, Endocrinology 85:492.

Kowi, J., 1970, ACTH and the metabolism of adrenal cell cultures. Rec. Prog. Horm. Res. 26:623.

Kortiz, S. B., Girija, B., and Schwartz, E., 1977, ACTH action on adrenal steroidogenesis, Ann. New York Acad. Sci. 297:329.

Liddle, G. W., Island, D., Rinfret, A. P., Forsham, P. H., 1954, Factors enhancing the response of the human adrenal to corticotropin. Is there an adrenal growth factor? J. Clin. Endocrinol. Metab. 14:839.

Liles, S., and Ramachandran, J., 1977, Regulation of Δ^5-3β hydroxysteroid dehydrogenase isomerase activity in adrenocortical cell cultures by ACTH, Biochem. Biophys. Res. Comm. 79:226.

Long, J. A., 1975, Zonation of the mammalian adrenal cortex, in: "Handbook of Physiology", Section 7, Volume 6, p. 13, R. R. O. Greep and E. B. Astwood, eds., Williams and Wilkins, Baltimore, MD.

Lostroh, A. J., and Li, C. H., 1957, Stimulation of the sex accessories of hypophysectomized male rats by non-gonadotropic hromones of the pituitary gland, Acta Endocrinol. 25:1.

Madhwa Raj, H. G., and Moudgal, N. R., 1970, Hormonal control
    of gestation in the rat, Endocrinology 86:874.
Malamed, S., 1975, Ultrastructure of the mammalian adrenal
    cortex in relation to secretory of function in: "Handbook
    of Physiology", Section 7, Volume 6, p. 25, R. O. Greep
    and E. B. Estwood, eds., Williams and Wilkins, Baltimore.
Manuelidis, L., and Mulrow, D., 1974, Aldosterone production by
    adrenal cultures via dibCAMP and the reversibility of ACTH
    and dibCAMP induced changes, Endocrinology 95:728.
Masui, H., and Garren, L. D., 1970, The mechanism of action of
    adrenocorticotrophic hormone stimulation of DNA polymerase
    and thymidine kinase activity in adrenal glands, J. Biol.
    Chem. 245:2627.
Masui, H., and Garren, L. D., 1971, Inhibition of replication
    in functional mouse adrenal tumor cells by adrenocortico-
    trophic hormone mediated by adrenosine 3'5' cycle mono-
    phosphate, Proc. Natl. Acad. Sci. USA 68:3206.
Means, A. R., Dedman, M. R., Tash, J. S., Tindal, D. J.,
    Vansickle, M., Walsh, M. J., 1980, Regulation of the testes
    sertoli cell by follicle stimulating hormone, Ann. Rev.
    Physiol. 42:59.
Moudgal, N. R., Jagannadha Rao, A., Maneckjee, R., Murlidhar,
    K., Venkatramiah, M., Sheela Rani, C. S., 1974, Gonado-
    tropins and their antibodies, Rec. Prog. Horm. Res. 30:47.
Muller, A. F., Riondel, A. M., Manning, E. L., 1956, Effect of
    corticotrophin on secretion of aldosterone, Lancet 2:1021.
Muller, J., 1970, Decreased aldosterone production by rat
    adrenal tissue in vitro due to treatment with 9α fluro-
    cortisol dexamethasone and adrenocorticotrophin in vivo,
    Acta Endocrinol. (kbh) 63:1.
Muller, J., 1978, Suppression of aldosterone biosynthesis by
    treatment of rats with adrenocorticotrophin: Comparison
    with glucocorticoid effects, Endocrinology 103:2061.
Nieschlag, E., (ed.), 1975, Immunization with hormones in repro-
    duction research, North Holland, Amsterdam.
Nussdorfer, G. G., Mazzocchi, G., Robba, C., Belloni, A. S.,
    Rebuftat, D., 1977, Effects of ACTH and dexamethasone on
    the zona glomerulosa of the rat adrenal cortex: an
    ultrastructural sterological study, Acta. Endocrinol. (kbh)
    85:608.
O'Hare, M. J., and Neville, A. M., 1973, Morphological responses
    to corticotropin and cyclin AMP by adult rat adrenocortical
    cells in monolayer culture, J. Endocrinol. 56:529.
Payet, N., Isler, H., 1976, Adrenal Glomerulosa mitotic
    stimulation by posterior pituitary hormones, Cell Tiss.
    Res. 172:93.

Payne, A. H., Downing, J. R., and Wong, K. L., 1980, LH recep-
     tors and testosterone synthesis in two distinct populations
     of Leydig cells, Endocrinology 106:1424.
Peytremann, A., Nicholson, W. E., Brown, R. D., Liddle, G. W.,
     and Hardman, J. G., 1973, Comparative effects of angioten-
     sin and ACTH on cyclic AMP and steroidogenesis in isolated
     bovine adrenal cells, J. Clin. Invest. 52:835.
Purvis, J. L., Canick, J. A., Mason, J. I., Estabrook, R. W.,
     and McCarthy, J. L., 1973, Lifetime of adrenal cytochrome
     P-450 as influenced by ACTH, Ann. New York Acad. Sci.
     212:319.
Purvis, K., Clausen, O. P. F., and Hansson, V., 1978, Functional
     characteristics of rat Leydig cells, Ann. Biol. Anim.
     Biochem. Biophys. 18:595.
Purvis, K., Cusan, L., and Hansson, V., 1981, Regulation of
     steroidogenesis and steroid action in Leydig cells, J.
     Steroid Biochem. 15:77.
Purvis, K., Clausen, O. P. F., and Hansson, V., 1980, Effects
     of age and hypophysectomy on responsiveness of rat Leydig
     cells to LH/hCG, J. Reprod. Fertil. 60:77.
Quadri, S. K., and Spies, H. G., 1966, Inhibition of spermato-
     genesis and ovulation in rabbits with antiovine LH rabbit
     serum, Proc. Soc. Expt. Biol. Med. 123:809.
Ramachandran, J., and Suyama, A. T., 1975, Inhibition of repli-
     cation of normal adrenocortical cells in culture by
     adrenocorticotropin, Proc. Natl. Acad. Sci. USA 72:113.
Ramachandran, J., Jagannadha Rao, A., and Liles, S., 1977,
     Studies on the trophic action of ACTH, Ann. New York Acad.
     Sci. 297:336.
Rybak, S. M., and Ramachandran, J., 1982, Mechanism of induction
     of Δ^5-3β-Hydroxysteroid dehydrognease-isomerse activity in
     rat adrenocortical cells by corticotropin, Endocrinology
     111:427.
Sairam, M. R., Jagannadha Rao, A., and Li, C. H., 1974, Termina-
     tion of pregnancy in the rat by the antiserum to β subunit
     of ovine interstitial cell stimulating hormone, Proc. Soc.
     Expt. Biol. Med. 147:823.
Sairam, M. R., Jagannadha Rao, A., and Li, C. H., 1975, The use
     of antiserum to rat prolactin to evaluate its role as
     luteotropin in the hamster, Acta Endocrinol. 79:351.
Suyama, A. T., Long, J. A., and Ramachandran, J., 1977, Ultra-
     structural changes induced by ACTH in normal adrenocortical
     cells in culture, J. Cell Biol. 72:757.
Schafer, G., Helstein, A. F., Hilz, H., 1982, Steroidogenic
     capacity of isolated mouse Leydig cells does not decrease
     with age, Endocrinology 110:1362.

Smith, P. E., 1927, The disabilities caused by hypophysectomy
    and their repair, J. Ann. Med. Assoc. 88:158.
Smith, P. E., 1930, Hypophysectomy and replacement therapy in
    the rat, Ann. J. Anat. 45:205.
Steinberger, E., and Steinberger, A., 1972, The testis: Growth
    vs. function in: "Regulation of Organ and Tissue Growth"
    p. 299, R. G. Goss, ed., Academic Press, New York.
Tepperman, J., Engel, F. L., Long, C. N. H., 1943, A review of
    adrenal cortical hypertrophy, Endocrinology 32:373.

DISCUSSION

NICHOLSON: Does fasting influence in any way the effects of
unilateral adrenalectomy and could any of the differences
observed between hypophysectomized and antiserum treated
animals be due to their nutritional status? I ask this
question because hyopphysectomized rats do not gain weight.

RAO: Yes, it is a good possibility, although we have no
data.

ROMMERTS: You showed that LH antiserum increased the number
of undifferentiated Leydig cells and decreased the number of
differentiated Leydig cells, but you did not show what was
different in these Leydig cells.

RAO: This classification was based on the size, shape of the
cell, nucleus and the quantity of cytoplasm in each cell.
This was done using morphometric studies.

MEANS: Have you screened the sera from anti-ACTH treated rats
for the presence of anti-idiotype antibody production?

RAO: No, it has not been done, but the serum from each rat
has been checked for presence of antibodies to ACTH.

TAYLOR: 1. Have you ever administered purified ACTH to
hypophysectomized animals to see whether ACTH might stimulate
growth in that setting? 2. Your data suggested that the
antibody-induced block of the ACTH effect upon the adrenal
was less complete than that induced by hypophysectomy. Might
it be that one needs less ACTH to have a "trophic" effect
upon the adrenal than to stimulate corticosterone production?
If so, then one might need a more complete neutralization of
ACTH to see adrenal regression.

RAO: 1. No, we have not done that, although others have shown that it causes increase in size and weight of the adrenals. 2. Although for reasons unknown, the effects of immunoneutralization are not always complete. Also it is possible that continued suppression of endogenous hormones may alter the natural feedback regulation and more hormone may be secreted into circulation as a result.

RITZÉN: In various syndromes of congenital adrenal hyperplasia (e.g. 21-hydroxylase deficiency), the adrenals are exposed to high concentrations of ACTH. This clearly causes adrenal hyperplasia. Would that not imply that in vivo, ACTH causes increased cell proliferation in the adrenal cortex?

RAO: The situation in a clinical case can be different. I can quote one study in this connection (Jailer, 1957). Adrenal weight maintenance activity was detected in plasma of patients with Cushing's syndrome due to bilateral adrenal hyperplasia but not in plasma of patients with Cushing's syndrome.

LABRIE: What was the time course of action of anti-LH serum on plasma testosterone levels, especially in view of the relatively small inhibitory effect observed?

RAO: The antiserum was administered once daily for 8 days to adult male rats. We had to choose a minimal effective dose as complete atrophy of the testis (which will be the result if testosterone is very low) will cause problems in isolation of Leydig cells.

UTILIZATION OF LIPOPROTEIN-CARRIED CHOLESTEROL FOR STEROIDOGENESIS BY RAT LUTEAL TISSUE

Jerome F. Strauss, III, Laurie G. Paavola,[a]
Mindy F. Rosenblum, Toshinobu Tanaka, and
John T. Gwynne[b]

[a]Departments of Pathology and Gynecology,
University of Pennsylvania, School of Medicine
Philadelphia, PA 19104
[b]Department of Medicine, University of North
Carolina School of Medicine, Chapel Hill, NC

1. Introduction

Steroidogenic cells have the capacity to synthesize de novo the obligate precursor of their secretory products, cholesterol. However, it has become apparent that many glands rely upon extracellular sterol as substrate (Brown et al., 1979; Gwynne and Strauss, 1982; Strauss et al., 1981). This seems to be particularly true of tissues which secrete large quantities of steroid, such as the corpus luteum.

Extracellular cholesterol is transported in the form of lipoproteins, complex structures which consist of a hydrophobic core containing esterified cholesterol and triglycerides and an outer layer containing phospholipid, free cholesterol and protein (Osborne and Brewer, 1977). Traditionally, these particles have been classified according to their hydrated densities, but they may also be categorized according to their lipid and apolipoprotein composition. The main cholesterol carrying lipoproteins in the blood are low density (LDL) and high density (HDL) lipoproteins; the predominant lipoprotein class depends upon the species in question. In man, LDL carry most of the cholesterol, whereas in rodents HDL are most abundant. LDL and HDL differ with respect to their lipid and protein composition. Moreover, each of these classes, defined by their hydrated densities, are heterogenous comprised of particles which have different contents of lipid and apolipoprotein, and even different apolipoproteins. The protein composition is important because the apolipoproteins are recognized by cell surface receptors and various enzymes, and hence determine the function of the particles.

Lipoproteins interact with cells in three different ways which promote cholesterol movement: (a) "collisional exchange"; (b) pinocytosis and non-receptor mediated endocytosis; and (c) receptor-mediated absorptive endocytosis (Gwynne and Strauss, 1982). Collisional exchange does not usually lead to net cholesterol uptake by cells, but does facilitate the rapid equilibration of lipoprotein and cellular lipids. Cells can accumulate cholesterol through pinocytosis and non-receptor-mediated endocytosis of lipoproteins. Like collisional exchange, these processes are not lipoprotein specific, and the amount of cholesterol taken up is directly related to the lipoprotein concentration. Receptor-mediated interactions are, in contrast, both saturable and lipoprotein specific. Under normal circumstances, the receptor-mediated pathways appear to be, quantitatively, the predominant means by which steroidogenic cells accumulate extracellular cholesterol.

Two apparently distinct receptor-mediated mechanisms for uptake of lipoprotein cholesterol have been described in steroidogenic tissues. One recognizes apolipoprotein B, the apolipoprotein of LDL, as well as apolipoprotein E, an arginine-rich apolipoprotein found in certain subclasses of HDL. The LDL receptor has been purified from bovine adrenal cortex (Schneider et al., 1982). It is an acidic glycoprotein of 164,000 molecular weight which requires calcium for lipoprotein binding. The other receptor-mediated system recognizes HDL, probably apolipoprotein A-I, a major apolipoprotein of this density class. The metabolism of LDL by cells has been well characterized (Goldstein and Brown, 1977). It involves, in sequence, the binding of lipoproteins to receptors located in specialized regions of the plasma membrane, called coated pits; the rapid internalization of the lipoprotein-receptor complex; and the processing of the internalized LDL by lysosomal enzymes. The lipoproteins are degraded and the receptors are recycled to the cell surface. Far less is known about the metabolism of apolipoprotein E-poor HDL. The steroidogenic glands of all species thus far studied can utilize LDL-carried cholesterol as a substrate for hormone synthesis, at least under certain circumstances. In contrast, the ability to use HDL-carried cholesterol by a receptor system other than that specific for apolipoproteins B and E appears to be relatively unique to rodents (Gwynne and Strauss, 1982).

The delivery of extracellular cholesterol to steroidogenic cells, as well as to those cells which do not secrete steroids, results in several metabolic consequences. They include the coordinate inhibition of de novo cholesterol synthesis and the stimulation of cellular cholesteryl ester storage (Goldstein and Brown, 1977). The extent to which these metabolic responses occur is governed by cellular sterol balance, which is determined by the availability of exogenous cholesterol, on one hand, and the rate of cellular sterol utilization, on the other (Schuler et al., 1981b). Thus, it appears that the availability of intracellular free cholesterol is closely monitored by cells and alterations in the size of the free sterol pool result, by mechanisms which are not well understood, in changes in sterol synthesis and esterification.

In this chapter we will review data which support the concepts (1) that luteal tissue uses lipoprotein-carried cholesterol as a substrate for hormone synthesis; (2) that lipoprotein-cholesterol uptake by lutein cells is receptor-mediated; (3) that the availability of exogenous cholesterol plays a role in the coordinate regulation of de novo sterol synthesis and sterol ester storage in these cells; and (4) that lipoprotein accumulation is regulated by tropic hormones. We will focus our attention on the utilization of HDL-carried cholesterol by rat ovarian cells.

2. Evidence that Lipoprotein-Carried Cholesterol is a Primary Substrate for Steroidogenesis

We have employed four different systems including in vivo, in vitro and in situ organ perfusion models to examine the importance of extracellular cholesterol as a substrate for luteal steroidogenesis. In the first system, ovarian function was examined after circulating lipoprotein levels were lowered by treating rats with certain drugs such as 4-aminopyrazolo (3,4-d) pyrimidine (4-APP) or large doses of estrogen. 4-APP is an adenine analogue which inhibits the secretion of lipoproteins from the liver (Christie et al., 1979; Schuler et al., 1981b). Treatment of immature PMSG-hCG-primed rats with this agent (10-12.5 mg/kg body wt) lowered

Table I. Effects of Estrogen-Induced Hypocholesterolemia on Luteal Function

	Estrogen-treated	Controls	p value
Plasma cholesterol (mg/dl)	37.7 ± 1.1	56.5 ± 2.0	< 0.001
Ovarian wt (mg/ovary)	81.3 ± 6	78.7 ± 5.7	N.S.
Plasma progesterone (ng/ml)	496 ± 67	550 ± 43	N.S.
Plasma 29 α-hydroxypregn-4-en-one	111 ± 13	120 ± 17	N.S.
Ovarian free cholesterol (nmol/mg wet wt)	4.25 ± 0.44	4.17 ± 0.36	N.S.
Ovarian cholesterol ester (nmol/mg wet wt)	5.05 ± 0.60	10.5 ± 1.65	< 0.001

PMSG-hCG-primed immature rats were treated with estradiol (10 mg/kg) in the propylene glycol vehicle on Day 6 post-hCG and killed 24 hr later. Plasma and ovarian sterols and steroids were quantitated. Values are means ± S.E. for N = 6 - 14 rats in each treatment group. N.S. = p > 0.05.

plasma cholesterol concentrations from the normal level of 50 mg/dl to < 15 mg/dl within 24 hr. Forty-eight hr after the start of 4-APP treatment, plasma progesterone levels had declined significantly compared to vehicle-treated controls. The luteinized ovaries also failed to accumulate cholesteryl esters while receiving 4-APP. These alterations in plasma steroids and ovarian lipids were observed despite a compensatory increase in ovarian cholesterol synthesis as indicated by a more than 10-fold rise in activity of 3-hydroxy-3-methyl-glutaryl Coenzyme A reductase (HMG-CoA reductase), the rate-limiting enzyme in cholesterol biosynthesis, and a notable increase in the incorporation of ^{14}C-acetate into sterols and progestins by enzymatically dispersed cells prepared from the ovaries of the 4-APP-treated animals. Under normal circumstances, the activity of HMG-CoA reductase in the luteinized ovaries at the time of maximal steroidogenic activity is quite low, an indication that exogenous cholesterol is a major substrate (Schuler et al., 1979). Dispersed cells prepared from ovaries of 4-APP-treated animals retained the ability to respond to LH or db cAMP in short incubations, but their basal and stimulated rates of progesterone secretion were much less than those of control cells, reflecting the depletion of endogenous steroid precursor (i.e., cholesteryl esters).

The effects of 4-APP administration upon ovarian sterol levels and plasma progestin concentrations were reversible in that plasma cholesterol concentrations were restored to normal after treatment was stopped with a concomitant return of ovarian sterol ester and plasma progestins to control values. Moreover, an intravenous infusion of total human serum lipoproteins to animals receiving 4-APP elevated circulating cholesterol levels and restored plasma progesterone concentrations to normal within 12 hr. The infusion of lipoproteins also suppressed ovarian HMG-CoA reductase activity and promoted storage of cholesteryl esters. Because 4-APP is a toxic drug which may have actions other than inhibition of hepatic lipoprotein secretion, it is essential to demonstrate that supplemental lipoproteins are capable of reversing the effects of this drug. These findings reveal that in the face of severe deprivation of extracellular cholesterol, the steroidogenic activity of luteinized rat ovaries is compromised beyond the capacity of the tissue to make metabolic adjustments to correct the substrate deficiency.

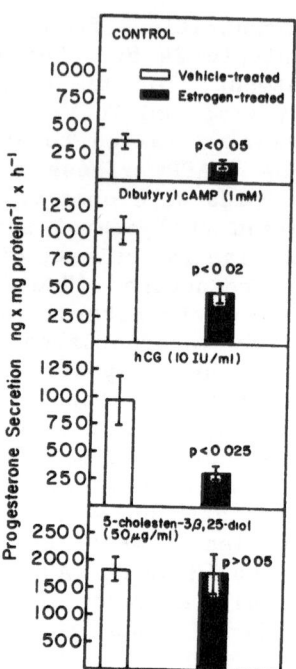

Figure 1. Effect of estrogen-induced hypocholesterolemia on progesterone secretion by dispersed luteal cells. Enzymatically dispersed cells were prepared from ovaries of rats treated with estradiol or vehicle on Day 6 post hCG and killed 24 hr later. Cells were incubated with the indicated additions for 1 hr and progesterone secretion was determined. 5-Cholesten-3β, 25-diol was added in 10 ul of ethanol. The ethanol vehicle was added to all other tubes. Values presented are means ± S.E. of 3 separate experiments in which each in vitro treatment was studied in triplicate. Significant differences between the function of cells from ovaries of estradiol-treated and control rats were determined by Student's t test.

Another means of pharmacologically lowering lipoprotein cholesterol levels in the rat is through the administration of large doses of estrogen (Kovanen et al., 1979). This treatment enhances hepatic catabolism of lipoproteins, which may explain the hypocholesterolemia. When PMSG-hCG-primed rats were given a single subcutaneous injection of estradiol in propylene glycol (10 mg/kg body wt) on Day 6 post-hCG, plasma cholesterol levels declined by 40% within 24 hr (Table I). While this was not accompanied by a fall in plasma progestins, ovarian sterol ester contents were significantly reduced. As a result, dispersed cells prepared from ovaries of estrogen-treated rats produced less progestin in vitro in the basal or stimulated state (Fig. 1). Estrogen treatment did not adversely affect steroidogenic enzymes since dispersed cells from ovaries of treated rats produced as much progesterone as those of controls when presented with 25-hydroxycholesterol, an exogenous substrate which readily enters the steroidogenic substrate pool (Toaff et al., 1982). The interpretation of these findings is that a moderate reduction in the supply of extracellular sterol caused alterations in ovarian sterol balance such that less cholesterol was esterified in order to provide substrate (free cholesterol) for the steroidogenic machinery.

A second experimental system which has revealed the importance of extracellular cholesterol as a substrate for steroidogenesis is primary cultures of luteinized granulosa cells (Schuler et al., 1979; Rosenblum et al., 1981). Granulosa cells isolated from follicles of gonadotropin-primed immature rats secreted large quantities of progestin when cultured in serum-containing medium, even in the presence of a potent inhibitor of de novo sterol synthesis, Compactin. These cells also accumulated numerous cytoplasmic inclusions which displayed the cross-formée under polarized light, indicating the presence of cholesteryl ester in the smectic liquid crystalline state. When cells were placed into medium supplemented with lipoprotein-deficient serum, progestin production fell off markedly within 24 hr, and cytoplasmic lipid droplets were depleted. These changes occurred despite increased cellular de novo sterol synthesis as evidenced by elevated HMG-CoA reductase activity and enhanced incorporation of ^{14}C-acetate into cellular sterols and secreted progestins (Fig. 2). Addition of human serum lipoproteins to cells cultured in lipoprotein-deficient medium restored progestin production; stimulated the accumulation of sterol esters as indicated by repletion of the cytoplasm with anisotropic inclusions and enhanced incorporation of ^{14}C-acetate and ^{14}C-oleate into the fatty acyl moieties of sterol esters; and reduced endogenous sterol formation as assessed by inhibition of ^{14}C-acetate labeling of cellular sterols and secreted progestins. Thus, the responses of luteinized cells in culture to lipoprotein deprivation were identical to those of the ovary in vivo in response to 4-APP treatment.

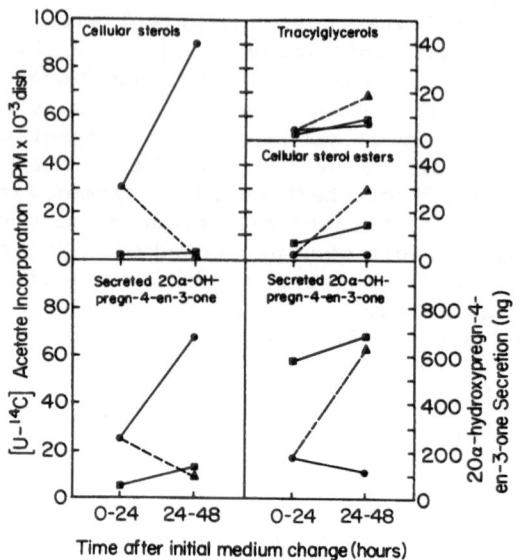

Figure 2. Effect of lipoproteins on [U-^{14}C] acetate metabolism and progestin secretion by cultured luteinized granulosa cells. The experiment was initiated after cells were grown for 48 hr in medium containing 10% human male serum. Some cultures were maintained in medium supplemented with 10% serum (closed squares), while others were changed to medium containing 10% lipoprotein-deficient serum (closed circles). After 24 hr, medium was changed again and some of the cultures growing in lipoprotein-deficient medium received 600 ug of cholesterol in the form of a total human serum lipoprotein preparation (closed triangles). The volume of incubation medium was 1.5 ml. [U-^{14}C] Acetate (50 µM, 2.85 µCi/ml of incubation medium) was added to some dishes after the initial medium change and to others 24 hr after the initial medium change. Incubations with [^{14}C] acetate were for 24 hr. Radioactivity incorporated into cellular lipids and secreted steroids was determined. 20 α-Hydroxypregn-4-en-3-one secreted into the medium was measured by radioimmunoassay. Values presented are averages obtained from three dishes in each treatment group.

A third system which we have utilized to study the role of exogenous cholesterol as a substrate is short term incubations of enzymatically dispersed cells (Schuler et al., 1981a). Collagenase-dispersed cells prepared from ovaries of PMSG-hCG-primed rats increased secretion of progestins when

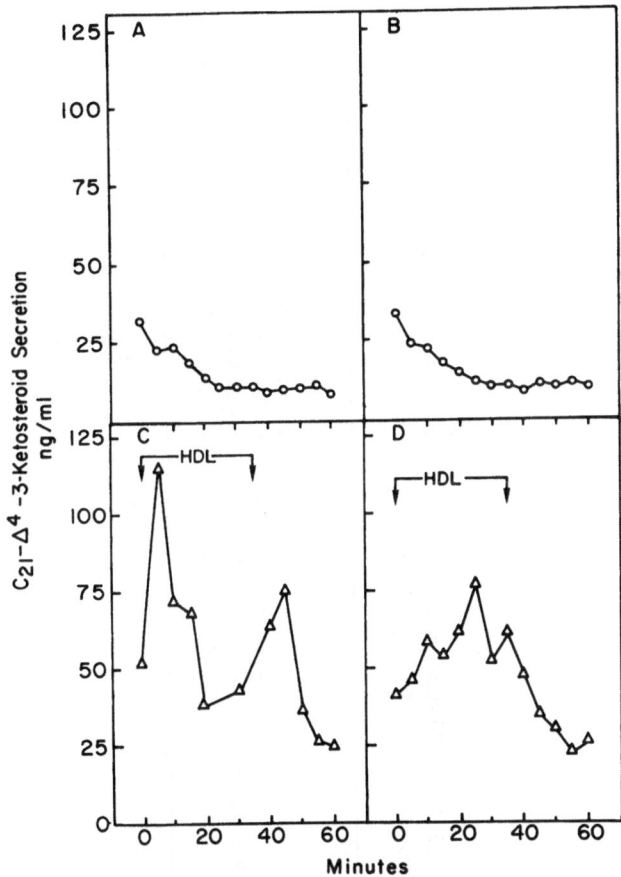

Figure 3. Effect of human HDL on steroid secretion by the perfused rat ovary. Animals were pretreated for 3 days with 4-APP (10 mg/kg) to reduce endogenous ovarian steroid precursors. After the rats were anesthetized and the perfusion sites prepared, ovaries were perfused for 15 min with oxygenated Krebs-Ringer bicarbonate buffer (KRB), pH 7.4, containing 2 mg/ml glucose to wash out blood. Perfusate containing 2% bovine serum albumin with or without 0.7 mg human HDL protein/ml was then introduced for a 30 min period at a perfusion rate of 1.5 ml/min. The venous effluent was collected at 5 min intervals for analysis of progesterone and 20 α-hydroxypregn-4-en-3-one by radioimmunoassay. The values presented are the sum of these two steroids. Panels A and B are results from control perfusions, panels C and D, from perfusions in which HDL was added.

Table II. Metabolism of $[1,2,6,7-{}^{3}H]$-Cholesteryl Linoleate Reconstituted into Human HDL by Perfused Rat Ovaries

Treatment	Perfusion no.	Ovarian wt (mg)	Radioactivity in venous effluent dpm $\times 10^{-6}$	Radioactivity in progesterone & 20 α-hydroxy-pregn-4-en-3-one dmp $\times 10^{-4}$	% Conversion
Reconstituted ^{3}H-HDL	1	91.8	7.14	19.4	2.72
	2	75.5	3.86	17.49	4.53
Reconstituted ^{3}H-HDL & "cold" HDL	3	55.6	9.87	10.91	1.11
	4	101.3	7.77	8.51	1.09

Animals were pretreated with 4-APP (10 mg/kg) for 3 days prior to the experiment which was performed on Day 6 post-hCG treatment. The ovaries were first perfused with KRB for 30 min as described in the legend for Fig. 3 and then for a 20 min period with KRB containing 18 ug/ml (9.6×10^5 dpm) reconstituted HDL or reconstituted HDL and 333 ug/ml of unlabeled HDL at a rate of 1.5 ml/min. The venous effluent was collected for analysis of radioactive products. The reconstituted particles were prepared from a mixture of delipidated HDL apolipoprotein; egg phosphatidylcholine; free cholesterol; cholesteryl linoleate; and tripalmitin according to the method of Hirz and Scanu (1970). The reconstituted particles were isolated at a density of 1.125 g/ml and contained a weight ratio of protein to sterol of 2:1. The reconstituted HDL had a specific activity of 5077 dmp/nmol of cholesteryl linoleate. The venous effluent was extracted with 6 vol of chloroform/methanol (2:1, vol/vol). The organic phase was dried under nitrogen and the residue subjected to thin-layer chromatography on Whatman K-5 plates using a solvent system of hexane/ethyl acetate 7:3 (vol/vol). Areas where ^{3}H-progesterone and [3]H-20 0-hydroxypregn-4-en-3-one migrated were located with the use of authentic standards and taken for liquid scintillation counting using Biofluor (New England Nuclear) as a counting medium.

incubated in the presence of human or rat HDL. The stimulatory effects of these lipoproteins were apparent within 30 min of incubation and were more marked when the cells were challenged with db cAMP. The basal and stimulated steroidogenic activity of the freshly dispersed cells was not sensitive to the inhibitor of de novo cholesterol synthesis, Compactin, during a one hr incubation. HDL also augmented sterol ester synthesis by the cells as indicated by increased incorporation of ^{14}C-oleate into this lipid fraction. These observations point out that even in relatively short term incubations, luteinized rat cells are dependent upon a supply of exogenous cholesterol for expression of maximal steroidogenic activity. This fact has not been recognized by many investigators who utilized such dispersed cell systems to study the control of steroid synthesis.

The fourth system we have employed to study the role of exogenous cholesterol in corpus luteum function is the perfused ovary in situ. In this system lipoproteins can be directly introduced into the arterial circulation of the ovary and secretory products can be collected from the venous drainage of the organ. After animals were pretreated with 4-APP to reduce ovarian stores of preformed steroid precursor (i.e., cholesteryl esters), the introduction of human HDL into the perfusate resulted in a prompt increase in progestin secretion (Fig. 3). The stimulation of steroid secretion under these conditions was due, at least in part, to the delivery of HDL-carried cholesterol since ^{3}H-cholesteryl linoleate reconstituted into human HDL by the method of Hirz and Scanu (1970) was converted into ^{3}H-progesterone and ^{3}H-20 α-hydroxy-pregn-4-en-3-one (Table II). The metabolism of the labeled sterol carried by HDL was inhibited by the inclusion of an excess of unlabeled HDL in the perfusate, suggesting that the labeled cholesteryl ester was being utilized by a saturable process.

3.   Effects of Hypercholesterolemia on Ovarian Function, and Estimation of the Rate of Uptake of Extracellular Cholesterol by Luteinized Rat Ovaries

In vivo, utilization of circulating cholesterol as a substrate by luteinized rat ovaries appears to be by a saturable process (Schuler et al., 1981b). Elevation of plasma cholesterol concentrations by feeding animals a diet enriched with cholesterol, or by intravenous infusions of rat or human serum lipoproteins did not increase plasma progestins or ovarian sterol ester stores; nor did it alter activities of

enzymes involved in de novo sterol synthesis or sterol esterification (Fig. 4). These findings suggest that at the normal
circulating cholesterol concentration of about 50 mg/dl, the
ovarian sterol uptake mechanism is working at a maximum. If
this conclusion is valid, by treating immature PMSG-hCG-primed
rats with aminoglutethimide, a drug which inhibits cholesterol
side chain cleavage, and as a result stimulates the storage
of the unmetabolized sterol as cholesteryl esters, it might
be possible to obtain a crude estimate of the amount of
extracellular sterol taken up hourly by a luteinized rat
ovary (Schuler et al., 1981b). When aminoglutethimide was
administered to PMSG-hCG-primed rats on Day 7 post-hCG over a
12 hr period, the ovaries accumulated sterol ester at a rate
of 220 nmol/ovary/hr. Assuming that de novo sterol synthesis
was minimal at this time, which is reasonable in view of the
low HMG-CoA reductase activities, and that most of the cholesterol accumulated was esterified when aminoglutethimide was
administered, this figure should represent the amount of
extracellular cholesterol taken up by the ovary. It is worth
noting that the uptake of this amount of cholesterol from the
circulation is comensurate with the needs of the luteinized
ovaries for steroid hormone precursor (Horikoshi and Wiest,
1971).

4.   The Mechanism of HDL Uptake by Rat Luteal Cells

The different experimental systems described above have
been utilized to probe mechanisms by which extracellular
cholesterol is accumulated by the luteinized rat ovary. In
vitro, lipoproteins affected the function of rat lutein cells
in a dose-dependent and saturable fashion. For example, HDL
stimulated progestin synthesis by primary cultures of granulosa cells (Rosenblum et al., 1981; Schreiber et al., 1982)
and collagenase dispersed luteal cells (Schuler et al.,
1981a; Azhar and Menon, 1981) in a saturable manner. These
observations suggest that HDL were interacting with lutein
cells by a receptor-mediated process.

In support of this contention, specific uptake of HDL by
luteinized ovarian tissue was demonstrated following the
intravenous administration of human and rat ^{125}I-labeled HDL
to immature PMSG-hCG-primed rats pretreated with 4-APP to
reduce endogenous lipoprotein levels (Christie et al., 1981;
Strauss et al., 1982). Ovarian lipoprotein uptake was time
dependent, reaching a maximum within 15 min after administration of the label. The injection of a bolus of unlabeled

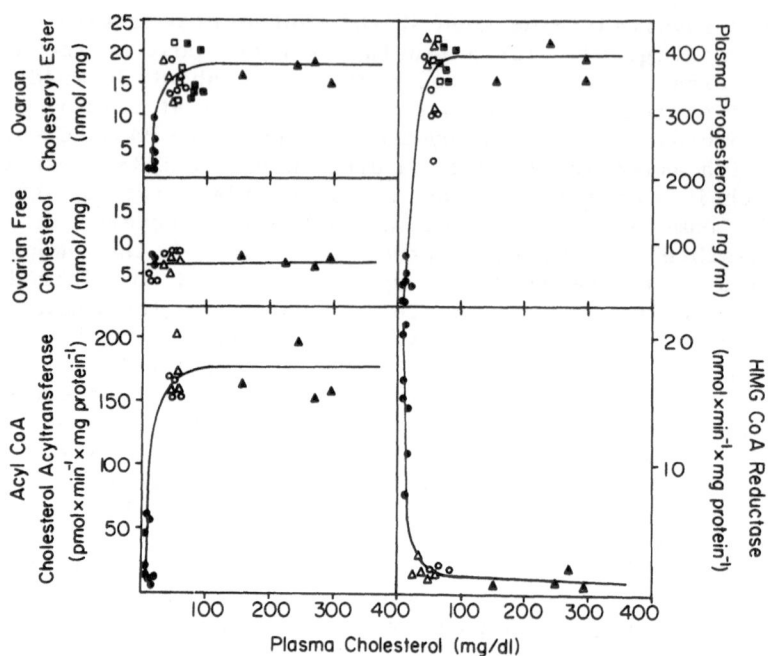

Figure 4. Relationships between blood cholesterol concentrations and ovarian sterol metabolism. PMSG-hCG primed rats were subjected to one of the following treatments and were killed on Day 7 post-hCG; 4-APP (10 mg/kg/day) (closed circles) or the vehicle (open circles) on Days 4-6 post-hCG; a cholesterol supplemented diet (closed triangles) or a control diet (open triangles) between Days 4-6 post-hCG; intravenous injections of total rat lipoprotein preparations (~ 5 mg of sterol) (closed squares) or saline vehicle (open squares) 12-14 hr before killing. Levels of plasma progesterone, ovarian free and esterified cholesterol and ovarian HMG-CoA reductase and acylcoenzyme A:cholesterol acyltransferase (ACAT) activities in individual rats are plotted against the plasma cholesterol level at the time of killing.

human HDL immediately prior to the infusion of labeled HDL significantly reduced ovarian uptake, whereas administration of unlabeled human LDL did not.

Uptake of human ^{125}I-labeled HDL by luteinized ovaries could also be observed upon introduction of labeled lipoproteins into the arterial circulation of perfused ovaries (Fig. 5). The ovarian uptake of lipoproteins delivered in this fashion was time dependent, and reached a maximum after 15 min of perfusion, a time course similar to that observed following the systemic injection of labeled HDL. The inclusion of unlabeled human HDL in the perfusate significantly suppressed accumulation of labeled HDL by the ovaries, suggesting a saturable and lipoprotein-specific uptake mechanism. A similar pattern of results were obtained when animals were pre-treated with 4-APP prior to the experiment, although the amount of ^{125}I-HDL accumulated by the ovaries was several-fold higher than with untreated animals.

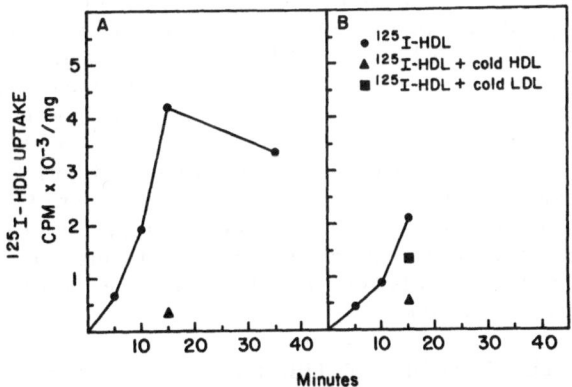

Figure 5. Uptake of human ^{125}I-labeled HDL by perfused rat ovaries. After animals were anesthetized and the perfusion sites prepared, the ovaries were perfused with a sequence of KRB containing 2 mg/ml glucose for 3 min and then KRB + ^{125}I-HDL (0.25 µg HDL protein, 10^6 cpm per ml) for 5-30 min at a rate of 1.5 ml/min. After the termination of the HDL infusion, the ovaries were perfused for 3 min with KRB to wash out label from the vascular space. In some instances 87 µg/ml of unlabeled human HDL or human LDL were included in the perfusion medium with the radiolabeled HDL. At the end of the experiment the ovaries were removed, trimmed of adherent tissue, weighed and counted using a γ-spectrometer. At all time points < 2% of the radioactivity accumulated by the ovaries was extractable with chloroform/methanol and > 95% of the radioactivity was precipitable by 10% trichloroacetic acid. These findings indicate that the ovaries had not selectively accumulated ^{125}I-labeled lipid or degradation products. Results from two separate experiments are presented. Each point represents a single perfusion.

Enzymatically dispersed lutein cells took up human ^{125}I-labeled HDL; there was a rapid phase of uptake, which was complete within 60 min, which was followed by a slower phase of lipoprotein accumulation (Schuler et al., 1981a). The uptake of labeled HDL by the cells could not be accounted for by pinocytosis; it was concentration-dependent and saturable with an apparent Km of 20 ug HDL protein/ml. The accumulation process was specific in that unlabeled human and rat HDL competed for uptake of human ^{125}I-labeled HDL by the cells, whereas unlabeled human LDL was much less effective as a competitor.

We have also described the binding of human ^{125}I-labeled HDL to membranes prepared from luteinized rat ovaries (Christie et al., 1981). The binding was saturable with a Kd of 54 µg HDL protein/ml at 4°C. Scatchard analysis indicated a single order of binding sites. Unlabeled human and rat HDL effectively competed for ^{125}I-labeled human HDL binding, whereas human LDL, bovine serum albumin and ovine FSH and LH did not. The HDL binding sites were apparently associated with the plasma membrane because the greatest specific binding activity was found in subcellular fractions containing the highest spefific activity of the plasma membrane marker enzyme, 5'-nucleotidase.

Unlike the binding of LDL to its receptor, the binding of human ^{125}I-labeled HDL to rat ovarian membranes did not require calcium, and lipoprotein binding was not affected by the polyanion, heparin. These characteristics, in addition to the previously described competition studies, distinguished the binding of human ^{125}I-labeled HDL to ovarian tissue from the binding of LDL to its receptor and support the concept of a discrete cell surface recognition site for this lipoprotein class on rodent steroidogenic cells. We should point out that the main lipoprotein preparation used in our studies was human HDL$_3$, which can be obtained essentially free of apolipoprotein E. This has allowed us to study the metabolism of HDL by pathways which did not involve a receptor recognizing LDL and apolipoprotein E-rich HDL.

5. Autoradiographic Studies of ^{125}I-HDL Uptake by Perfused Luteinized Ovaries

Data from autoradiographic studies provide further support for the presence of HDL binding sites on plasma

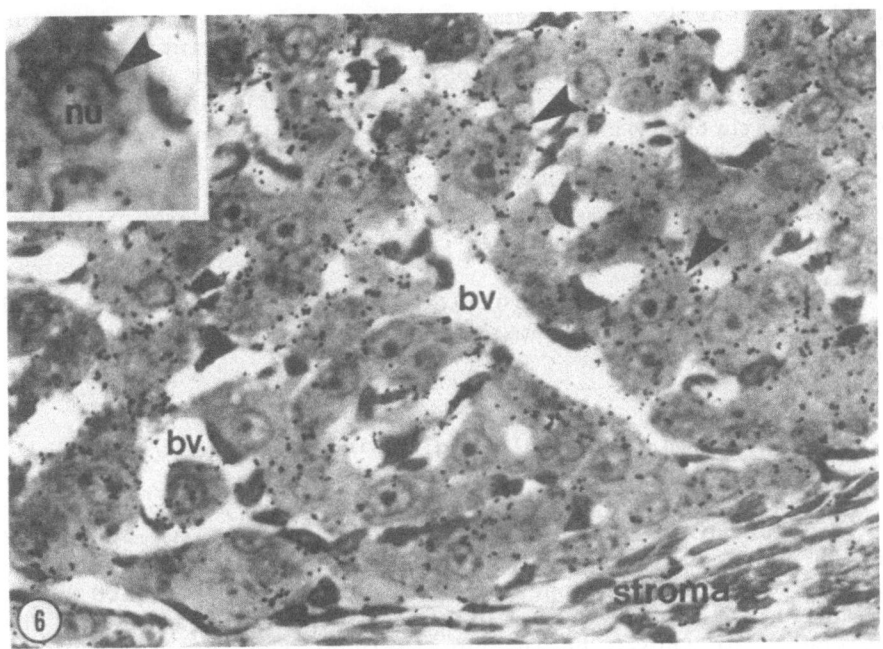

Figure 6. Light microscope autoradiograph showing uptake of human ^{125}I-labeled HDL by luteinized ovaries of immature rats on Day 6 after hCG injection. Following a 15 min perfusion with ^{125}I-HDL, silver grains are numerous over corpora lutea and sparse over cells of the stroma. Silver grains are associated primarily with the surfaces and cytoplasm of luteinized granulosa cells (arrowheads). The white spaces (bv) in the field represent blood vessel lumens emptied of blood by the perfusion. Magnification × 800.

Inset: Silver grains are often observed in a perinuclear location (arrowhead), suggesting the internalization of lipoprotein (nu, nucleus). Magnification × 1650.

membranes of rat luteal cells. After the perfusion of human ^{125}I-labeled HDL into the arterial circulation of luteinized ovaries, silver grains were detected by light microscopic autoradiography over the luteinized tissue (Fig. 6); few grains occurred over stromal cells, follicles or oocytes. Upon examination of tissue fixed with paraformaldehyde-glutar-aldehyde-cresol and embedded in glycomethacrylate, the silver grains could be clearly seen to be associated with luteal

cells, primarily the plasma membranes, after a 15 min perfusion. In addition, some grains appeared to be intracellular,
located in a peri-nuclear position. A similar distribution
of silver grains was found when rat ^{125}I-labeled HDL was
perfused through the ovaries for 15 min. The uptake of human
^{125}I-labeled HDL by the lutein cells was specific since the
labeling was markedly reduced by the inclusion of a 350-fold
excess of "cold" human HDL in the perfusion medium, but not
by a similar quantity of "cold" human LDL.

At the fine structural level, silver grains were found
associated with the plasma membranes, as well as in the cell
interior (Fig. 7).

6.   Catabolism of HDL by Luteinized Ovarian Cells

The fate of HDL components after they interact with
luteinized ovarian cells has not been completely mapped and
is the subject of considerable interest. With respect to the
apolipoproteins, it appears that they are taken into cells
and then degraded, to some extent, to smaller molecules. The
evidence for these conclusions includes the autoradiographic
observation of silver grains in the interior of luteal cells.
Other evidence of internalization is the fact that not all
human ^{125}I-labeled HDL taken up by enzymatically dispersed
luteal cells could be released by a brief exposure of the
cells to trypsin (Schuler et al., 1981a). A portion of the
radioactivity remained associated with the cells and, presumably, was internalized. The trypsin-releasable label was
assumed to be on the cell surface. This fraction reached a
plateau within 30 min of incubation, while the cell-associated
radioactivity not removed by trypsin continued to increase
with time.

Little cell-specific lipoprotein degradation could be
detected when collagenase-dispersed cells were incubated with
human ^{125}I-labeled HDL for a 2 hr period (Schuler et al.,
1981a). However, steroidogenesis and sterol ester storage
were clearly stimulated at this time. With primary cultures
of luteinized granulosa cells, degradation of human ^{125}I-
labeled HDL to trichloroacetic acid soluble products could be
demonstrated during a 24 hr period (Table III). Yet, the
amount of protein degraded was not associated with enough
cholesterol to meet the substrate needs of the cells for
steroidogenesis. It was estimated that the amount of sterol
delivered by HDL which was degraded could account for only 25%

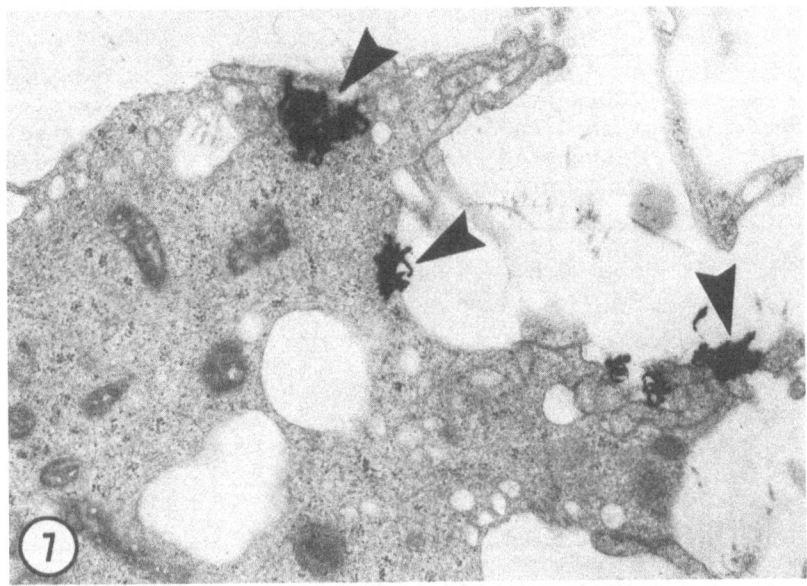

Figure 7. Detail of ^{125}I-HDL uptake by rat ovaries. The localization of silver grains (arrowheads) to the surface of luteal cells is confirmed by electron microscope autoradiography. Controls, in which excess "cold" HDL or LDL were given along with ^{125}I-HDL, verified the specificity of uptake shown in this autoradiogram. Magnification × 19000.

of the substrate utilized for hormone synthesis. From these observations it has been concluded that HDL may be internalized by rat luteal cells, but that simultaneous complete degradation of the HDL apolipoproteins is not required for the utilization of the HDL-cholesterol.

The metabolism of HDL-carried lipids by the luteinized ovarian cells has not been examined in any detail and it remains to be determined where and how HDL cholesteryl esters are hydrolyzed and how the sterol derived from these particles is transported to various organelles for further metabolism. It is likely that intracellular cholesterol transport proteins play a significant role in the latter process (Tanaka et al., 1982).

Table III. Catabolism of human ^{125}I-labeled HDL by Luteinized
Granulosa Cells

HDL Concentration μg/ml	20 α-hydroxy-pregn-4-en-3-one secreted μg/mg protein	HDL Degraded μg/mg protein	Sterol delivered by degraded HDL μg/mg protein
0	0.8	-	-
50	3.5	1.9	0.53
100	5	4.6	1.3
200	7.2	6	1.7
400	13	10	2.8

Granulosa cells were cultured in the presence of lipoprotein-deficient medium as described in the legend for Fig. 2 for 24 hr prior to the initiation of the experiment. The indicated concentrations of ^{125}I-HDL (specific activity: 325 cpm/ng) were added and progestin secretion and formation of trichloroacetic acid soluble products by the cells were determined during a 24 hr incubation. The weight ratio of sterol to protein in the HDL was 1 to 3.6. Values presented are means from duplicate cultures.

7. Gonadotropic Regulation of HDL Uptake

The uptake of ^{125}I-labeled HDL by rat ovarian tissue appears to be influenced by gonadotropic hormones and to be directly correlated with the steroidogenic activity of the cells (Strauss et al., 1982). This might be expected if lipoprotein-carried cholesterol is a primary substrate for steroidogenesis. Evidence for hormonal regulation of HDL uptake includes the observation of greater uptake of human and rat ^{125}I-labeled HDL by ovaries of PMSG-hCG-primed rats compared to immature unprimed animals. Moreover, uptake of human ^{125}I-labeled HDL by collagenase-dispersed cells prepared from ovaries of hypophysectomized immature rats could be increased by administration of a sequence of hormones which induced follicular growth and luteinization (Table IV). The ability of the dispersed cells to accumulate ^{125}I-labeled HDL in vitro was correlated with the plasma progestin levels at the time of killing. Uptake of HDL was low by cells from immature hypophysectomized animals. Following treatment with estradiol, or estradiol and FSH to induce follicular development, plasma progestin levels remained relatively low and only a modest increase in the capacity of cells to take up labeled HDL in a specific fashion was noted. However, after treatment with estradiol and FSH, a single injection of LH to induce luteinization produced, within 2 days, a significant increase in plasma progestin concentrations and enhanced the capacity of the dispersed cells to accumulate labeled HDL. Four days after the injection of LH, plasma steroid levels and cellular uptake of HDL had increased even further. The addition of prolactin treatments, starting on the day of LH injection, increased both plasma progestin levels and uptake of unlabeled HDL.

The changes in HDL accumulation in the latter study were apparently the result of an increase in the number of lipoprotein uptake sites and/or the rate of lipoprotein internalization since the concentration of HDL which promoted half-maximal cellular uptake was not markedly changed in response to hormone treatments. From these observations we conclude that (1) luteinization is attended by a significant increase in the ability of ovarian cells to take up HDL, and this occurs concomitantly with an increase in steroidogenic capacity; and (2) gonadotropins, primarily LH, regulate ovarian uptake of HDL.

8.   Utilization of LDL by Luteinized Ovarian Cells

In addition to utilizing cholesterol carried by HDL, luteinized rat granulosa cells in culture are able to employ human LDL to support progestin synthesis and sterol esterification (Schuler et al., 1979; Rosenblum et al., 1981; Schreiber et al., 1982). Human LDL stimulated these processes in a dose-dependent and saturable fashion, indicating a receptor-mediated mechanism. However, in vivo human LDL was a poor substrate for rat ovarian tissue (Anderson and

Table IV. Effect of Administration of Gonadotropic Hormones to Hypophysectomized Immature Rats on Uptake of Human ^{125}I-labeled DHL by Dispersed Ovarian Cells, and Plasma Sterol and Progestin Concentrations.

Treatment	Ovarian weight (mg/ovary)	^{125}I-HDL Uptake ng/μg DNA/2h	^{125}I-HDL Uptake (ng/ovary 2h)	K_{12} (μg HDL protein/ml)	Plasma cholesterol (mg/dl)	Plasma progestins Progesterone (ng/ml)	Plasma progestins 20 α-OH-P (ng/ml)
Unprimed	4.6 ± 0.4	1.79 ± 0.75	37.8 ± 17.6	14.6 ± 8.9	64 ± 5	1.7 ± 0.7	0.5 ± 0.2
E_4	6.2 ± 1.2	1.77 ± 0.17	39.9 ± 8.8	6.98 ± 3.2	52 ± 7	1.1 ± 0.3	1.2 ± 0.9
E_4F_2	16.4 ± 1.5	3.87 ± 1.81	249 ± 13	25 ± 8.4	54 ± 8	9.7 ± 3.5	4.3 ± 2.8
$E_4F_2L_2$	24.7 ± 1.8	12.17 ± 1.05	565 ± 61	19.7 ± 3.8	50 ± 5	19.3 ± 4.7	45 ± 9.8
$E_4F_2LP_2$	40.0 ± 5.3	32.74 ± 9.40	1596 ± 192	23.2 ± 12.7	46 ± 9	70.3 ± 11.5	82 ± 8.6
$E_4F_4L_4$	50.7 ± 8.0	32.79 ± 8.56	3400 ± 1156	48.5 ± 5.7	58 ± 7	54.6 ± 27.7	62.3 ± 7.6
$E_4F_2LP_4$	54.0 ± 9.2	51.38 ± 12.50	6064 ± 2021	30.4 ± 16.7	51 ± 6	198 ± 40	72.9 ± 7.3

Immature female rats, hypophysectomized on Day 21 of life, received the following treatments starting 4 days after surgery: Unprimed: propylene glycol; E_4: 1 mg estradiol in propylene glycol for 4 days; E_4F_2: 1 mg estradiol for 4 days followed by oFSH (2.8 ug B.I.D.) for 2 days; $E_4F_2L_2$: 1 mg estradiol for 4 days, 2 days of oFSH followed by oLH (60 μg), with killing 48 hr after LH treatment; $E_4F_2LP_2$: 1 mg estradiol for 4 days, 2 days of oFSH followed by oLH (60 μg) and prolactin (125 μg B.I.D.) for 2 days, starting on the day of LH treatment; $E_4F_4L_4$, except killing 96 hr after LH treatment; $E_4F_2LP_4$: Same as $E_4F_2LP_2$ except prolactin (125 μg B.I.D.) was administered for 4 days starting on the day of LH treatment. Animals were killed 12-24 hr after the last hormone treatment. Ovaries were removed and plasma collected for sterol and progestin assays. The ovaries were dispersed with collagenase and uptake of human ^{125}I-labeled HDL during a 2 hr incubation was determined. Uptake of ^{125}I-labeled HDL/ovary was estimated from the value for maximal specific uptake per aliquot of cells × the number of aliquots from the ovarian dispersion. Complete dispersion of the tissue has been assumed. HDL concentrations permitting half-maximal uptake (K_{12}) were estimated from Eadie-Hofstee plots of the specific binding data as a function of HDL concentration in the incubation medium. The following gonadotropins were used NIH-FSH-S11, NIH-LH-S22 and NIH-P-S12. Values presented are means ± S.E. for three separate experiments.

Dietschy, 1978), and ovarian uptake of human ^{125}I-labeled LDL
after intravenous administration was minimal compared to the
accumulation of labeled HDL (Strauss et al., 1982). The
apparent discrepancy between the in vitro and in vivo
observations can be explained, in part, by the failure of
human LDL to readily penetrate the vascular compartment and
reach the parenchymal cells. When human ^{125}I-labeled LDL was
perfused through the arterial circulation of luteinized
ovaries for 15 min, it was localized by autoradiography in
blood vessels with little labeling of the lutein cells. The
inclusion of excess "cold" human LDL in the perfusate did not
reduce this labeling, indicating the vascular accumulation
was non-specific. The large molecular weight (2.5 × 10^6
daltons) of LDL presumably hinders its movement from the
capillaries to the steroidogenic cells.

9.   Conclusions and Caveats

We have employed four different experimental systems in
our studies of lipoprotein cholesterol utilization by luteinized rat ovarian tissue. While each of the systems has
certain advantages, it should also be recognized that they
have drawbacks as well. For example, the pharmacologic
agents used to reduce levels of circulating lipoproteins in
vivo (4-APP and estradiol) may have had direct effects upon
the ovary or the hypothalamic-pituitary axis which could
complicate interpretation of the results. In the case of the
primary cultures of luteinized granulosa cells, it could be
argued that these cells do not express lipoprotein receptors
or lipoprotein metabolic pathways as they do in vivo. Factors
in serum supplementing the culture medium such as platelet
derived growth factor, or the confluency of the cultures,
might have influenced lipoprotein metabolism (Gwynne and
Strauss, 1982). The enzymatic treatment used to prepare
luteal dispersions may have altered the cell surfaces, including lipoprotein receptors, or cellular metabolism. Moreover,
the primary cultures of luteinized granulosa cells and the
enzymatically dispersed cell systems do not permit the study
of lipoprotein utilization as it occurs in the context of the
normal structural organization of the tissue (i.e., movement
of lipoproteins from the vascular space to the parenchymal
cells) as does the in situ perfused ovary. Nonetheless, the
four different systems have each provided convincing evidence
that extracellular cholesterol is utilized for steroidogenesis
and cholesteryl ester storage by rat luteal tissue.

The rat is not unique in the reliance of its luteal tissue on extracellular cholesterol as a substrate for steroidogenesis. Studies on primary cultures of human (Tureck and Strauss, 1982; Tureck et al., 1983) and porcine (Veldhuis et al., 1982) granulosa cells in our laboratory, as well as on human luteal explants (Carr et al., 1981) and bovine granulosa cells by others (Savion et al., 1982) revealed that extracellular cholesterol is required for the maintenance of maximal rates of steroidogenesis. In all of these cases, LDL-carried cholesterol was the preferred substrate. However, Savion et al. (1982) found that bovine HDL stimulated progestin secretion by bovine granulosa cells when added in relatively high concentrations. Whether this represents the operation of a HDL pathway similar to that described in rodent cells remains to be determined.

Although the ovarian cells from these several species utilize exogenous cholesterol as a substrate for steroidogenesis, the concept may not be universal and care must be taken before extending it to all steroidogenic cell types and to all species. For example, while the luteinized rat ovary and adrenal gland require extracellular cholesterol for maintenance of steroidogenesis, the rat testes seems to utilize, under normal circumstances, endogeneously synthesized cholesterol (Gwynne and Strauss, 1982). This may be due to the fact that the testes secrete lesser quantities of steroid than the adrenal cortex and luteinized ovarian tissue and, therefore, have a smaller requirement for substrate.

We have directed our attention to the study of metabolism of HDL by rat lutein tissue because HDL are the predominant cholesterol carriers in rat blood. The main lipoprotein preparation employed in our work, human HDL_3, has permitted us to study the utilization of HDL by a pathway different from that recognizing LDL and apolipoprotein E-rich HDL. The mechanism of cholesterol uptake from this subclass of HDL appears to involve specific binding sites at the cell surface. Luteinized cells are enriched with these binding sites, and it has been estimated that there may be 3×10^5 sites per lutein cell (Schuler et al., 1981). This would be in keeping with the substantial need of these cells for exogenous cholesterol for use in hormone synthesis. However, rat steroidogenic cells also have the capacity to utilize LDL and, presumably, apolipoprotein E-rich HDL by a mechanism which is distinct from that for HDL_3 (reviewed by Gwynne and

Strauss, 1982). Hence, the luteinized rat ovary probably expresses two distinct receptor-mediated pathways for lipoprotein-cholesterol accumulation. It is not yet known which of these is quantitatively most important for provision of substrate to the ovary in vivo. This situation does, however, permit the ovary access to cholesterol carried by all the lipoprotein classes. It is worth noting that certain rat HDL subclasses are rich in apolipoprotein E so that the presumed LDL receptor in this tissue may actually function to take up the apolipoprotein E-rich HDL. It is likely that uptake systems for both LDL and HDL are subject to similar controls, i.e., gonadotropins. Our studies suggest that the ability of ovarian cells to take up HDL is closely tied with their steroidogenic capacity. Indeed, the regulation of lipoprotein accumulation appears to be a focus of gonadotropin action which, heretofore, has been unappreciated. Presently we believe LH is the primary tropic hormone regulating lipoprotein uptake by the ovary, although roles for other hormones including prolactin in the uptake process or the subsequent metabolism of lipoprotein accumulated by the cells cannot be excluded at this time.

ACKNOWLEDGMENTS

The technical assistance of Ms. Kathi Porter and Mr. Glenn Boyd, and the aid of Ms. Janet Brennar in the preparation of the manuscript are greatly appreciated. Mindy F. Rosenblum was a fellow in Pediatric Endocrinology supported by Children's Hospital of Philadelphia. Toshinobu Tanaka has been supported by a grant from the Rockefeller Foundation.

REFERENCES

Andersen, J. M. and Dietschy, J. M., 1978, Relative importance of high and low density lipoproteins in the regulation of cholesterol synthesis in the adrenal gland, ovary and testis of the rat, J. Biol. Chem. 253:9024.

Azhar, S., and Menon, K. M. J., 1981, Receptor-mediated gonadotropin action in the ovary. Rat luteal cells preferentially utilize and are acutely dependent upon the plasma-lipoprotein-supplied sterols in gonadotropin-stimulated steroid production, J. Biol. Chem. 256:6548.

Brown, M. S., Kovanen, P. T., and Goldstein, J. L., 1979,
    Receptor-mediated uptake of lipoprotein-cholesterol and
    its utilization for steroid synthesis in the adrenal
    cortex, Recent Prog. Hormone Res. 35:215.
Carr, B. R., Sadler, R. K., Rochelle, D. B., Stalmach, M. A.,
    MacDonald, P. C., and Simpson, E. R., 1981, Plasma lipo-
    protein regulation of progesterone biosynthesis by human
    corpus luteum in organ culture, J. Clin. Endocrinol.
    Metab. 52:875.
Christie, M. H., Gwynne, J. T., and Strauss, J. F. III, 1981,
    Binding of human high density lipoproteins to membranes of
    luteinized rat ovaries, J. Steroid Biochem. 14:671.
Christie, M. H., Strauss, J. F. III, and Flickinger, G. L.,
    1979, Effect of reduced blood cholesterol on sterol and
    steroid metabolism by rat luteal tissue, Endocrinology
    105:92.
Goldstein, J. L., and Brown, M. S., 1977, The low-density lipo-
    protein pathway and its relation to arteriosclerosis,
    Annu. Rev. Biochem. 46:897.
Gwynne, J. T., and Strauss, J. F. III, 1982, The role of lipo-
    proteins in steroidogenesis and cholesterol metabolism in
    steroidogenic glands, Endocrine Rev. 3:299.
Hirz, R., and Scanu, A. M., 1970, Reassembly in vitro of a
    serum high density lipoprotein, Biochem. Biophys. Acta
    207:364.
Horikoshi, H., and Wiest, W. G., 1971, Interrelationships
    between estrogen and progesterone secretion and trauma-
    induced deciduomata. On causes of uterine refractoriness
    in the "Parlow rat", Endocrinology 89:807.
Kovanen, P. T., Brown, M. S., and Goldstein, J. L., 1979,
    Increased binding of low density lipoprotein to liver
    membranes from rats treated with 17 α-ethinyl estradiol,
    J. Biol. Chem. 254:11367.
Osborne, J. C. Jr., and Brewer, H. B. Jr., 1977, The plasma
    lipoproteins, Adv. Prot. Chem. 31:253.
Rosenblum, M. F., Huttler, C. R., and Strauss, J. F. III, 1981,
    Control of sterol metabolism in cultured rat granulosa
    cells, Endocrinology 109:1518.
Savion, N., Laherty, R., Cohen, D., Lui, G. -M., and
    Gospodarowicz, D., 1982, The role of lipoproteins and
    3-hydroxy-3-methylglutaryl coenzyme A reductase in proges-
    terone production by cultured bovine granulosa cells,
    Endocrinology 110:13.
Schneider, W. J., Beislegel, V., Goldstein, J. L., and Brown,
    M. S., 1982, Purification of the low density lipoprotein

receptor, an acidic glycoprotein of 164,000 molecular
weight, J. Biol. Chem. 257:2664.

Schreiber, J. R., Nakamura, K., and Weinstein, D. B., 1982,
Degradation of rat and human lipoproteins by cultured rat
ovary granulosa cells, Endocrinology 110:55.

Schuler, L. A., Langenberg, K. K., Gwynne, J. T., and Strauss,
J. R. III, 1981a, High density lipoprotein utilization
by dispersed rat luteal cells, Biochim. Biophys.
Acta 664:583.

Schuler, L. A., Scavo, L., Kirsch, T. M., Flickinger, G. L.,
and Strauss, J. F. III, 1979, Regulatioh of de novo
biosynthesis of cholesterol and progestins, and formation
of cholesteryl ester in rat corpus luteum by exogenous
sterol, J. Biol. Chem. 254:8662.

Schuler, L. A., Toaff, M. E., and Strauss, J. F. III, 1981b,
Regulation of ovarian cholesterol metabolism. Control of
3-hydroxy-3-methylglutaryl coenzyme A reductase and acyl
coenzyme A; cholesterol acyltransferase, Endocrinology
108:1476.

Strauss, J. F. III, MacGregor, L. C., and Gwynne, J. T., 1982,
Uptake of high density lipoproteins by rat ovaries in vivo
and dispersed ovarian cells in vitro. Direct correlation
of high density lipoprotein uptake with steroidogenic
activity, J. Steroid Biochem, 16:525.

Strauss, J. F., III, Schuler, L. A., Rosenblum, M. F., and
Tanaka, T., 1981, Cholesterol metabolism by ovarian
tissue, Adv. Lipid Res. 18:99.

Tanaka, T., Billheimer, J. T., and Strauss, J. F. III,
1982, Luteinized rat ovaries contain a sterol binding
protein similar to hepatic SCP_2. Abstracts, 64th Annual
Meeting of the Endocrine Society, San Francisco, CA
Abstract 402.

Toaff, M. E., Schleyer, H., and Strauss, J. F. III, 1982,
Metabolism of 25-hydroxycholesterol by rat luteal
mitochondria and dispersed cells, Endocrinology
111:1785.

Tureck, R. W., and Strauss, J. F. III, 1982, Progesterone
synthesis by luteinized human granulosa cells in
culture. The role of de novo sterol synthesis and
lipoprotein-carried sterol, J. Clin. Endocrinol. Metab.
54:367.

Tureck, R. W., Wilburn, A. B., Gwynne, J. T., Paavola, L. G.,
and Strauss, J. F. III, 1983, The role of lipoproteins in
steroidogenesis by human luteinized granulosa cells in
culture, J. Steroid. Biochem. in press.

Veldhuis, J. D., Klase, P. A., Gwynne, J. T., and Strauss,
    J. F. III, 1982, Low density lipoproteins (LDL) augment
    progesterone biosynthesis by swine granulosa cells in
    vitro: Relation of LDL effects to estrogen and gonadotro-
    pin action. Biol. Reprod. 26(Suppl. 1): 12.

DISCUSSION

NAOR: Since the rat luteal cell can utilize cholesterol
also via the LDL pathway, what determines which receptor-
mediated pathway is activated in the ovary or the adrenal?

STRAUSS: There is no question that the rat luteal cells
can utilize LDL. Rat steroidogenic cells appear to have
an LDL receptor identical to that found on fibroblasts
and the bovine adrenal cortex. It appears that tropic
hormones increase both LDL and HDL uptake simultaneously.
Thus, it seems that rats are gifted with two distinct
receptor-mediated systems for lipoprotein uptake and I would
assume that they are controlled by tropic hormones by similar
mechanisms. I think the HDL pathway is more significant
for cholesterol supply in vivo simply because HDL are the
predominant sterol carrier in this species, but I have no
data to directly support this belief.

SELSTAM: You showed a correlation between steroid production
and ability of cells to take up HDL for granulosa cells
and luteal cells. We have shown that a few hours after
ovulation there is a dramatic drop in steroid production.
Is this accompanied by a decrease in ability of cells to take
up HDL?

STRAUSS: We don't have any information at this time.
However, in the situation you describe, lipoprotein uptake
need not decline as the accumulated cholesterol could be
stored as cholesterol ester.

TAYLOR: Among the patients with homozygous familial hypercholesterolemia, are there any defects in ovarian steroidogenesis?

STRAUSS: There are no direct studies of ovarian function
in these patients. However, there have been reports of

successful pregnancies in affected women. Hence, I would assume that ovarian function is not markedly impaired. In such patients ovarian de novo sterol synthesis might be sufficient to supply steroid precursor. Alternatively, uptake of lipoproteins by non-receptor mediated pathways may provide precursors. I guess an HDL uptake system might also become functional, but that is speculation.

HAZUM: You have indicated that the HDL pathway is different from the LDL pathway. Do you know if the HDL receptors are recycled?

STRAUSS: The LDL receptors certainly appear to be recycled. I would bet that the same is true for the HDL binding sites, but we have no direct evidence for this at present.

HANSSON: You showed data indicating gonadotropin regulation of HDL uptake. Do you know anything about the mechanism for this effect?

STRAUSS: We do not see an acute effect of LH (1 hr) on HDL uptake. Our other studies have been performed after 12-24 hr of stimulation with LH/hCG, and in these experiments we see a stimulation of HDL uptake. I would assume this reflects an increase in receptor synthesis, but I have no direct evidence for this contention.

A MODEL SYSTEM FOR STUDYING THE EFFECTS OF HORMONES ON

LYSOSOMAL POLYPHOSPHOINOSITIDE METABOLISM

Mark A. Seyfred, Christine A. Collins,
and William W. Wells

Department of Biochemistry
Michigan State University
East Lansing, MI 48824-1319

1.   Introduction

Lysosomes, whose functions involve receptor mediated endocytosis, phagosome-lysosome fusion, exocytosis and auto-phagy, are generally believed to be under the influence of various extracellular stimuli. Rapid morphological changes of lysosomes are observed in response to these stimuli suggesting that a mechanism exists to signal primary lysosomes to participate in subsequent physiological events. Lysosomes from livers of starved rats (DeDuve, 1969) and those from livers perfused with glucagon or cAMP (Ashford and Porter, 1962; Deter and DeDuve, 1967; Mortimore et al., 1978; Saito and Ogawa, 1974) rapidly undergo remarkable structural trans-formations associated with autophagy. The stimulation of lysosomal membrane rupture under standard homogenization procedures is attributed to increased volume of the resulting autophagolysosomes. In our laboratory (Schroeder et al., 1974), it was observed that liver lysosomes from normal chickens exhibited a significant diurnal variation in fragility, suggesting dietary and hormonal influences on this process. We became interested in the possibility that lysosomal membrane protein phosphorylation/dephosphorylation reactions may be under hormonal regulation and might result in altered membrane function. In support of this concept, Zahlten et al. (1972) had reported that glucagon stimulated the net uptake of ^{32}Pi in vivo into proteins of rat liver microsomes, mitochondria and lysosomes. Accordingly, highly purified rat liver lysosomes were examined for membrane

391

phosphorylation activity (Wells et al., 1981; Collins and Wells, 1982). These studies demonstrated that a 14,000 dalton component was rapidly phosphorylated at an acid residue as an acylphosphate. We have tentatively proposed that it is a catalytic intermediate of a lysosomal membrane phosphotransferase or ATPase. A second ^{32}P-labeled component was a stable phosphomonoester that migrated in the 3,000 dalton range on 15% SDS polyacrylamide gels (Collins and Wells, 1982). In subsequent studies (Collins and Wells, 1983), the phosphorylated product was identified as phosphatidylinositol 4-phosphate (DPI). Thus, one of the enzyme activities we originally observed was phosphatidylinositol kinase (EC 2.7.1.67). The properties of the lysosomal membrane enzyme were very similar to those of phosphatidylinositol kinase from rat liver plasma membranes (Michell et al., 1967; Harwood and Hawthorne, 1969) and microsomes (Harwood and Harthorne, 1969). Phosphatidylinositol 4,5-bisphosphate (TPI), the product of DPI phosphorylation by a reaction catalyzed by DPI kinase, often accompanies DPI in biological membranes. However, we were unable to detect more than traces of labeled TPI even when substrate levels of DPI were added to lysosomal membrane preparations in vitro. Thus, if TPI is formed by lysosomal membranes in vivo, DPI kinase from the cytosol would most likely act at the outer lysosomal membrane surface.

Since the original discovery by Hokin and Hokin (1953), the inositolphosphatides have been extensively studied with regard to their participation in membrane events in response to hormones utilizing Ca^{2+} as a second messenger (Michell, 1975). These stimuli provoke the rapid turnover of phosphatidylinositol and the rapid incorporation of phosphate into phosphatidic acid and the phosphoinositides. The polyphosphoinositides, DPI and TPI, have been recently shown to be degraded by phospholipase C activity in iris smooth muscle stimulated by muscarinic agonists (Abdel-Latif et al., 1978); in synaptosomes (Griffin and Hawthorne, 1978); in erythrocytes (Buckley and Hawthorne, 1972; Allan and Michell, 1978); and in platelets (Shukla and Hanahan, 1982). Kirk et al. (1981) have observed that Ca^{2+} mobilizing hormones, vasopressin, angiotensin II and epinephrine acting at a α_1-receptors, provoke the rapid degradation of ^{32}P-labeled DPI and TPI in cultured hepatocytes. It has been postulated that the polyphosphoinositides play a special role in binding membrane calcium, contributing to their hydrophobicity. Thus, the activity of calcium dependent phospholipase C specific for polyphosphoinositides (Kemp et al., 1961) could result in a transition from a stable to an unstable lysosomal membrane configuration. Accordingly, the purpose of the present investigation was to determine whether primary cultured hepatocytes incorporate ^{32}Pi into DPI and TPI of lysosomes and whether such cells would serve as suitable models for investigating the effects of hormones on lysosomal membrane polyphosphoinositide metabolism.

2.   Experimental Procedures

Materials.   [^{32}P]-Orthophosphate, carrier free, was purchased from New England Nuclear or ICN. For studies of phosphatidylinositol kinase activity, [^{32}P]ATP was prepared by the method of Glynn and Chappell (1964) as modified by Reimann et al. (1971). Phosphatidylinositol and other phospholipid standards were obtained from Serdary Research Laboratories. Polyphosphoinositide standards were purchased from Sigma. Glass distilled organic solvents were obtained from MCB. Triton WR-1339 was from the Ruger Chemical Co. and Triton X-100 was from Research Products International. Percoll was a product of Pharmacia. An Aminex A-27 anion exchange HPLC column (250 × 4 mm) was obtained from BioRad.

Subcellular Fractionations. Membranes from Triton WR-1339 filled lysosomes were prepared from rat liver by the method of Leighton et al. (1968) as were previously reported (Collins and Wells, 1982). Plasma membranes and microsomes were prepared as described previously (Collins and Wells, 1982). Highly purified liver lysosomal membranes were compared with plasma membranes and microsomes for phosphatidylinositol kinase activity (Collins and Wells, 1983).

Characterization of Lysosomes. The following enzyme activities were measured to estimate the degree of contamination of the lysosomal membranes with other subcellular components. For lysosomes, acid phosphatase (Schroeder et al., 1976) and hexosaminidase (Sellinger et al., 1960); for mitochondria, fumarase (Hill and Bradshaw, 1969); for plasma membranes, alkaline phosphodiesterase, (Aronson and Touster, 1974); for microsomes, NADH-cytochrome c reductase (Fleischer and Fleischer, 1967); for peroxisomes, urate oxidase (London and Hudson, 1956); for Golgi, galactosyltransferase (Fleischer, 1974) was measured.

Phosphatidylinositol Kinase Determination. The assay mixture contained 50 mM Tris-HCl, pH 7.5, 30 mM MgCl$_2$, 2 mM [γ-^{32}P]ATP (20-100 cpm/pmol), and lysosome sample in a final volume of 0.1 ml. The final protein concentration was 1 mg/ml. The reaction was started by the addition of ATP-Mg^{2+} after a 5 min preincubation of the other components at 30°C. After extraction of lipids by the method of Schacht (1981), the chloroform phase was dried under N$_2$ and the residue suspended in a small volume of chloroform:methanol (2:1, v/v). The lipids were separated in silica gel H thin layer plates in the undirectional 2 solvent system of Hauser et al. (1971). The ^{32}P-labeled lipids were visualized by autoradiography and PI, DPI, and TPI standards were detected by staining with I$_2$. Areas of the thin layer plate containing radioactivity were scraped off into vials containing fluor for scintillation counting. In some experiments the combined chloroform extracts were washed twice with methanol:1N HCl (1:1, v/v) and counted directly to measure ^{32}P incorporation.

Protein Determination. Protein was determined by the method of Lowry et al. (1951) with bovine serum albumin as the standard.

Hepatocyte Isolation. Hepatocytes from normal rats were isolated by the method of Seglen (1976) as modified by Kurtz and Wells (1981). Typically, 2.0 - 3.5 × 10^8 cells of 85 - 95% viability were obtained. The cells were suspended at a concentration of 10^6 cells/ml in low phosphate (0.1 mM) Dulbecco's modified Eagle's medium (DME) containing 20 mM HEPES and 1% bovine serum albumin at a pH of 7.3. Cell suspensions of 30 - 50 ml were placed in 490 cm^2 tissue culture roller bottles which were flushed with a 3 sec burst of CO$_2$, sealed and rotated at 2 rpm at 37°C. Under these conditions, the cells remained well suspended and exhibited no loss in viability as judged by trypan blue exclusion over a 3 hr period.

Hepatocyte Incubations. Carrier free ^{32}Pi was added to the cell suspensions at a concentration of 5 - 10 μCi/10^6 cells. At various times of incubation up to 90 min, the cells were transferred to 40 ml conical centrifuge tubes and sedimented at 75 × g for 3 min. The separated cells were resuspended in 3 ml of homogenizing fluid consisting of 250 mM sucrose; 10 mM sodium pyrophosphate, 5 mM EDTA and 50 mM Tricine buffer, pH 8.0.

Isolation of Lysosomes on Percoll Gradients. The cell suspension was homogenized using a Tekmar SDT Tissumizer operating at 65 volts for 60 sec at 0-4°C. This temperature was maintained throughout the preparation. Cell breakage was in excess of 95% as judged by phase contrast microscopy. The homogenate was centrifuged at 750 × g for 10 min. The supernatant was removed and the pellet was washed in 1.0 ml of homogenizing buffers and recentrifuged at 750 × g for 10 min. The supernatants were combined and centrifuged at 15,000 × g for 20 min. The supernatant was removed and discarded. The pellet was gently resuspended in 1.0 ml of homogenizing buffer and mixed with 11.5 ml of a 35% (v/v) Percoll solution in 250 mM sucrose, 5 mM EDTA, 10 mM sodium pyrophosphate and 10 mM Tricine buffer, pH 8.0 at an initial density of 1.080. A self-generating gradient of Percoll was formed by centrifuging at 40,000 × g for 45 min using a 40K rotor in a Spinco model L-2 centrifuge (Pertoft et al., 1978). The gradient was fractionated by injecting 2M sucrose into the bottom of the tube and collecting 0.5 ml fractions from the top. These fractions were analyzed for protein and marker enzymes as previously described (Collins and Wells, 1982). Fractions which had a 14.7-fold increase in hexosaminidase specific activity over that of the whole homogenate were used for further analysis. The major contaminating organelles were peroxisomes with lesser amounts of mitochondria and microsomes. Plasma membranes were absent based on alkaline phosphodiesterase activity.

Analysis of ^{32}P Labeled Phospholipids. The total phospholipid fraction was isolated by the method of Schacht (1981) as described previously (Collins and Wells, 1983). The radioactive lipids were deacylated by the method of Kates (1972), and the polar fraction was evaporated and dissolved in 20 mM ammonium borate and 100 mM ammonium formate, pH 9.5. The deacylated products were analyzed by high performance liquid chromatography (HPLC) on a 250 × 4 mm BioRad Aminex A-27 anion exchange column using a modification of the ion exchange chromatography procedure described by Dittmer and Wells (1969). A 60 ml linear gradient of 20 mM ammonium borate : 100 mM ammonium formate, pH 9.5 to 20 mM ammonium borate : 750 mM ammonium formate, pH 9.5 at a flow rate of 0.6 ml/min was used to elute the deacylated products. Fractions (1.5 ml) were collected and inorganic phosphate which coeluted with L α-glycerol phosphate was extracted from fractions 21 - 24 by adding 0.4 ml of 2% ammonium molybdate

in 2N H_2SO_4 to each fraction. Isobutanol : benzene (1:1, v/v)
(1.9 ml) was added and the mixture was vortexed for 15 sec.
The phosphomolybdic acid which partitions into the upper phase
was removed and the extraction was repeated twice. The
fractions were evaporated in a hood by heating at 150°C.
After the addition of 1.0 ml of water to each fraction, the
samples were evaporated twice to assure removal of the excess
salts. The residues which remained were digested with 0.3 ml
of 14% H_2SO_4 ; 12% $HClO_4$ (2:1, v/v) for 90 min at 180°C. The
fractions were analyzed for their phosphate content by the
method of Ames (1966). Radioactivity in the samples was
measured by Cerenkov radiation.

3.   Results

       Lysosomal   Membrane   Phosphatidylinositol   Kinase   The
typical purity of lysosomes prepared by the method of Leighton
et al. (1968) is shown in Table I. Hexosaminidase and acid
phosphatase were 51.2 and 59.7-fold purified over the crude
homogenate, whereas the fraction was estimated to be contamin-
ated 1.3% by mitochondria, 6.6% by plasma membranes and 4.0%
by microsomes.

       A comparison of liver lysosomal membrane, plasma membrane
and microsomal membrane phosphatidylinositol kinase, assayed
as previously described (Collins and Wells, 1983) is shown in
Table II. Using added phosphatidylinositol as substrate, the
specific activities of the kinase from all three preparations
were similar. However, the plasma membrane preparation was
strongly inhibited by Triton X-100 (0.4%) in the absence of
exogenous substrate.

       Lysosomal   Fractions   from   Cultured   Primary   Rat
Hepatocytes. The total phospholipid from the lysosomal
fraction of hepatocytes incubated with ^{32}Pi for 60 min was
deacylated, and the polar deacylation products were compared
with those obtained from deacylated phospholipid standards
(Fig. 1A). Fractions were analyzed for radioactivity as
shown in Fig. 1B. It can be seen that all major phospholipids
incorporated ^{32}P with the possible exception of phosphatidyl
serine, and that both DPI and TPI deacylation products
were significantly labeled. A time course study of ^{32}P
incorporation into the lysosomal phosphoinositides (Fig. 2)
from hepatocytes of rats starved for 24 hr indicated a rapid
incorporation of ^{32}P into the deacylation products of the

Table I. Characteristics of Purified Triton-Filled
Lysosomes[a]

Component	Relative specific activity in lysosome fraction	% Contamination of lysosomes by organelles
Acid phosphatase (lysosomes)	59.7	--
Hexosaminidase (lysosomes)	51.2	--
Fumarase (mitochondria)	0.06	1.3
Alkaline phosphodiester- ase (plasma membrane)	2.02	6.6
NADH-cytochrome c reduc- tase (microsomes)	0.02	4.0
Urate oxidase (peroxisomes)	negligible	--
Galactosyl transferase (Golgi)	negligible	--
Estimated % contamination by defined organelles		11.9

[a]Lysosomes were prepared from Triton WR 1339-injected rats
by the sucrose floatation method of Leighton et al., 1968.
The enzyme assays were conducted as described in Methods.
The percent of contaminating organelles in the lysosome
fraction was calculated as described by Leighton et al.,
1968 and is the product of the percent of homogenate
protein contributed by the organelle and the relative
specific activity of the marker enzyme for that organelle
in the lysosome fraction.

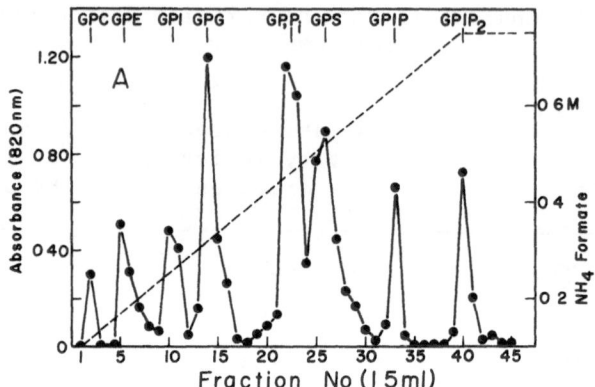

Figure 1A. Separation of the polar deacylation products of standard phospholipids on an Aminex-27 anion exchange column (250 × 4 mm) by HPLC as described under Methods. The products were eluted by a linear gradient of ammonium formate (0.1 M - 0.75 M) with a constant proportion of 20 mM ammonium borate, pH 9.5.

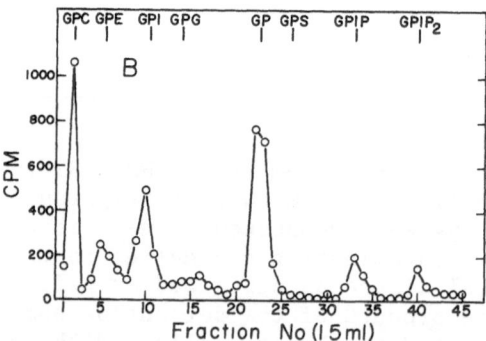

Figure 1B. Incorporation of ^{32}Pi into deacylation products of the lysosomal phospholipids from rat hepatocytes incubated for 60 min under conditions described under Methods.

Table II. Activity of PI Kinase from Lysosomes, Plasma
Membrane and Microsomes[a]

Additions	Lysosomes	Plasma membranes	Microsomes
		nmol/min/mg protein	
None	0.79	1.46	0.63
0.4% Triton X-100	1.40	0.48	1.31
0.4% Triton X-100 + 1 mM PI	2.38	2.07	1.98

[a]PI kinase assays were carried out for 1 and 2 min at 30°C as
described in Methods. The initial rate of reaction was determined in the presence of added detergent and substrate as indicated, with enzyme protein at 1 mg/ml for each sample. Adopted
from Collins and Wells, 1983, by permission of J. Biol. Chem.

[b]The results are the mean of 2-4 determinations.

polyphosphoinositides.   The   combined   evidence   suggests
that both DPI and TPI are located on lysosomal membranes.
In addition there is a rapid incorporation of ^{32}Pi into
each   polyphosphoinositide   before   incorporation   into
PI itself, suggesting that they are derived from non-
labeled phosphatidylinositol by way of the action of
membrane bound PI kinase and a cytosolic DPI kinase.
Alternatively, DPI and TPI labeled elsewhere could
have migrated to the lysosomal membrane bound to a carrier
protein.

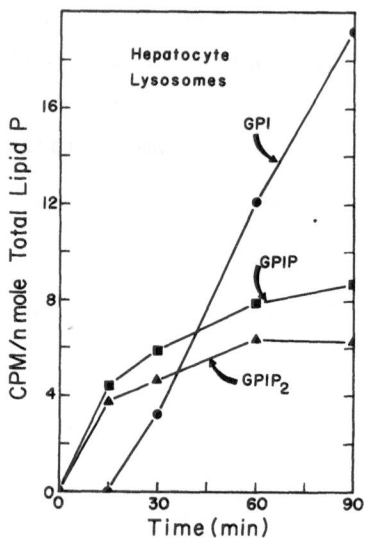

Figure 2. Time course of ^{32}Pi incorporation into the phosphoinositides isolated from a Percoll gradient enriched lysosomal fraction from cultured hepatocytes isolated from a rat starved for 24 hr as outlined under Methods.

4.   Discussion

     In the early studies of phosphatidylinositol kinase localization by Michell et al. (1967) and Harwood and Hawthorne (1969), lysosomal fractions were not considered active enough to postulate the occurrence of a polyphosphoinositide metabolic pathway. Contributing to this previous viewpoint were the differences in purity of the liver lysosomal fractions and the failure to detect the polyphosphoinositides in previous phospholipid analyses of lysosomes (Wherrett and Huterer, 1972; Henning and Heidrich, 1974;

Hostetler and Poorthius, 1978). By the more sensitive method of ^{32}P incorporation catalyzed by PI kinase and HPLC analysis of polar deacylation products, it was possible to detect these minor components under both in vitro (DPI) and cell culture conditions (DPI and TPI).

From our earlier study of the phosphatidylinositol kinase reaction with lysosomal membranes without added detergent or substrate, the product, DPI, was very stable (Collins and Wells, 1983). However, in the presence of 0.4% Triton X-100, greater activity was observed, but the product was degraded by either phospholipase C or phosphomonoesterase activity under the conditions of the assay, i.e., high Mg^{2+} at a pH of 7.5. Studies of the degradation of lysosomal DPI and TPI in the intact cell have not been concluded. However, phospholipase C activity specific for phosphatidylinositol (Takenawa and Nagai, 1981) and when tested for polyphosphoinositides as well (Kemp et al., 1961), is located in rat liver cytoplasm. This activity is activated by Ca^{2+} and it is possible that the modulation of intracellular Ca^{2+} levels in response to hormonal stimulation could provoke the breakdown of lysosomal membrane polyphosphoinositides into diglyceride and the polar head groups, inositol 1,4-bisphosphate and inositol 1,4,5-trisphosphate. These products could be rapidly degraded as demonstrated for erythrocytes (Downes et al., 1982).

An analogy appears to exist between liver lysosomal membranes and adrenal gland chromaffin granules with respect to a phosphatidylinositol kinase system (Phillips, 1973; Muller and Kirshner, 1975; Lefebvre et al., 1976). This is of interest since chromaffin granules are known to fuse with the plasma membrane upon stimulation of the secretion process. Thus, whether the polyphosphoinositides of lysosomal membranes play an important role in the fusion functions of lysosomes is a question that is worthy of further inquiry. For example, hormones that mobilize Ca^{2+} in hepatocytes such as vasopressin, angiotensin II, and epinephrine acting at α_1-receptors stimulate the rapid degradation of whole liver cell polyphosphoinositides (Kirk et al., 1981). From the work of others (Takizawa and Hayashi, 1980), it might be speculated that critical levels of polyphosphoinositides bound to Ca^{2+} as a hydrophobic membrane component would contribute to membrane stability. The lysosomal membrane fluidity could then be enhanced by the action of a hormone stimulated phospholipase C activity that catalyzed formation of 1,2-diacylglycerol and the release of the polar head groups

into the cytosol. Alternatively, phospholipase A_2 action on
TPI for example, would produce lysotriphophoinositide which
would participate in membrane Ca^{2+}-sensitive univalent cation
channel formation as shown by Hayashi et al. (1978, 1981).

To further investigate the role of polyphosphoinositides
in lysosome function, the primary cultured hepatocyte, which
has been shown to be responsive to hormones, should provide a
useful model.

ACKNOWLEDGMENTS.   We gratefully acknowledge the technical
assistance of Mrs. Lynn Farrell during some of the studies
reported herein. We are indebted to Mrs. Carol Fenn for her
expertise in preparing the manuscript. This work was
supported by grant AM 10209 from the United States Public
Health Services.

REFERENCES

Abdel-Latif, A. A., Akhtar, R. A., and Smith, J. P., 1978,
    Studies on the role of triphosphoinositide in cholinergic
    muscarinic and α-adrenergic receptors function of iris
    smooth muscle, in: "Cylitols and Phosphoinositides,"
    W. W. Wells, F. Eisenberg Jr., eds., pp. 121-143, Academic
    Press, New York.
Allan, D., and Michell, R. H., 1978, A calcium-activated poly-
    phosphoinositide phosphodiesterase in the plasma membrane
    of human rabbit erythrocytes, Biochim. Biophys. Acta,
    508:277.
Ames, B. N., 1966, Assay of inorganic phosphate, total phosphate
    and phosphatases, Meth. Enzymol., 8:115.
Aronson, N. N., Jr. and Touster, O., 1974, Isolation of rat
    liver plasma membrane fragments in isotonic sucrose, Meth.
    Enzymol., 31:90.
Ashford, T. P., and Porter, K. R., 1962, Cytoplasmic components
    in hepatic cell lysosomes, J. Cell Biol., 12:198.
Buckley, J. T., and Hawthorne, J. N., 1972, Erythrocyte membrane
    polyphosphoinositide metabolism and the regulation of cal-
    cium binding, J. Biol. Chem., 247:7218.
Collins, C. A., and Wells, W. W., 1982, Characterization of
    endogenous protein phosphorylation in isolated rat liver
    lysosomes, J. Biol. Chem., 257:827.

Collins, C. A., and Wells, W. W., 1983, Identification of phosphatidylinositol kinase in rat liver lysosomal membranes, J. Biol. Chem., 258:2130.

DeDuve, C., 1969, The lysosome in retrospect, in: "Lysosomes in Biology and Pathology," J. T. Dingle, H. B. Fell, eds., pp. 3-40, North-Holland Publishing Co., Amsterdam.

Deter, R. L., and DeDuve, C., 1967, Influence of glucagon, an inducer of cellular autophagy, on some physical properties of rat liver lysosomes, J. Cell. Biol., 33:437.

Dittmer, J. C., and Wells, M. A., 1969, Determination of individual phospholipids by selective hydrolysis, Meth. Enzymol. 14:516.

Downes, C. P., Mussat, M. D., and Michell, R. H., 1982, The inositol triphosphate phosphomonesterase of the human erythrocyte membrane, Biochem. J., 203:169.

Fleischer, B., 1974, Isolation and characterization of golgi apparatus and membranes from rat liver, Meth. Enzymol., 31:180.

Fleischer, S., and Fleischer, B., 1967, Assay of DPNH or succinate-cytochrome c reductase activity, Meth. Enzymol., 10:427.

Glynn, I. M., and Chappell, J. B., 1964, A simple method for the preparation of ^{32}P-labeled adenosine triphosphate of high specific activity, Biochem. J. 90:147.

Griffin, H. D., and Hawthorne, J. N., 1978, Calcium-activated hydrolysis of phosphatidyl-myo-inositol 4-phosphate and phosphatidyl-myo-inositol 4,5-bisphosphate in guinea-pig synaptosomes, Biochem. J., 176:541.

Harwood, J. L., and Hawthorne, J. N., 1969, The properties and subcellular distribution of phosphatidylinositol kinase in mammalian tissues, Biochim. Biophys. Acta, 171:75.

Hauser, G., Eichberg, J., and Gonzalez-Sastre, F., 1971, Regional distribution of polyphosphoinositides in rat brain, Biochim. Biophys. Acta, 248:87.

Hayashi, F., Sokabe, M., and Amakawa, T., 1981, Carbamylcholine-effect on inositol phospholipids in acetylcholine receptor membrane from Narke japonica, Proc. Japan Acad., 57:Series B, 48.

Hayashi, F., Sokabe, M., Takagi, M., Hayashi, K., and Kishimoto, U., 1978, Calcium-sensitive univalent cation channel formed by lysotriphosphoinositide in bilayer lipid membranes, Biochim. Biophys. Acta, 510:305.

Henning, R., and Heidrich, H. G., 1974, Membrane lipids of rat liver lysosomes prepared by free-flow electrophoresis,

Biochim. Biophys. Acta, 345:326.

Hill, R. L., and Bradshaw, R. A., 1969, Fumarase, Meth. Enzymol. 13:91.

Hokin, M. R., and Hokin, L. E., 1953, Enzyme secretion and the incorporation of ^{32}P into phospholipids of pancreas slices, J. Biol. Chem., 203:967.

Hostetler, K. Y., and Poorthuis, B. J. H. M., 1978, Acidic phospholipids and lysosomal bis(monoacylglycerl) phosphate synthesis: The role of phosphatidylinositol and lysophosphatidylglycerol, in: "Cyclitols and Phosphoinositides," W. W. Wells, F. Eisenberg Jr., eds., pp. 585-597, Academic Press, New York.

Kates, M., 1972, Mild alkaline deacylation of phosphatides and glycolipids, in: "Techniques of Lipidology: Isolation, Analysis and Identification of Lipids," pp. 558-559, North-Holland Publ. Co., Amsterdam.

Kemp, P., Hubscher, G., Hawthorne, J. N., 1961, Phosphoinositides. 3. Enzymic hydrolysis of inositol-containing phospholipids, Biochem. J., 79:193.

Kirk, C. J., Creba, J. A., Downes, C. P., and Michell, R. H., 1981, Hormone-stimulated metabolism of inositol lipids and its relationship to hepatic receptor function, Biochem. Soc. Transact., 9:377.

Kurtz, J. W., and Wells, W. W., 1981, Induction of glucose-6-phosphate dehydrogenase in primary cultures of adult rat hepatocytes. Requirement for insulin and dexamethasone, J. Biol. Chem., 256:10870.

Lefebvre, Y. A., White, D. A., and Hawthorne, J. N., 1976, Diphosphoinositide metabolism in bovine adrenal medulla, Can. J. Biochem., 54:746.

Leighton, F., Poole, B., Beaufay, H., Baudhuin, P., Coffey, J. W., Fowler, S., and DeDuve, C., 1968, The large-scale separation of peroxisomes, mitochondria, and lysosomes from the livers of rats injected with triton WR-1339, J. Cell. Biol., 37:482.

London, M., and Hudson, P. M., 1956, Purification and properties of solubolized uricase, Biochim. Biophys. Acta, 21:290.

Lowry, O. H., Rosebrough, N. J., Farr, A. L., and Randall, R. J., 1951, Protein measurement with the Folin phenol reagent, J. Biol. Chem., 193:265.

Michell, R. H., Harwood, J. L., Coleman, R., and Hawthorne, J. N., 1967, Characteristics of rat liver phosphatidylinositol kinase and its presence in the plasma membrane, Biochim. Biophys. Acta, 144:649.

Mortimore, G. E., Ward, W. F., and Schworer, C. M., 1978, Lysosomal processing of intracellular protein in rat liver and

its general regulation by amino acids and insulin, in:
"Protein turnover and lysosomal functions," H. L. Segal,
D. J. Doyle, eds., pp. 67-87, Academic Press, New York.

Muller, T. W., and Kirshner, N., 1975, ATPase and phosphatidylinositol kinase activities of adrenal chromaffin
vesicles, J. Neurochem., 24:1155.

Pertoft, H., Warmegard, B., and Hook, M., 1978, Heterogeneity
of lysosomes originating from rat liver parenchymal cells,
Biochem. J., 174:309.

Phillips, J. H., 1973, Phosphatidylinositol kinase. A component of the chromaffin-granule membrane, Biochem. J., 136:
579.

Reimann, E. M., Brostrom, C. O., Corbin, J. D., King, C. A., and
Krebs, E. G., 1971, Separation of regulatory and catalytic
subunits of the cyclic 3,'5'-adenosine monophosphate-
dependent protein kinase(s) of rabbit skeletal muscle,
Biochem. Biophys. Res. Commun., 42:187.

Saito, T., and Ogawa, K., 1974, Lysosomal changes in rat
hepatic parenchymal cells after glucagon administration,
Acta Histochem. Cytochem., 7:1.

Schacht, J., 1981, Extraction and purification of polyphosphoinositides, Meth. Enzymol., 72:626.

Schroeder, H. R., Gauger, J. A., and Wells, W. W., 1976, On
lysosomal fragility and induction of liver hexose-monophos-
phate dehydrogenases in the fasted-refed rat, Arch.
Biochem. Biophys., 172:206.

Schroeder, H. R., Lawler, J. R., and Wells, W. W., 1974, Effect
of dietary galactose on lysosomal enzymes in the chick,
J. Nutr., 104:943.

Seglen, P. O., 1976, Preparation of isolated rat liver cells,
Meth. Cell Biol., 13:29.

Sellinger, O. Z., Beaufay, H., Jacques, P., Doyen, A., and
DeDuve, C., 1960, Tissue fractionation studies 15. Intracellular distribution and properties of β-Galactosidase
in rat liver, Biochem. J., 74:450.

Shukla, S. D., and Hanahan, D. J., 1982, AGEC (Platelet Activating Factor) induced stimulation of rabbit platelets:
Effects on phosphatidylinositol, di- and tri-phosphoinosi-
tides and phosphatidic acid metabolism, Biochem., Biophys.
Res. Commun., 106:697.

Takenawa, T., and Nagai, Y., 1981, Purification of phosphatidyl-
inositol-specific phospholipase C from rat liver, J. Biol.
Chem., 256:6769.

Takizawa, T., and Hayashi, K., 1980, Calorimetric study of Ca^{2+}
binding to triphosphoinositide, Rep. Prog. Polymer Physics
in Japan, 23:25.

Wells, W. W., Collins, C. A., and Kurtz, J. W., 1981, Metabolic
    regulation of lysosome activity, in: "Lysosomes and Lyso-
    somal Storage Diseases," J. W. Callahan, J. A. Lowden,
    eds., pp. 17-30, Academic Press, New York.
Wherrett, J. R., and Huterer, S., 1972, Enrichment of bis-
    (monoacylglyceryl) phosphate in lysosomes from rat liver,
    J. Biol. Chem., 247:4114.
Zahlten, R. N., Hochberg, A. A., Stratman, F. W., and Lardy, H.
    A., 1972, Glucagon-stimulated phosphorylation of mitochon-
    drial and lysosomal membranes of rat liver in vivo, Proc.
    Natl. Acad. Sci. USA, 69:800.

DISCUSSION

NAOR: Farese's work on ACTH action suggests a role for DPI
and TPI in mediating membrane events to mitochondria function,
could you comment on the possible similarity of his data to
yours?

WELLS: Our results have been obtained with highly purified
lysosomal membranes of rat liver origin, so it is difficult
to compare with their studies. Mitochondrial membranes are
not known to possess polyphosphoinositides, although we have
some preliminary evidence that they are there in very small
quantities. Since stimulated adrenal steroidogenesis could
involve rate limiting precursor cholesterol mitochondrial
membrane transport, the relative quantity of DPI and TPI
might very likely affect the membrane fluidity or hydrophobicity and therefore cholesterol transport. Farese's effect was
sensitive to cycloheximide, but it would be important to
assess the direct effect of cycloheximide on polyphosphoinositide metabolizing enzymes.

NICHOLSON: It is also possible to see autophagic processes
on hormonal withdrawal from sex-steroid dependent tissues such
as mammary glands. Do you envisage that this process works
through a common mechanism to that observed for hormone-
induced autophagy?

WELLS: We have no direct data to answer your question at
this time because the polyphosphoinositide pathway in lysosomal membrane has only recently been appreciated. However,
I would speculate that a similar mechanism may be involved in
all functions of lysosomes that involve fusion processes.

HOLLOW FIBERS: THEIR APPLICATIONS TO THE STUDY OF

MAMMALIAN CELL FUNCTION

W. C. Hymer[a], M. Angeline[a], M. Chu[b], R. Grindle-
land[c], J. Harkness[a], J. Hatfield[a], E. Hibbard[a],
K. Kovacs[d], G. Mansur[a], A. Mastro[a], K. Motter[a],
J. Parsons[e], C. Phelps[a], B. Ruskin[a], A. Signorel-
la[a], W. Taylor[a], M. Thorner[f], G. Tindall[g], and
D. Wilbur[h]

[a]Department of Biochemistry, Microbiology, Molecular and Cell Biology, The Pennsylvania State
   University, University Park, PA
[b]Roswell Park Memorial Institute, Buffalo, NY
[c]Ames Research Center, Moffett Field, CA
[d]Department of Pathology, University of Toronto,
   Toronto, Canada
[e]Department of Anatomy, University of Minnesota,
   Minneapolis, MN
[f]Department of Internal Medicine, University of
   Virginia, Charlottesville, VA
[g]Department of Neurosurgery, Emory Univeristy,
   Atlanta, GA
[h]Department of Anatomy, University of South Carolina
   Charlestown, SC

1.   Introduction

The purpose of this report is to summarize our experi-
ences with hollow fibers; especially their applications with
regard to the study of target cell responsiveness, the general
theme of this book.

The use of hollow fibers in cell culture and transplantation has a brief but interesting history. The unique properties of the ultrafiltration membranes that make up the hollow

fiber lie at the heart of their potential application to biological science. These ultrafiltration membranes are cast from a variety of polymer solutions. They consist of a very thin (0.1 - 1.5 μm) dense "skin" of fine, controlled pore structure which open to a thicker (50 - 250 μm) open-celled spongy layer of the same polymer (Fig. 1). Hollow fibers with pore sizes which exclude molecules of 500, 1000, 5000, 10,000, 30,000, 50,000, 100,000 and 300,000 mol. wt. are comercially available from Amicon Corp., Danvers, MA. In general, two sizes of hollow fibers are available; one with an internal diameter of 500 μm, the other 1100 μm. Important morphological features of the fibers are the porous nature of the outer aspects of the wall and the rigid character of the inner lumen surface (Fig. 1).

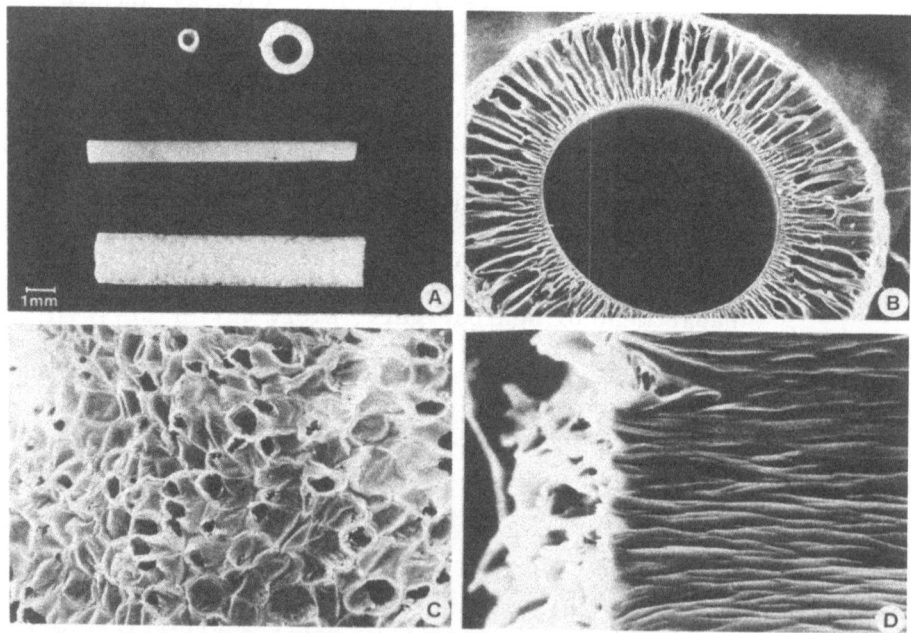

Figure 1. Morphological features of XM-50 hollow filters. (A) Light micrograph of "thin" (500 μm I.D.) and "thick" (1100 μm I.D.) fiber. (B) Scanning electron micrograph (SEM) of fiber in cross section. (C) SEM of outer capsule wall. Note porous nature. Inflammatory cells penetrate the capsule via these pores. (D) SEM of inner aspect of fiber lumen. Cells "grow" on this surface.

Knazek et al. (1972) were the first to show that mammalian cells could attach to the outer surface of the hollow fiber and grow in vitro. Furthermore, choricarcinoma cells growing on the fiber surface secreted hCG through the fiber wall into the lumen where the hormone was subsequently pumped into a reservoir. In this configuration the hollow fiber mimicked a capillary. This same group later showed that hollow fibers were useful for culturing pituitary cells to obtain sizeable quantities of rat and human prolactin (PRL) (Knazek, 1974; Knazek and Skyler, 1976). Knazek has listed the advantages of this approach in culturing cells:

1.   Cell densities attained are similar to growth of solid tissues in vivo.

2.   Cells are maintained in a more physiological state with regard to nutrient supply, waste removal, and pH control.

3.   Hormone secretion rates from cells grown on artificial capillaries are higher than from those grown in dishes.

4.   Hormones can be recovered from the perfusate without disturbing the culture (medium changes are known to alter hormone release rates).

Shortly after Knazek's reports, an important conceptual development in the use of hollow fibers occurred, viz, their implantation into animals. This approach was used primarily by workers studying diabetes. Implant studies began shortly after it was first shown that pancreatic beta cells from neonatal rats, when grown on the surface of hollow fibers in vitro according to the Knazek procedure, released immunoreactive insulin into the medium for at least one month. Release was dependent upon the concentration of glucose in the culture medium (Chick et al., 1975). Implantation of beta cell-containing artificial capillary units into diabetic rats were subsequently found to result in lowered glucose and elevated insulin in the blood of the recipient (Tze et al., 1976; Chick et al., 1977; Sun et al., 1977). Fibers of the XM-50 series were used in these studies. XM-50 fibers are made of a polyvinyl-chloride-acrylic co-polymer and exclude molecules greater than 50,000 mol. wt. It was pointed out by these investigators that antibody molecules circulating in the bloodstream would not reach the tissue by virtue of the sieving properties of the fiber. In theory, the pancreatic implant was immunologically privileged.

In 1978 we reported that dispersed pituitary cells
implanted into the cerebral ventricles of hypophysectomized
rats resulted in growth of the recipient (Weiss et al.,
1978). However, the key disadvantage to this experimental
approach was that the cells could not be recovered for subsequent study. In view of the pancreatic transplant data, the
possibility of developing an implantable "artificial pituitary
hollow fiber unit" seemed exciting. It soon became obvious,
however, that employing the strategy of Knazek and others,
i.e., placing the cells on the outside of the fiber, resulted
in a unit that was far too large for implantation into the
rat's brain. Accordingly, we adopted the strategy of placing
the pituitary cells inside the hollow fiber unit. This was
easily accomplished by inserting a cell-filled 10 µl Hamilton
syringe into the fiber lumen. After loading, we found that
the fiber unit could be sealed by squeezing the ends with a
heated forceps. Finally, dipping the fiber ends in a hot
melt wax ensured complete closure.

Before embarking on implantation studies using the
hollow fiber technology, we felt it was essential to document
that pituitary hormones released from encapsulated cells
could, in fact, diffuse through the pores in the hollow fiber
membrane and be detected in the medium outside the fiber. In
two separate experiments, $25 - 400 \times 10^3$ cells were plated in
35 mm dishes in either encapsulated (7 µl/XM-50 capsule) or
unencapsulated form. The results indicated that after three
days in culture (a) that PRL was released from the encapsulated cells into the medium; (b) that the capsule did not
adversely affect PRL cell function since the levels of
released hormone were similar between the two treatments
and (c) that the quantity of released hormone was related
to cell number (Fig. 2). In a related experiment, five
capsules, each containing 1.4×10^6 cells, were perifused
in a microchromatography column with M199 containing 0.1%
BSA at a rate of 0.5 ml/min. At selected intervals buffer
containing 1 mM dibutyryl cyclic AMP was perifused through
the encapsulated cells. Results (Fig. 2) showed (a) that
GH was released from the encapsulated cells and (b) that
cAMP was an effective FH secretagogue for pituitary GH cells
in this configuration.

2.   Morphology of Implanted Pituitary Cells

The data in Fig. 2 demonstrated that pituitary hormones
can indeed diffuse through the pores and walls of the hollow

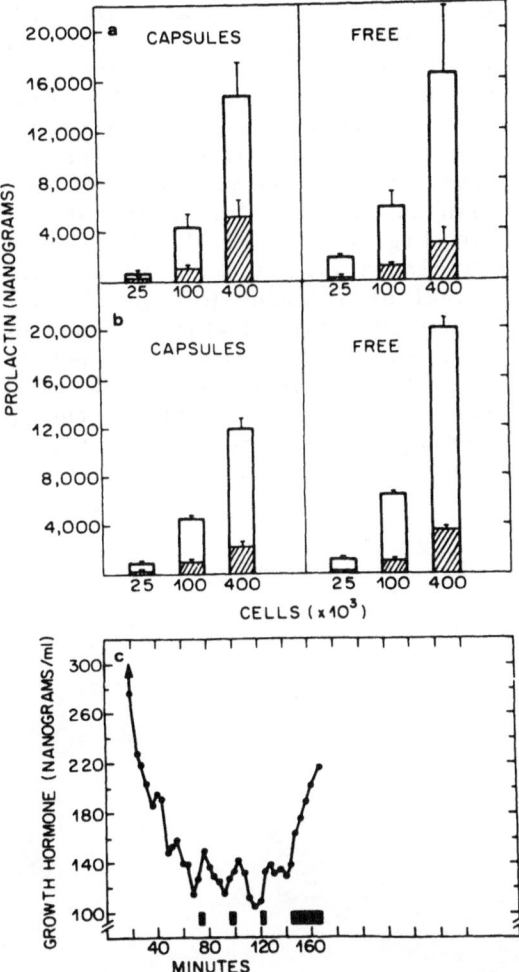

Figure 2. Comparison of PRL release from encapsulated pituitary cells vs unencapsulated cells in vitro (experiments A,B).
Open bars = released hormone; hatched bars = intracellular
hormone. Culture conditions: 3 days in α-MEM + 20% horse
serum. Four dishes/group. (C) Release of GH from 5×10^6
encapsulated pituitary cells maintained in perifusion. Solid
bars indicate time and length of exposure to 1 mM dibutyryl
cyclic AMP.

fibers when cells are loaded inside the fiber. We next
sought to define the morphology of the encapsulated pituitary

cells before and after their implantation into the rat. A scanning electron micrograph of freshly trypsinized and encapsulated rat pituitary cells reveals their surface features and relative position to the fiber lumen immediately prior to implantation (Fig. 3). Our previous finding that hypophysectomized rats grew after intracerebroventricular injection of pituitary somatotrophs provided the rationale for choosing the brain as the site for implantation of the hollow fiber. Shown in Fig 4 is (1) the loading of the hollow fiber, (2) its implantation, and (3) placement and extent of lesion after removal of a "thin" (500 μm ID) or "thick" (1100 μm ID) fiber 39 days post-implantation. Histological sections of the brain have shown that the fiber penetrates into or through the lateral ventricle in > 95% of the implants. Additional areas with lesions include the parietofrontal cortex (capsule entrance), anterior dorsal hippocampus, dorsal caudate-putamen nuclear complex and lateral septal nucleus.

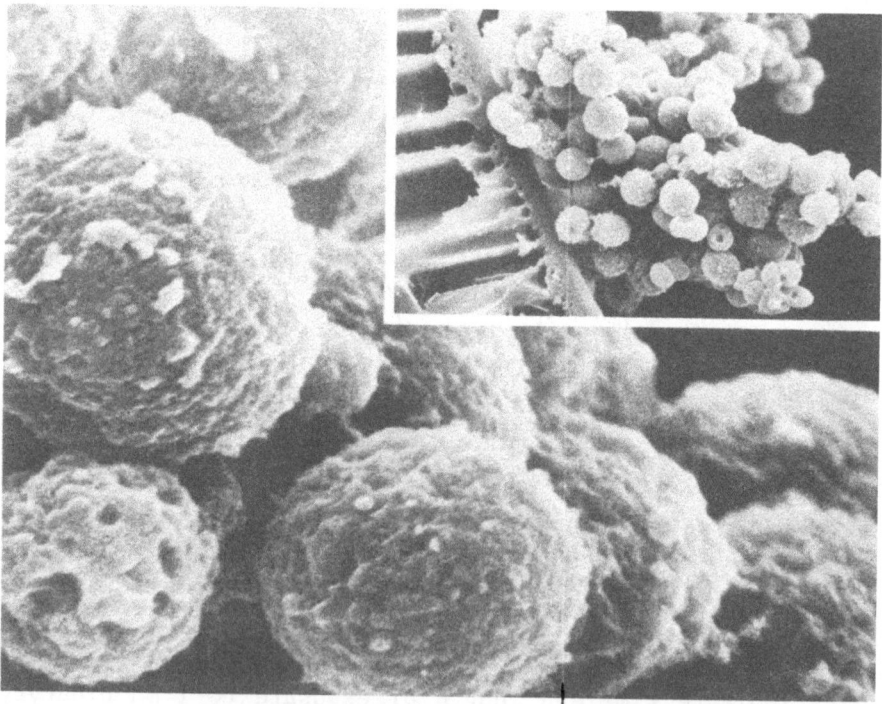

Figure 3. Scanning electron micrographs of freshly dispersed and encapsulated rat pituitary cells. These cells were not implanted. Insert. Cells in relation to fiber lumen.

In our experience surgical mortality averages < 5% (based on ~ 1000 rats). Recipients appear normal in appearance, mobility, and eating and drinking habits.

At the level of the scanning electron microscope, encapsulated and implanted pituitary cells show signs of (a) aggregation, (b) spreading over the lumen surface, (c) deposition of fibrous material (basement membrane?) between cells and lumen surface and (d) blebbing at the cell surface suggestive of exocytosis (Fig. 5). At the immunocytochemical level, all of the anterior pituitary cell types have been detected seven days post-implantation. The size and relative staining intensity of the cells at this time is similar to that of the zero time controls (compare Figs. 6 and 7). Somatotrophs, corticotrophs and mammotrophs have been seen 40 days post-implantation. Our impression is that the glycoprotein-hormone containing cells are less healthy after 40 days, but this issue requires further study. Transmission electromicroscopic study of the encapsulated cells has proven difficult due to technical problems associated with infiltration of the plastic into the hollow fiber itself. Nevertheless, preliminary results document that ultrastructural integrity of the implanted cells is maintained; a key test of viability (Fig. 8). In sum, these morphological data (Fig. 3-8) document viability of encapsulated and implanted pituitary cells.

It is not the purpose of this report to review the extensive literature regarding pituitary cell morphology after transplantation to various ectopic sites. Suffice it to say that the combined efforts of many workers in the 1950's and 1960's documented mammotroph survival in such sites as the kidney capsule, anterior chamber of the eye, subcutaneous tissue, etc. Of course, the classic experiments of Halasz (Halasz et al., 1963, 1965) led to the identification of the well-known "hypophysiotropic zone." Knigge has recently reopened the issue of graft morphology and shown quite nicely that pituitaries grafted to the third ventricle of hypophysectomized rats retain their normal complement of cells as identified by immunocytochemistry (Knigge, 1980). Our morphological findings are entirely consistent with those of Knigge's. Evidence for function of the pituitary hollow fiber unit is offered in the following sections.

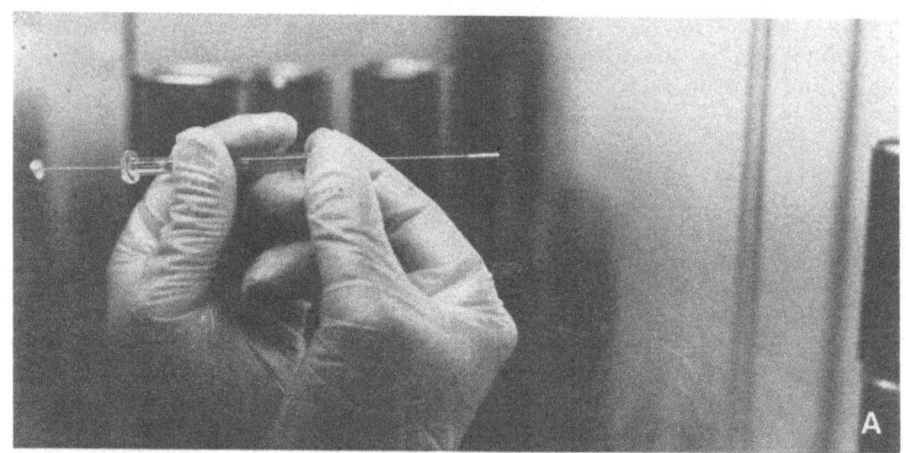

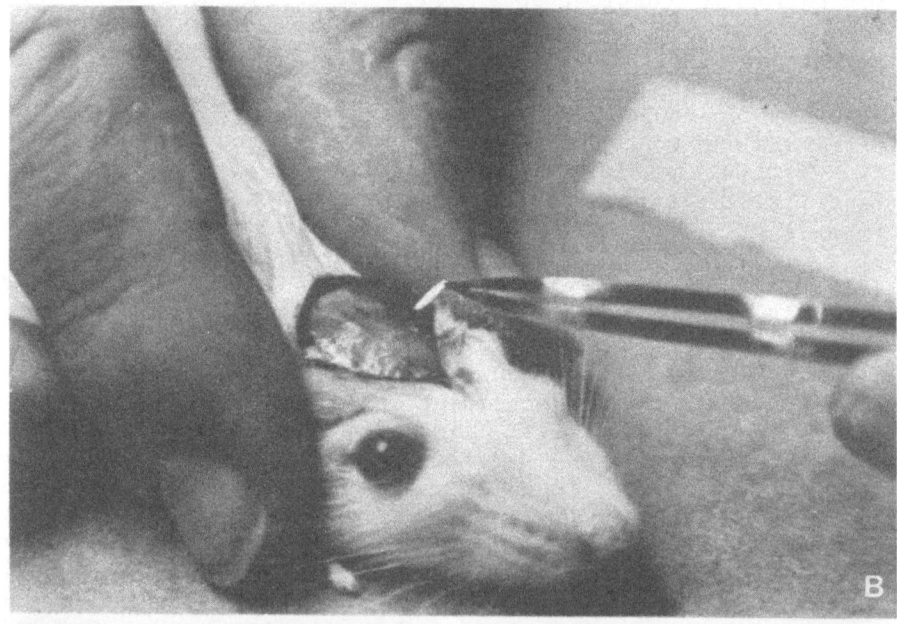

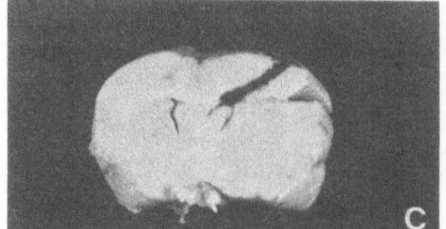

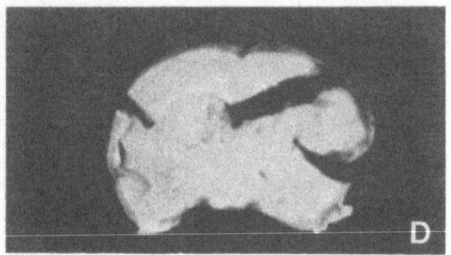

3.   Somatotroph Function Using Hollow Fiber Technology

3.1. Donor: Rat Pituitary Cells

      Recipient: Hypophysectomized Rats

3.1.1. Rationale

In 1978 we reported that implantation of acutely dispersed pituitary cells into the lateral ventricles of hypophysectomized rats resulted in restoration of growth for periods of 1 - 3 months (Weiss et al., 1978). However, this experimental approach was limited since it did not permit recovery of the implanted cells for subsequent study in vitro. Accordingly, we wanted to find out if pituitary cells encapsulated in hollow fibers were capable of restoring growth of the hypophysectomized rat (see Hymer et al., 1981a for additional detail).

3.1.2. Materials and Methods

Anterior pituitary glands of 20 - 30 rats were dissociated aseptically (Hymer et al., 1973) concentrated by centrifugation, and resuspended in small volumes of M199 or MEM to achieve a final concentration of $250 - 500 \times 10^3$ cells/µl. Loading of cells into the hollow fiber was as discussed above. Fibers which are 10 mm long can receive ~ 2 µl of cell suspension (thin fibers) or ~ 8 µl (thick fibers). Animals receiving hollow fibers were usually male rats hypophysectomized at ~ 150 gm. See part 2 for description of implantation procedure.

←

Figure 4. (continued) Fiber loading and implantation procedure. (A) Cells are loaded into fiber using 10 µl Hamilton syringe. Ends are subsequently heat sealed and wax coated (not shown). (B) Fiber being implanted intracranially (angle intensified for photographic purposes. (C) Lesion produced by thin fiber. (D) Lesion produced by thick fiber.

3.1.3. Results and Discussion

Growth rates of animals receiving intracranial implants was rapid during the first two weeks and slower thereafter (Fig. 9). Final body weights in the experimental group were

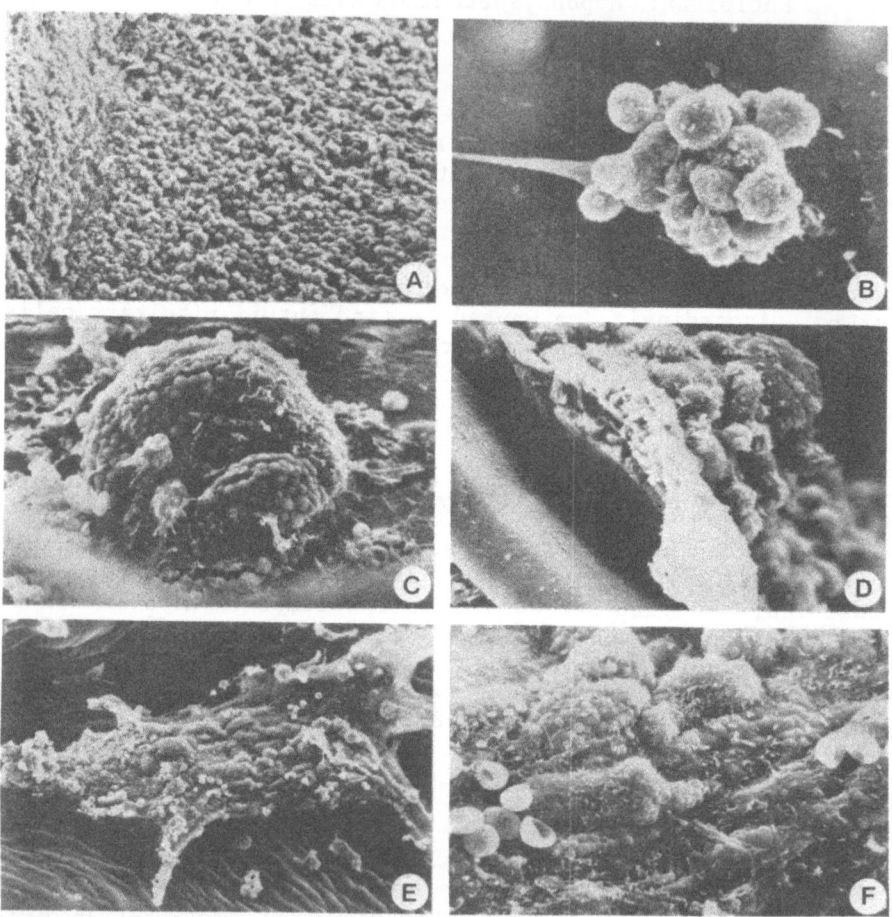

Figure 5. Scanning electron micrographs of rat pituitary cells 8 - 39 days post implantation. (A) Densely packed cells within capsule. (B) Cell cluster. (C) Surface features suggestive of exocytosis. (D) Aggregated cells partially retracted from inner lumen surface. (E) Pituitary cell aggregate attached to inner surface. (F) Enlargement of (E) showing secretion granules on cell surface.

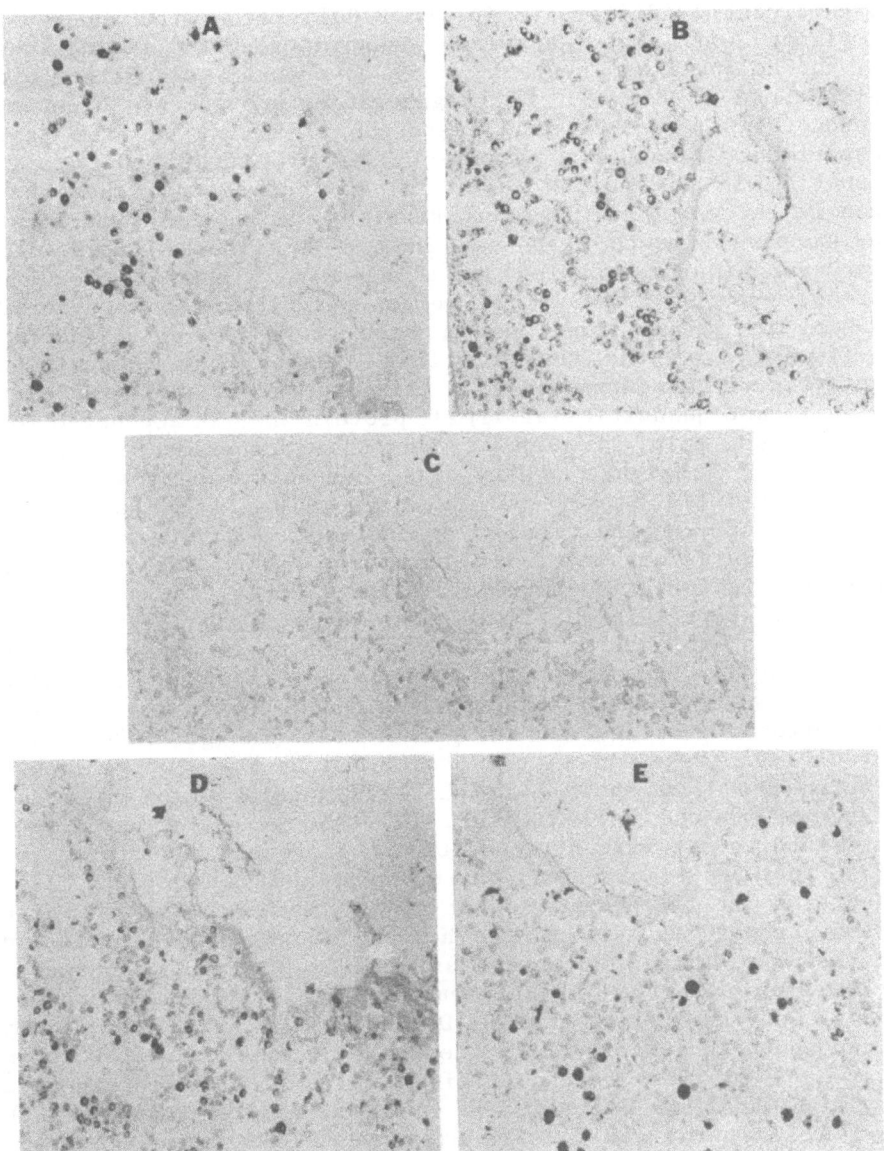

Figure 6. Immunocytochemical appearance of sectioned pituitary cells which have been encapsulated, but not implanted. Panel C shows extent of non-specific staining with normal rabbit serum. All antisera used at final dilution of 1:100. (A) ACTH, (B) PRL, (D) GH, (E) LH.

significantly different (p < 0.001) from the controls implanted with empty capsules. Scanning electron micrographs of the hollow fiber contents seven days post-implantation are also shown in Fig. 9. Cell aggregation and surface blebbing (exocytosis?) were common features. The results from this experiment showed two important things: first, that cells function in the hollow fiber in vivo and second, that they can be recovered for in vitro studies. In another experiment we compared growth responses induced by fibers loaded with syngeneic (Sprague-Dawley) or allogeneic (Fisher 344 rat and sheep) pituitary cells. As before, growth rates were rapid during the first three weeks; each group was significantly different from the controls (Fig. 10A). Body composition analysis of the carcasses from this experiment indicated that significant quantities of lipid, protein and ash accounted for the weight gain in each of the three experimental groups (Fig. 10B). Weights of thyroids, adrenals, and testes were also stimulated in several instances (Fig. 10C). Especially interesting were the signs of gonadotropin activity in recipients implanted with syngeneic pituitary cells. However, since testes weights varied between 218 and 1500 mg, the result was not statistically significant. The recent study by Knigge may provide an explanation for this variability in that pituitary grafts in the third ventricle which contained PRL cells also had elevated testes weights, but those grafts with sparse mammotroph densities had atrophic testes (Knigge, 1980). The results of these experiments described by Fig. 10 are important since they show: (1) that allogeneic pituitary cells function in the hollow fiber, (2) that weight gains can be ascribed to significant depositions of protein and lipid, and (3) that corticotrophs, thyrotrophs and mammotrophs also function in the fiber. What is the mechanism(s) by which somatotrophs function in the hollow fiber? Hypothalamic and anterior pituitary hormones, as well as arginine vasopressin have been detected in ventricular fluid (Knigge and Joseph, 1974; Schroeder et al., 1976; Dogterom et al., 1978). TRH has been shown to restore GH in the renal pituitary graft both in vivo and in vitro (Giannattasio et al., 1979). As suggested by the model in Fig. 11, TRH would stimulate release of GH which, in turn, could leave major vessels leaving the brain to promote its peripheral growth effects. In the early transplantation periods, somatostatin (SIF) levels surrounding the capsule would be low as suggested by the observations of Hoffman and Baker (1977) which indicate that hypophysectomy induces depletion of medium eminence somatostatin. It seems possible that some of the GH diffusing out of the capsule would eventually reach these SIF producing neurons to activate

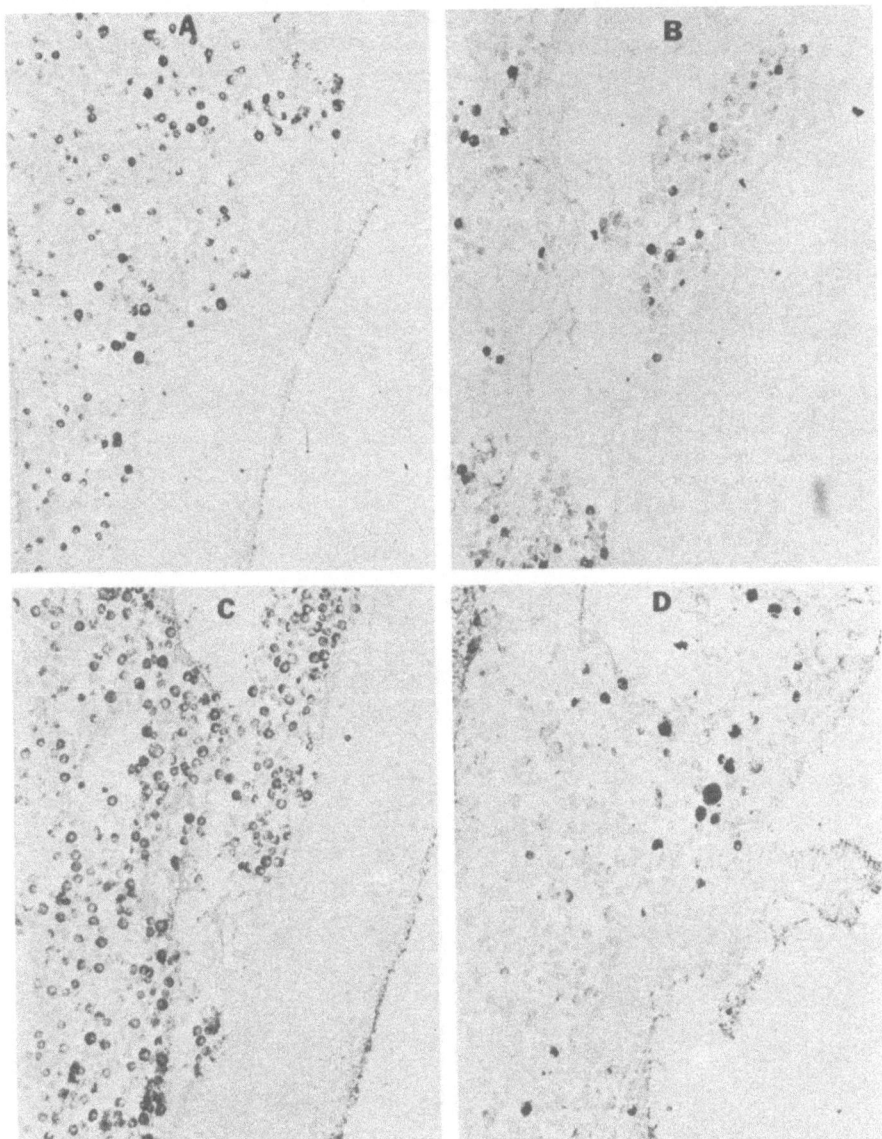

Figure 7.   Immunocytochemical   appearance   of   rat   pituitary
cells implanted into hypophysectomized rats and recovered 7
days later.   All pituitary cell types are present and are
similar in size and staining intensity to zero time controls
(Fig. 6).   (A) ACTH, (B) PRL, (C) GH, (D) LH.

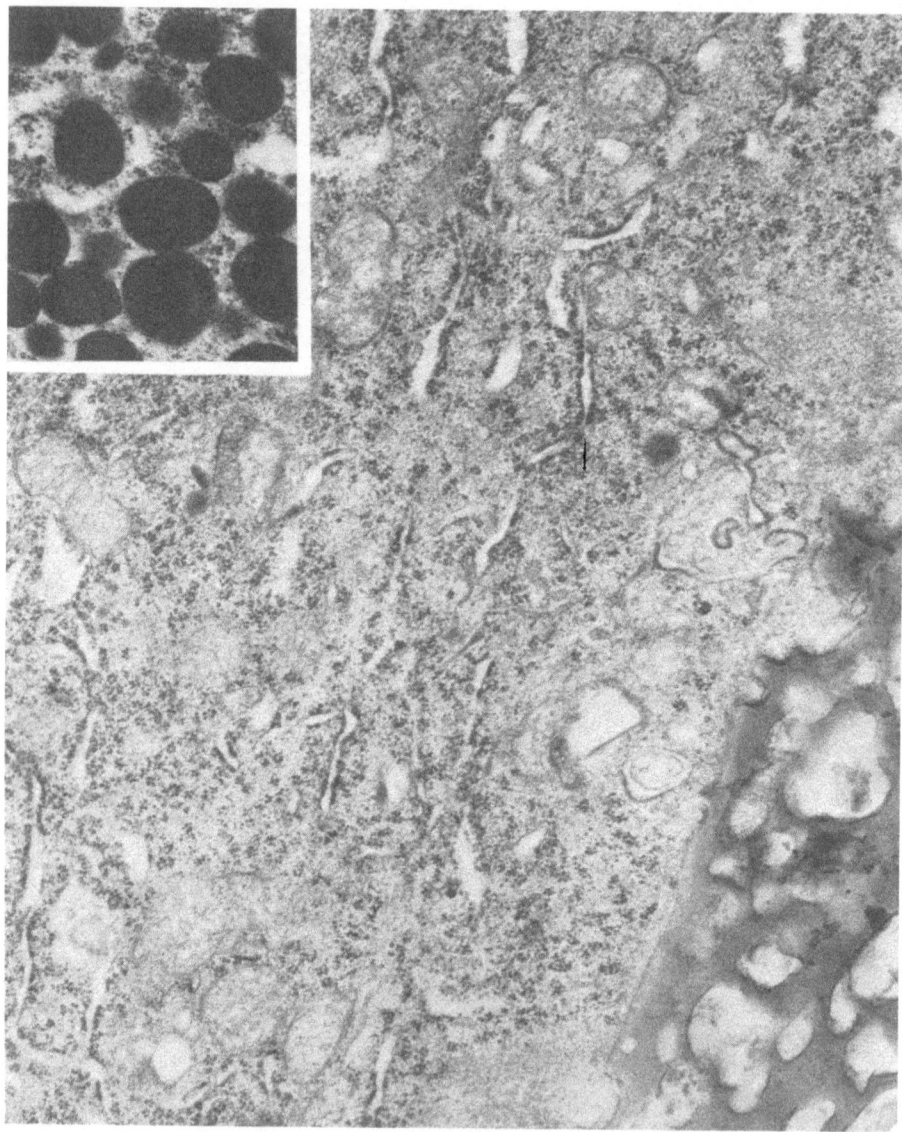

Figure 8. Transmission electron micrograph of a portion of a cell which has been implanted using the hollow fiber technology (8 days post implantation). Intracellular organelles are well preserved, implying cell viability. <u>Insert</u>: PRL secretion granules. Porous material in corner of micrograph is capsule matrix.

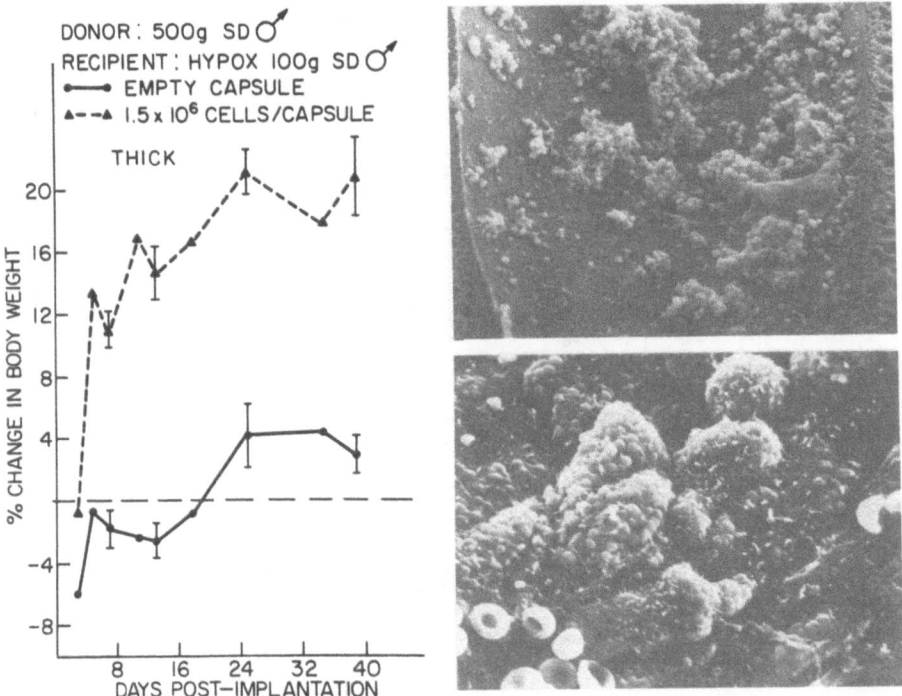

Figure 9. Left. Weight gain response of hypox animals receiving cell-filled or vehicle-filled capsules intracranially (n = 10/group). Top right: SEM of capsule removed from experimental group 7 days post implantation (× 250). Bottom right: Surface of cells showing features of exocytosis (× 2400).

SIF synthesis and release. Eventually then, the somatotrophs would come under regulation by SIF and the recipients would stop growing.

3.2.   Donor: Rat, Bovine Pituitary Cells

        Recipient: Intact Rats

3.2.1. Rationale

        In marked contrast to hypophysectomized rats, intact rats receiving pituitary cells in the brain ventricles exhibit

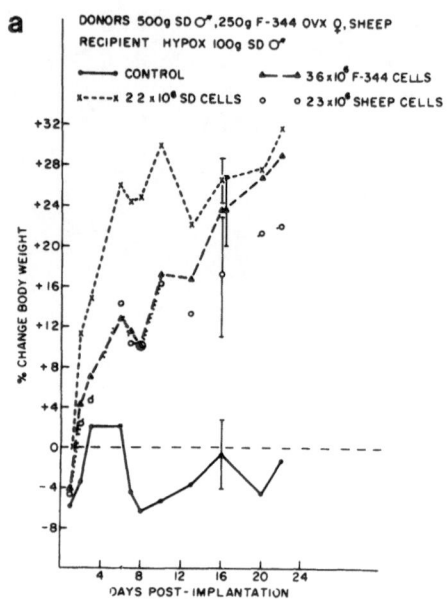

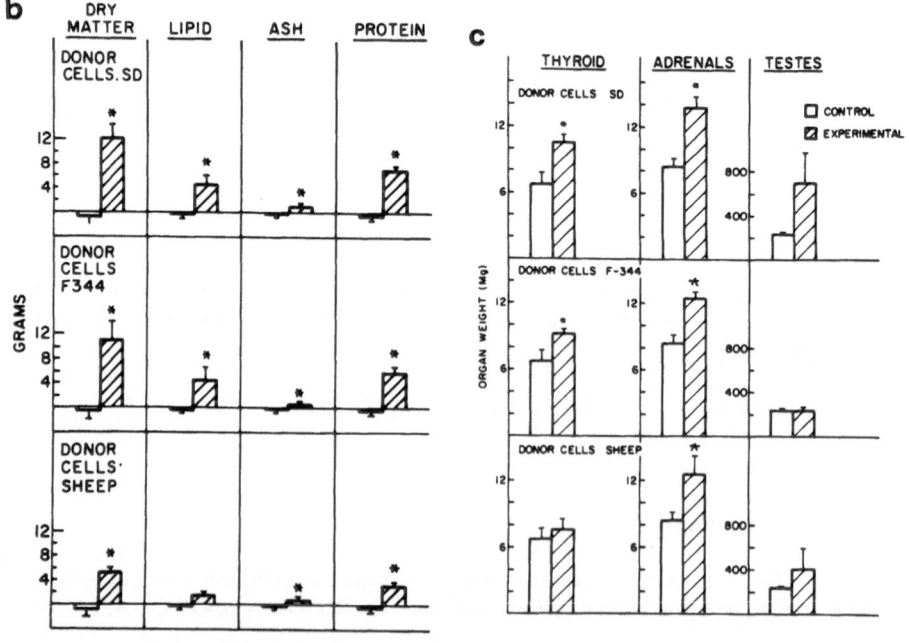

significantly suppressed growth as early as 12 days post-implantation (Kelsey et al., 1981). In this experimental paradigm, growth suppression is probably mediated via the host pituitary. Thus, pituitaries from the cell implanted group weigh 25 - 46% less than those from the vehicle-injected group, have 30 - 40% less protein; and contain 50 - 70% less growth hormone and 22 - 47% less prolactin. With the hollow fiber technology, we were interested to find out if growth suppression could be induced by the encapsulated cells. Finally, we were interested to find out what would happen when allogeneic pituitary cells were used.

3.2.2. Materials and Methods

Rat pituitary glands were dissociated into single cells, loaded into hollow fibers, and implanted intracranially according to the procedures described in section 2. Bovine pituitary tissue, obtained within 30 min after the animal was killed, was dissociated in medium containing collagenase I (Sigma; 0.3%) plus 0.1% BSA and antibiotics by periodic agitation of the tissue at 37°C for a total of two hours. Cell viability was > 90%. Recipients were 34 - 45 day old male and female rats of the Sprague Dawley (SD) and Fischer 344 (F-344) strain.

3.2.3. Results and Discussion

Consistent with our previous study (Kelsey et al., 1981), encapsulated rat pituitary cells suppressed growth of the intact recipient by 10 - 15% up to four weeks post-implantation (Fig. 12A). On the other hand, encapsulated bovine pituitary cells actually stimulated weight gain by 5 - 10% in the same experiment. The differential response

---

Figure 10.   (A) Growth responses obtained from hollow fibers containing syngeneic (Sprague-Dawley, Fischer 344) rat or allogeneic (sheep) pituitary cells. Each group caused significantly more growth than controls (empty fibers), but within group comparisons showed no significant differences. (B) Body composition analyses of carcasses in experiment represented in panel A. * = p < .05. (C) Weights of endocrine glands in experiment represented by panel A.

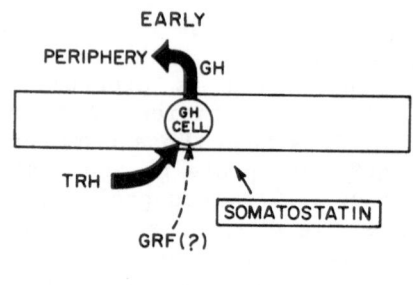

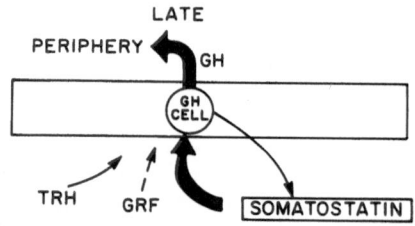

Figure 11. Model to explain GH release from the encapsulated
and implanted somatotroph. In this model, the somatotroph
is under positive control of TRH (or GRF) early after
implantation while later, GH secretion is controlled by
somatostatin.

induced by the encapsulated rat and bovine pituitary cells
in terms of weight gain was also reflected in a second experiment in which the recipient animal was a F-344 female rat
(Fig. 12B). As before, rat pituitary cells suppressed weight
gain of the F-344 recipients. In this case, suppression was
related to cell dose. On the other hand, implantation of
bovine cells slightly stimulated weight gain, but this gain
was not dependent upon cell dose (Fig. 12B, bottom). The
animals represented by the growth curves in Fig. 12B were
analyzed, at autopsy, for endocrine weight changes. As seen
by the data in Fig. 12C, pituitary glands from animals receiving rat pituitary cells were significantly smaller than
controls, whereas pituitaries from the bovine cell implanted
group was significantly increased. A similar profile was
seen in the adrenal glands where suppression was found with
the rat pituitary cell implants, while stimulation was seen
with the bovine group.

What is the mechanism(s) by which this interesting result might be explained? In the case of the rat - rat system, growth hormone released from the implants could act (1) either at the level of the somatostatin-producing neurons in positive fashion or (2) directly at the level of the pituitary somato-troph. In either case, the end result would be suppression of somatotrophs in the host pituitary. In the case of the rat-bovine system, however, we would suggest that the bovine growth hormone molecule is not recognized at the level of either the host pituitary and/or somatostatin neuron. It will be interesting to characterize the pituitary of the host in this case to determine if somatotroph function is actually increased.

3.3. Donor: Mouse Pituitary Cells

Recipient: Snell (dw/dw) and Ames (df/df) Female Mice

3.3.1. Rationale

The dwarf mutation in mice, originally described by Snell in 1929, results in adults which rarely exceed 1/3 the body weight of their normal littermates. Pituitaries of these animals lack somatotrophs and quantifiable GH as determined by bioassay, RIA, or electrophoresis (Bartke, 1979). Recent studies however, indicate that the GH gene is probably still present in these glands (Phillips et al., 1982). That the growth lesion therefore probably involves control of GH gene expression can be inferred from the results of other studies which clearly show that animal growth can be reinitiated after GH injections or transplantation of pitui-tary tissue (Bartke, 1979; Carsner and Reynolds, 1960). The purpose of the experiment described in this section was to find out if intracranial implantation of encapsulated mouse pituitary cells could restore growth of the dwarf mouse (see Hymer et al., 1981b for additional details).

3.3.2. Materials and Methods

Thin XM-50 hollow fibers, 6 mm in length, were loaded with 1.5 µl of pituitary cell suspension (~ 400,000 cells/capsule) prepared from normal ICR-derived outbred mice. Recipients were either Snell (dw/dw) or Ames (df/df) female mice 1 - 5 months old. Implantation procedures were exactly as described previously.

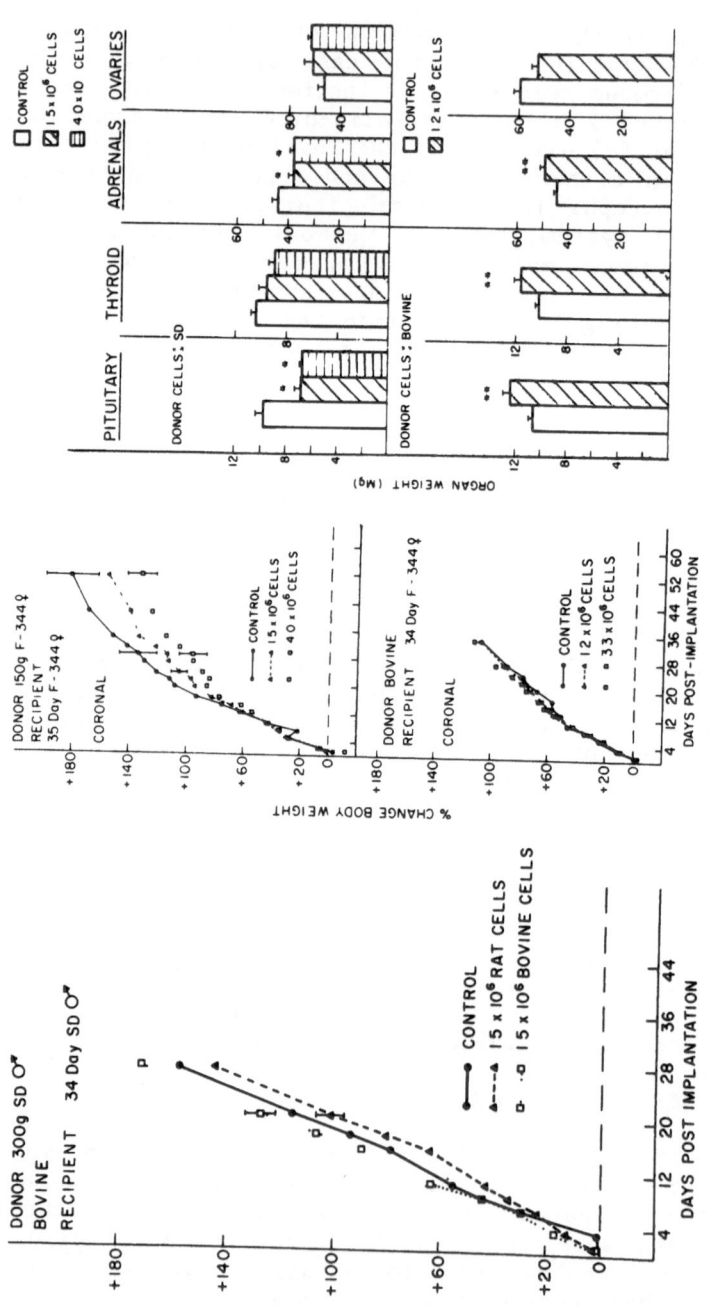

3.3.3. Results and Discussion

Animals receiving cell-filled capsules showed an average weight gain of 125% 110 days post-implantation (Fig. 13, p < 0.001). A majority of the experimental animals exhibited centripetal deposition of adipose tissue as well as loss of abdominal muscle tone and body hair. The percentage of lipid in the carcass of the experimental animal was $26.7 \pm 3.3\%$ vs $11.7 \pm 0.3\%$ for controls (p < .01). Long bone lengths, as well as organ weights (liver, kidneys, heart) were all significantly greater in the experimental group. This result suggested that growth hormone and ACTH cells were probably both functioning in the hollow fiber. (In other studies we had shown that 1 mg of corticosterone injected three times a week for 54 days resulted in a significant weight gain due to obesity as well as hair loss.) We were particularly interested to try thyroxine (T_4) supplementation in this pituitary hollow fiber model since (a) growth responses of dwarf mice injected with T_4 + GH is greater than that observed with either hormone alone (Bartke, 1965; Lister, 1977) and (b) T_4 stimulates fat mobilization (Turakulov et al., 1975). Injection of T_4 (3.5 µg/injection - 3 ×/week) was found to markedly enhance the growth response of the pituitary-implanted animals (Fig. 14). In marked contrast to the mice in Fig. 13, T_4 injection prevented hair loss and obesity. These results obviously document function of mouse somatotrophs in the hollow fiber configuration.

4.   Prolactin Function Using Hollow Fiber Technology

4.1.   Donor: Rat Pituitary Cells

Recipient: Intact Rats/Ovariectomized Rats

4.1.1. Rationale

The obvious marker to demonstrate GH cell function in

Figure 12. Left panel. Growth responses of normal, intact 34 day old Sprague-Dawley male rats implanted with either syngeneic (rat) or allogeneic (cow) pituitary cells. Middle panel. Growth responses of normal, intact 34 day old Fischer 344 female rats implanted with syngeneic (rat) or allogeneic (cow) pituitary cells. Right panel. Endocrine gland weights of Sprague-Dawley intact recipient female's receiving encapsulated syngeneic (rat) or allogeneic (cow) pituitary cells 28 days post implantation. * = p < .01.

hollow fibers in vivo is animal growth (discussed in section 3). The marker to demonstrate PRL cell function is less obvious. Since end points such as mammary gland responses may not possess the sensitivity required to demonstrate mammotroph function in vivo, we have used a more indirect approach; viz. testing of the hollow fiber in vitro after its removal from the animal.

4.1.2. Materials and Methods

Donor rats were 50-60 day old female Fischer 344 (F-344) rats. In some cases they were ovariectomized 7 - 10 days prior to use; in others they were implanted subcutaneously

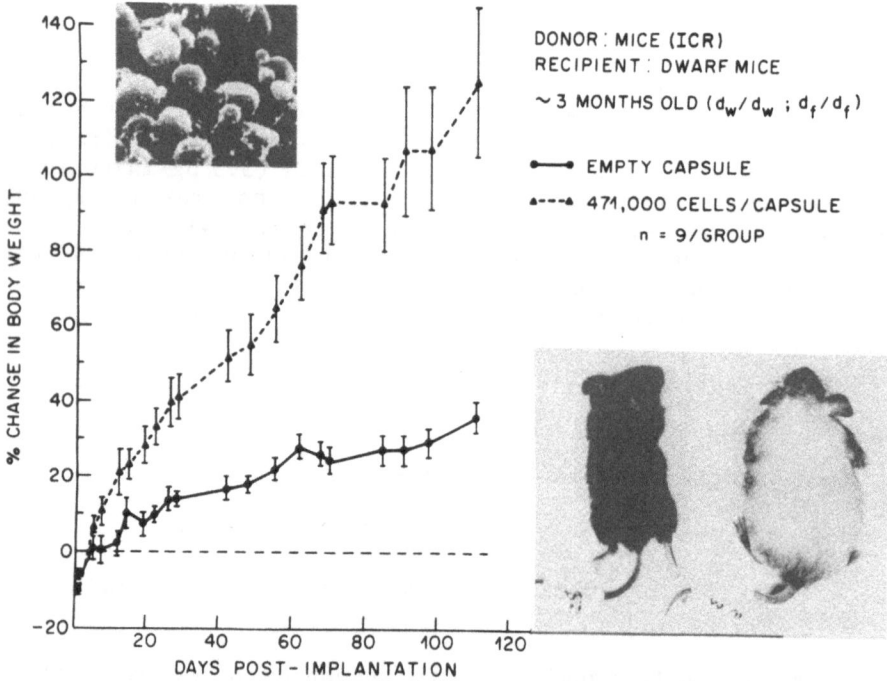

Figure 13. Weight gain response of dwarf mice implanted with empty or cell-filled capsules. Inserts: appearance of control and experimental animal 110 days post implantation. Scanning electron micrograph of cells in fiber taken from animal 110 days post implantation.

with a single silastic capsule containing 7 mg of DES. The number of pituitary cells/capsule ranged 150,000 to 250,000, depending upon the experiment. Recipients were also F-344 female rats of the same age range. Implantation sites were usually intracranial; occasionally they were in the leg ("triad") region where the capsule lies next to the femoral artery and vein. In some cases the recipients were ovariect-omized and treated with estrogen (see text).

Capsules removed from the animals were cultured in medium containing MEM + 20% horse serum as described previously (Wilfinger et al., 1979). In some cases capsules were placed in a 2.0 cm^3 microchomatography column (Biorad, Inc.) and

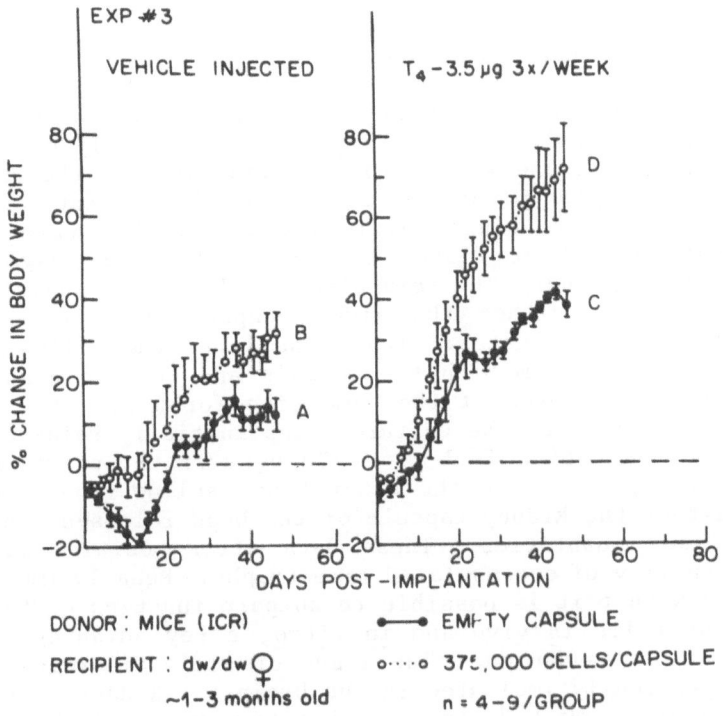

Figure 14. Weight gain responses of dwarf mice implanted with mouse pituitary fiber units. A = group A, empty capsule-alkaline saline injected; B = group B, cell capsules-alkaline-saline injected; C = group C, empty capsules-T$_4$ injected; D = group D, cell capsules-T$_4$ injected.

perfused at a flow rate of 0.5 ml/min with M199 + 0.1% BSA + 25 mM Hepes, pH 7.4. PRL released into the medium was assayed either by standard RIA or by the NB-2 lymphoma bioassay procedure (Tanaka et al., 1980).

In one experiment, cells from ovariectomized rats were encapsulated (250,000/capsule) and either implanted (head, triad) into F-344 female rats or placed in culture. One half of the experimental groups received E_2 (20 µg/day/4 days) in vivo or 1 ng/ml of culture medium. After four days the capsules were sliced open and boiled in sample gel electrophoresis buffer containing 2% SDS for 5 min. Electrophoresis of the protein extract was then done in 12.5% SDS gels under reducing conditions (Mittra, 1980).

4.1.3. Results and Discussion

We were interested to compare the in vitro release of PRL from encapsulated pituitary cells previously maintained in culture vs those which had been implanted in the rat. To do this, 150,000 pituitary cells were loaded into each of 18 hollow fibers using sterile technique. Six were placed in individual 35 mm dishes and cultured for 14 days using standard technique. The remaining 12 fibers were individually implanted into either the kidney capsule (n = 6) or head (n = 6) of littermates. Two weeks later the hollow fibers were recovered from both the animals and culture dishes and all fibers perifused at the same time for 6 hr. As seen in Fig. 15, cells from the culture group initially released high levels of PRL which fell to ~ 250 ng over the course of the perifusion period. On the other hand, hollow fibers removed from either the kidney capsule or the head released considerably lower quantities. These data offer positive evidence for viability of encapsulated mammotrophs. Equally important, they show that it is possible to compare function of the same group of cells in vivo and in vitro, a key advantage to the hollow fiber technique. The issue of prolactin release from cells previously implanted in the brain vs. kidney is reasonably complex. We had expected that kidney capsule site would favor hyperprolactinemic cells. Why it did not (relative to the intracranial site) requires further study.

The pituitary gland is a well known target for estrogenic hormones both in terms of prolactin cell hypertrophy/hyperplasia as well as prolactin synthesis/secretion. Since

prolactin release from encapsulated cells implanted intracranially is low (Fig. 15), we wondered if exogenously
administered estrogen might not activate such cells; i.e.,
would the target cells still respond in this ecotropic site?
Several protocols were tried. In one, pituitary cells from
ovariectomized (7 days) female rats were encapsulated and
implanted into ovariectomized littermate recipients. At the
time of implantation the recipients were also injected subcutaneously with a single injection of 500 μg polyesterdiol
phosphate (a long-acting estrogen) or vehicle. In three
separate experiments, fibers were removed from the rats
at 5, 7 and 12 days post-implantation followed by prolactin
release measurements over a 9 day culture period. In two
of three experiments, the results showed that the encapsulated
cells had responded to the estrogen (Fig. 16). However, 12
days post-implantation of the effect had dissipated. In a
similar experiment, we also compared the response of the in
situ pituitaries of the control and experimental groups, en-
capsulating them in hollow fibers, and finally culturing under

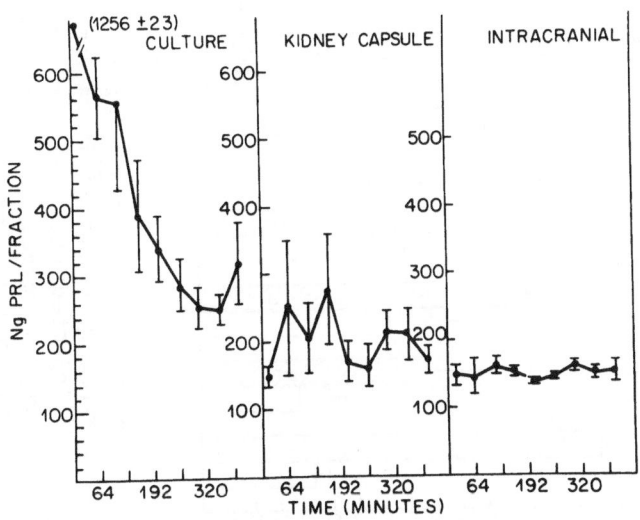

Figure 15. Kinetics of in vitro PRL release from encapsulated rat pituitary cells previously in culture or implanted
in the kidney capsule or intracranially for 14 days. Cells
(150,000/capsule) were implanted into intact F-344 female
rats. See text for additional details.

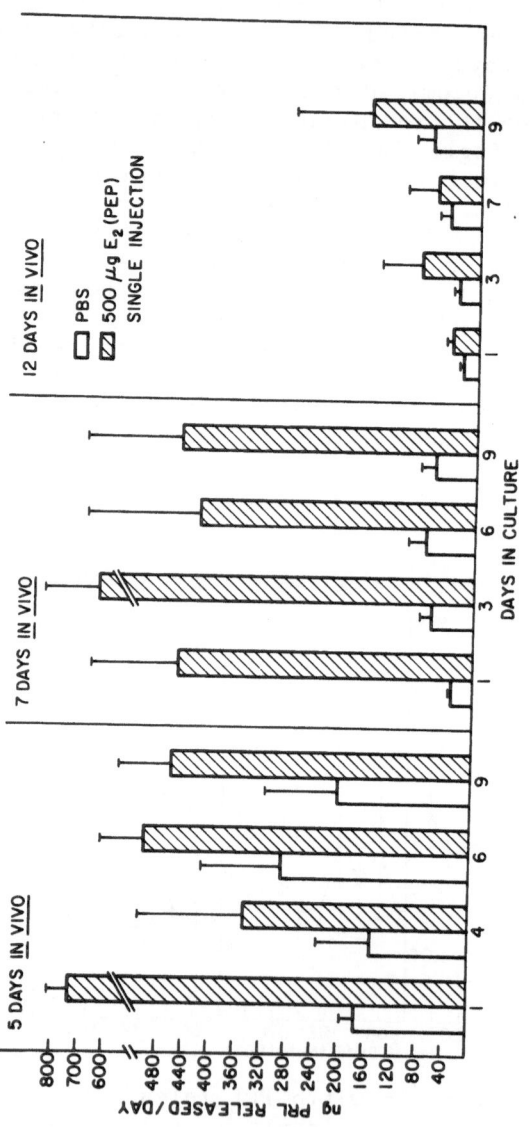

Figure 16. In vitro release of PRL from pituitary cells previously implanted intracranially into ovariectomized rats and injected one time with polyestradiol phosphate, a long acting estrogen. Data represent total PRL secreted into culture medium over a 9 day period.

conditions identical to the ectopic cells. Cell concentrations in capsules from the ectopic and in situ sites were the same. The results showed (a) that the ectopic cells again responded to the estrogen, (b) that the in situ cells responded to the estrogen and (c) that the estrogen effect was maintained over the 9 day culture period in the case of the ectopic, but not the in situ cells. In summary, these data document that prolactin cells, encapsulated in hollow fibers, live and respond to stimulatory molecules in vivo.

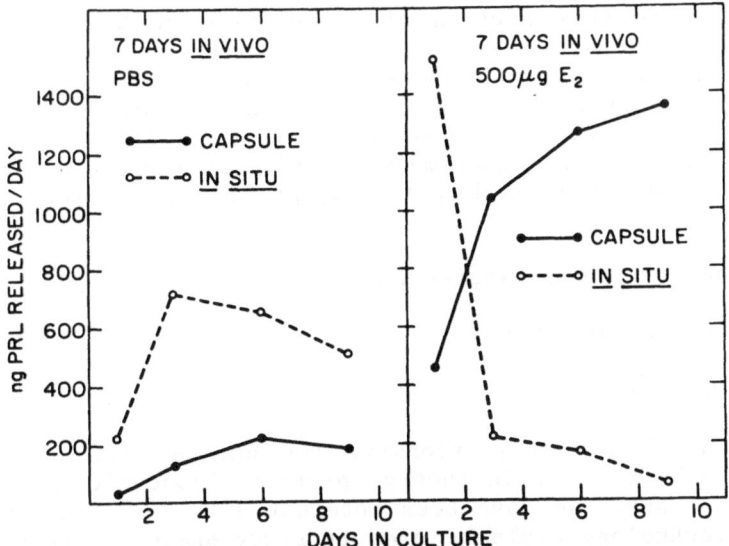

Figure 17. In vitro release of PRL from pituitary cells encapsulated and subsequently implanted into ovariectomized rats for one week. One group received a single injection of E_2 (right panel) whereas the other received vehicle (left panel). Subsequent PRL release in vitro from the E_2 treated group was significantly higher than corresponding control (closed circles). At the end of the 7 day post implantation period, the in situ pituitary glands were dissociated and numbers equal to those originally implanted were encapsulated in hollow fibers prior to culture. In this case, signs of E_2 stimulation were apparent early, but not late, in the culture period (open circles).

In a preliminary experiment, we have compared gel electrophoresis profiles of proteins contained in encapsulated cells implanted in vivo vs those cultured in vitro. While the profiles show general overall similarities, important differences are apparent (Fig. 18). For example, several protein species in the PRL cleavage area of 16.1 - 17.2 K are present in cells maintained in vivo, but not in vitro. Furthermore, a 14.1 K species dominates in cells recovered from the head. Whether these proteins are newly synthesized is an area of current investigation. These results point out the advantages of using the hollow fiber technology in the study of processing of the PRL molecule (Mittra, 1980).

The results of the numerous experimental approaches described in this section offer positive evidence that rat pituitary prolactin cells function after encapsulation in hollow fibers. The hollow fiber technique uniquely permits comparisons of prolactin cell function in vivo vs in vitro. Our ongoing research is directed toward this later goal in an effort to sort out experimental artifacts induced by current methodologies employed in pituitary prolactin research.

4.2.   Donor: Human Pituitary Cells

Recipient: Rats

4.2.1. Rationale

As discussed previously, the unique construction of hollow fibers will, in theory, protect allogeneic cells from immune attack. We have been interested to see if the hollow fiber technology could be used to study human pituitary cell function in the rat. Prior to the advent of a specific radio-immunoassay for prolactin, a significant percentage of human pituitary tumors were considered to be non-functional. However, with the ability to reliably measure hormone in serum, it has been estimated that 40% of all human pituitary tumors are indeed prolactinomas and are therefore the most common pituitary tumors currently recognized in man (Faglia et al., 1980). Meaningful questions relating to the physiology, cell biology and biochemistry of this tumor tissue could be asked if it were possible to keep human pituitary tumor cells alive in the rat. Our efforts in this direction must still be considered highly preliminary; yet the results to date do

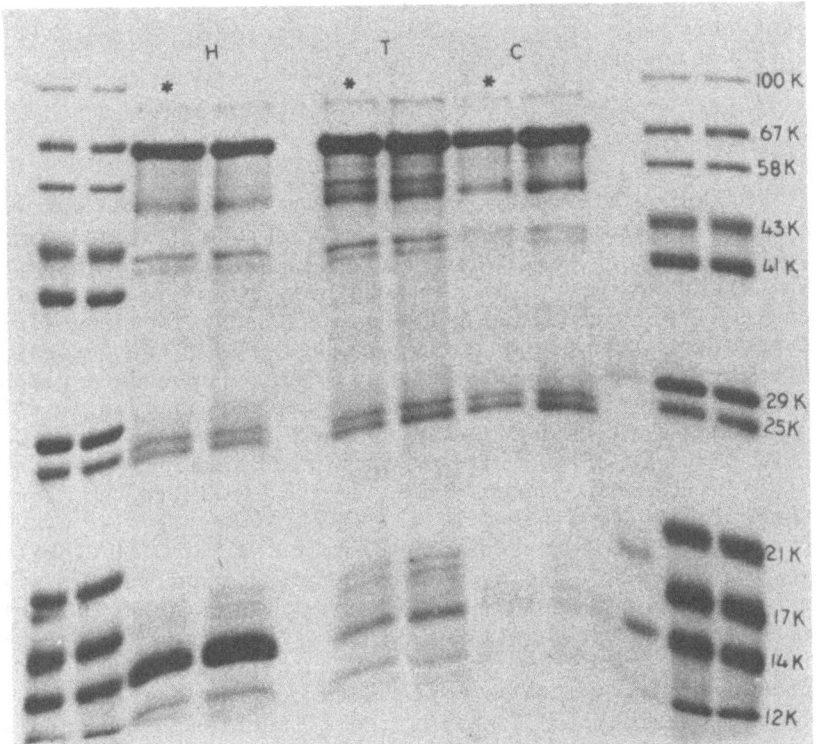

Figure 18. Gel electrophoresis profiles of proteins extracted from pituitary cells which have been encapsulated and either implanted (F-344 female rats) or maintained in culture. Cells (250,000/capsule) were implanted either in the head (H), tirad (T), or cultured (C) in αMEM + 20% horse serum for 4 days. Rats were given 20 µg of E_2/day/4 days (*) or oil vehicle (no mark). Cultures contained either E_2 at 1 ng/ml (*) or vehicle (no mark). Electrophoresis in 12.5% SDS gels under reducing conditions (Mittra, 1980). Mol. wt. standards (2 left lanes and 2 right lanes) are phosphorylase (100 K), BSA (67 K), catalase (58 K), ovalbumin (43 K), alcohol dehydrogenase (41 K), carbonic anhydrase (29 K), chymotrypsinogen (25 K), soybean trypsin inhibitor (21 K), myglobin (17 K), ribonuclease A (14 K), and cytochrome c (12 K). Third lane from right are radiolabeled mol. wt. marker proteins.

suggest this may represent a feasible approach. Some of these results are now briefly summarized.

4.2.2. Materials and Methods

Human pituitary tissue removed at surgery was cut into ~ 2 mm^3 fragments and shipped at ambient temperature to University Park in sterile M199 containing 5% horse serum and antibiotics. During shipment (< 24 hr), tumor cells are often liberated from the tissue pieces into the surrounding fluid. Contaminating red blood cells in this fluid can be easily removed by a simple one-step centrifugation procedure through Ficoll-Hypaque. The tissue can be dispersed into single cells by incubation in M199 containing 0.3% collagenase and 0.5% BSA for 1 hr at 37°C. After this period, exhaustive washing of the pieces in enzyme-free medium followed by gentle mechanical dispersion with a Pasteur pipette is usually sufficient to liberate additional tumor cells. Cell viability ranges 70 - 90%. Yields vary depending upon sample size; however it is not uncommon to harvest 30 - 40 × 10^6 cells from 50 mg of tissue (i.e., total yield from tissue plus medium). The encapsulation and implantation of hollow fibers containing human pituitary tumor cells is done exactly as described previously. To assess cell function, human prolactin is measured in rat serum by a specific and sensitive hPRL radioimmunoassay. In certain experiments, cells were recovered from the capsules; deposited onto microscope slides with a Cytospin; and evaluated for DNA content by microdensitometry.

4.2.3. Results and Discussion

In our experiments to date, most of the recipient animals have been Fischer 344 female rats ~ 50 days of age. Blood samples from 95 rats bearing empty hollow fibers (head) yield an average value of 5.1 ± 0.3 ng "hPRL"/ml rat serum when measured by radioimmunoassay using the reagents for the hPRL kit. This represents the amount of material in rat serum which cross reacts with the hPRL antibody.

In three separate experiments we have addressed the issue of implant site on subsequent cell function (Fig. 19). In one experiment, cells placed intracranially released more hormone into the blood than equivalent numbers implanted subcutaneously. In this case, hPRL was detected in the rat blood 100 days post-implantation (Fig. 19A). In a second experiment (Fig. 19B) cells in the subcutaneous site released hPRL in approximately linear fashion into rat blood for 32 days after post-implantation, whereas equal numbers in the head apparently released little hormone. Finally, the results of the third experiment (Fig. 19C) suggest that implant site made little difference on the experimental outcome.

While these data are consistent with the conclusion that human prolactin cells can release hormone into the bloodstream of the recipient host, it is impossible to generalize about an optimum implant site. It seems likely that each tissue sample will have its own peculiar characteristics that will, in turn, account for a good deal of this variability. For example, one might argue that the tissue in the first experiment (Fig. 19A) was not under dopaminergic control, whereas that of the second (Fig. 19B) was.

The data in Fig. 20 document that release of hPRL from fibers implanted intracranially is also variable. Note that in the first four experiments (panels, Fig. 20), hormone release tends to have a positive slope, in the next it is negative and in the final four, levels of hPRL are no different than the preimplantation values. What accounts for this variable release pattern? It seems likely that tissue variation, being absolute, is probably the major contributor. Since recipients are all of one strain, sex, and defined age (50 - 60 days), variation induced by this component should be minimal. Capsule placement could also account for some experimental variability, but the reader will recall that we had shown previously that common ventricular lesions were produced in 95% of a large number of brains examined.

It is obvious that the issue of human pituitary cell survival within the hollow fiber in vivo is critical to data interpretation. In a few of the experiments represented in Fig. 20 this has, in fact, been done. An example of cell quality after tissue dissociation (63 yr female, serum PRL = 156ng/ml) is given in Fig. 21A and B. These cells were encapsulated in hollow fibers, but not implanted. The cells are well preserved (H & E, Fig. 21A) and occasional PRL cells can be identified in serial sections of this same preparation by immunocytochemistry (Fig. 21B). An example of cell quality

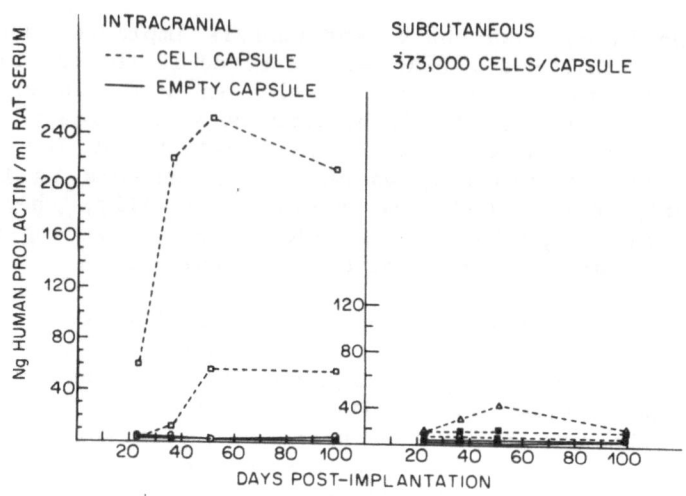

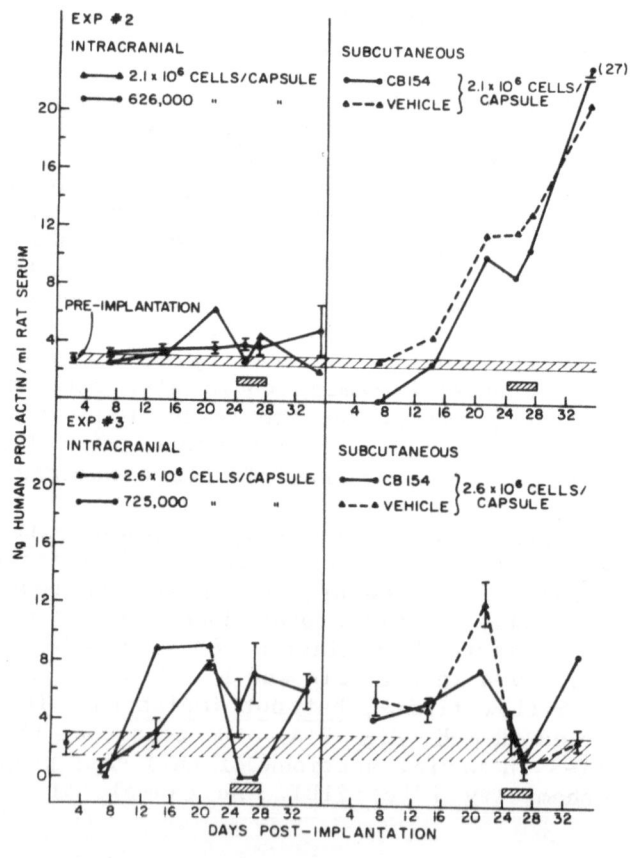

after tissue dissociation from another patient (24 yr female, serum PRL = 738 ng/ml) is given in Fig. 21C and Fig. 21D. In this case the cells were encapsulated in hollow fibers and implanted into the brains of F-344 female rats. The presence of viable cells seven days post-implantation (H & E, Fig. 21C) are obvious. Note that after this relatively short implantation time the cells are largely single. Also note the presence of inflammatory cells in the capsule walls. Recall that the pituitary cells are protected from these inflammatory cells by virtue of the membrane lining the fiber lumen. That some of the cells in this preparation contain prolactin is shown in Fig. 21D. Approximately one third of the cells are mammotrophs. It is interesting that they tend to be concentrated along one edge of the fiber lumen. In this latter case, we were unable to detect hPRL in the rat serum (Fig. 20, 6th panel), yet viable, hormone containing cells are obviously present in the fiber (Fig. 21D). One can speculate that cells in this case come under dopaminergic control of the brain.

We have been able to compare the morphology of human pituitary cells before they are implanted with those after implantation in two additional experiments. In the first case (30 yr female, 536 ng/ml), cells which were encapsulated but not implanted showed good viability (Fig. 22A) and some prolactin cells when stained immunocytochemically (Fig. 22B). However, 35 days post-implantation, many of the cells appear necrotic (Fig. 22C) and relatively few show the presence of immunoreactive prolactin in their cytoplasm (Fig. 22D). The secretion data from these same cells (Fig. 20, panel 1) offer

---

Figure 19. Release of human PRL into rat serum from encapsulated and implanted human prolactinoma cells. In experiment 1 (top), cells from a 33 yr male with serum PRL > 5,000 ng/ml were implanted into 60 day old SD male rats. Some rats received empty fibers (o——o). Note that cells implanted intracranially released more hormone than those implanted subcutaneously. In experiment 2 (middle), cells from a 39 yr female with serum PRL 286 ng/ml were implanted into F-344 female rats (50 days old). In this case, PRL release was greater from the subcutaneous site. Hatched line indicates level of "hPRL" reacting material in preimplantation rat serum. Small hatched bar at days 24 - 28 indicate treatment period with CB-154. In experiment 3 (bottom) cells from a 63 yr female with serum PRL 156 ng/ml were implanted into F-344 female rats (50 days old).

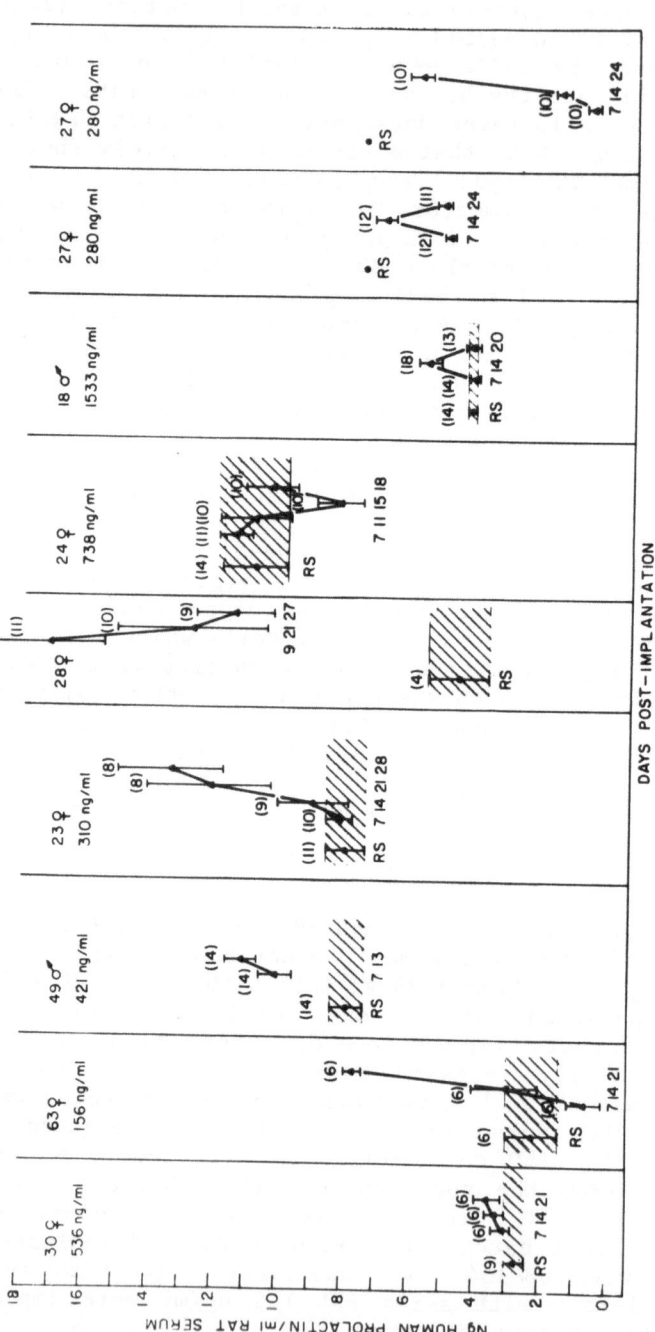

little evidence for cell function. Taken together, the negative secretion data for this experiment could easily be accounted for by cell death. In the second experiment (23 yr female, 310 ng/ml) cells which were encapsulated but not implanted showed good viability (Fig. 23A) as well as immuno-reactivity in several cases (Fig. 23B). However, after 66 days in the rat's head, the cells were obviously viable (Fig. 23C). They had aggregated along fibrous cords and their histology was not unlike human pituitary tissue. The cells in this preparation were also larger than those contained in the initial starting material. The secretion data (Fig. 20, panel 4) from these cells tend to support the idea that the fibers in this experiment contained viable, functioning cells. However, by 45 days post-implantation hPRL levels had returned to baseline in this experiment (data not shown in Fig. 20).

In summary, these morphological findings show that viable, hormone containing human prolactin cells are present in hollow fibers 8 (Fig. 21) and 66 (Fig. 23) days post-implantation. They also suggest that the variability in secretion data (Fig. 20) can probably be accounted for, at least in part, by cell death (Fig. 22). Obviously more extensive work is required before definitive conclusions can be drawn.

In a few experiments, we also have attempted to determine the extent of cell division in the encapsulated and implanted human pituitary cells. Measurements of individual cellular DNA contents were made on cells prepared from acutely dissociated pituitary tissue ("START" samples) and on cells recovered from capsules (~ 100,000 cells each) which had been maintained for 1 to 22 days in vitro (in αMEM containing 20% horse serum) or in vivo (implanted intracranially). Cells were deposited on microscope slides using a cytocentrifuge, fixed overnight at 4°C in formaldehyde fumes, and processed for the Feulgen reaction, specific for DNA, using a 50 minute hydrolysis (5 N HCl at 20°C) period. DNA content/cell was determined using a scanning integrating microdensitometer (Vickers M85),

←───

Figure 20. Release of hPRL from human pituitary cells encapsulated and implanted intracranially into F-344 female rats. Hatched bar represents cross-reacting material in rat serum prior to implantation. Patient information given at top of each panel.

with light source set at 570 nm. Three hundred cells per slide were measured, when cell recovery was adequate. Percentages of cells in S + G$_2$ phases were determined as those having DNA contents greater than two standard deviations greater than the mean; i.e., S + G$_2$ estimates are conservative. The results from five such experiments plus average "start" values from five post-mortem samples, are given in Table 1. Generally, the high DNA synthetic rates encountered among "start" samples from surgical samples was not maintained in culture, either in vitro or in vivo: synthesis did continue however, at levels approximating or exceeding average post

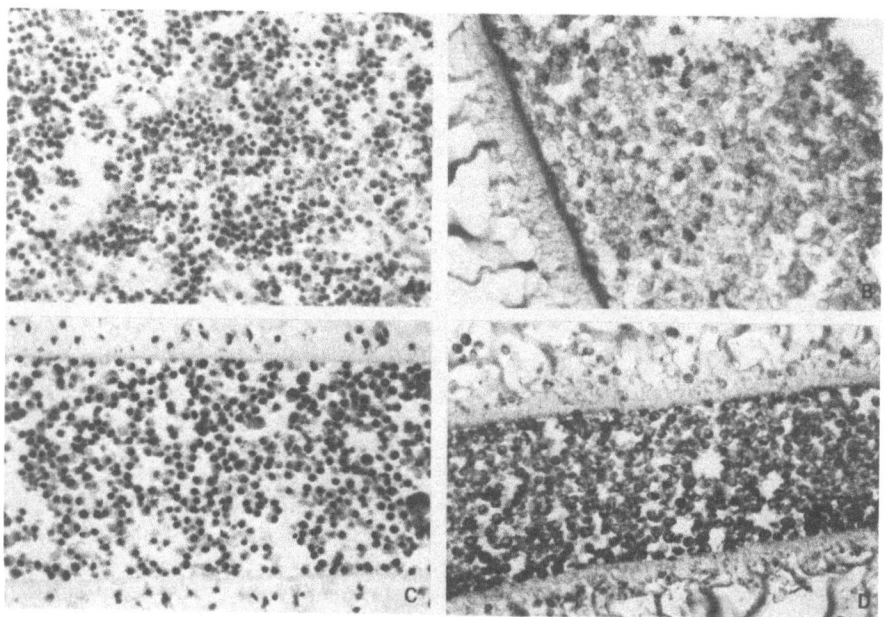

Figure 21. Morphology of human pituitary cells pre- and post-implantation. (A) Encapsulated cells from 63 yr female, serum PRL = 156 ng/ml stained by H & E. (B) Same sample as panel A, but stained by immunocytochemistry for PRL. Occasional PRL cells are identified in this specimen. Cells in A and B were not implanted. (C) Encapsulated cells from 24 yr female, serum PRL = 738 ng/ml, 8 days post implantation (H & E). Pituitary cells are well preserved. Note inflammatory cells in capsule wall. (D) Same specimen as in C, but stained by immunochemistry. Many PRL cells are present in this preparation.

Tabel 1.   Nuclear DNA Contents of Dissociated and Encapsulated (XM-50) Human Pituitary Cells _in vitro_ and _in vivo_.

Tissue	% of Cells in Initial cell suspension with > 2 C content[b]	Time in vitro (days)[c]	% > 2 C	Time in vivo (days)	% > 2 C (C) [d]	(E)
Post Mortem:[e]						
67 ♂	17.7	-	-	1	8.7	17.3
				2	6.8	6.4
				6	4.0	-
				22	-	5.7
62 ♂	9.6	-	-	1	31.0	2.0
				5	6.0	2.0
				12	4.5	2.0
Biopsy:						
72 ♂ chromo-phobe adenoma	73.7	-	-	20	30.8	-
68 ♀ breast cancer	18.0	12	8.7	7	2.9	-
		15	9.3			
65 ♂ prostate cancer	12.0	-	-	1	1.0	5.0
				2	4.3	5.0
				5	4.3	6.0
				12	12.0	3.6

[a]Tissue, obtained either at post mortem or surgery (biopsy), was shipped to University Park in sterile M199 containing 5% horse serum and antibiotics. Post mortem interval = < 6 hrs. Tissues were dissociated with collagenase (see text). Cells XM-50 capsule ranged 100,000 - 200,000.

[b]Percentages are given for numbers of cells in a sample having DNA contents > 2 standard deviations from the mean 2 C amount. Numbers of cells measured was 300 in each case.

[c]Capsules maintained in αMEM + 20% horse serum at 37°C in 95% air; 5% CO_2.

[d]Capsules implanted intracranially into intact F-344 ♀ rats (50-60 days old). Animals (E) were injected with 500 µg of estradiol benzoate or (C) control vehicle one time after capsule implantation.

[e]In an additional 5 post-mortem samples, the percentage of cells in the initial suspension with > 2 C content was: 49 ♂, 10.0%; 56 ♂, 9.2%; 59 ♂, 8.0%; 70 ♂, 6.0%; 77 ♂, 5.3%. In some of these cases cells were implanted into rats.

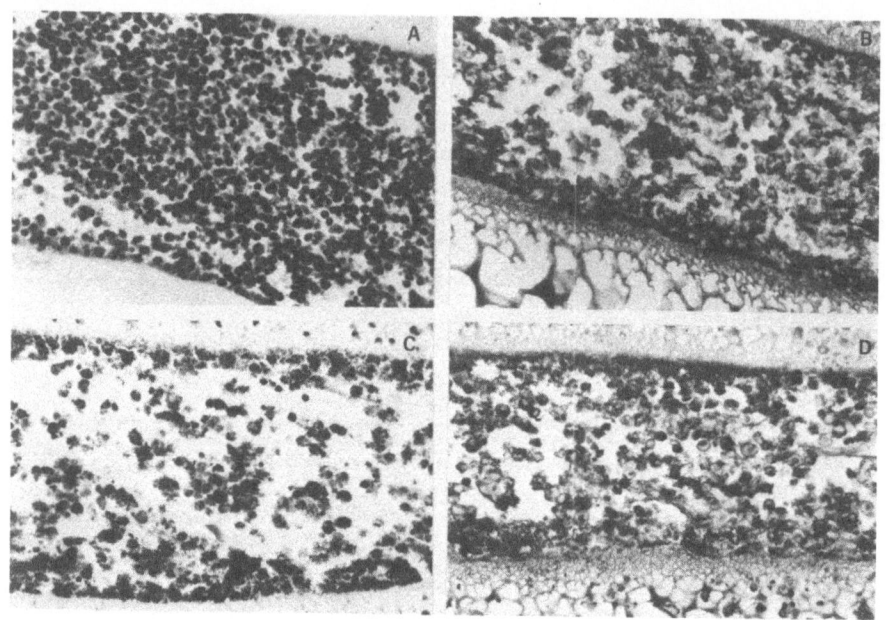

Figure 22. Morphology of human pituitary cells pre (panels A, B) and post (panels C, D) implantation (35 days). Patient = 30 yr female, PRL 536 ng/ml. Cells show good viability (H & E, panel A) with PRL immunoreactivity (panel B) prior to implantation. However, 35 days post implantation cells are necrotic (H & E, panel C), but still appear to contain immunoreactive hormone (panel D).

mortem values. In cases where the recipient rat was treated with estrogen, significantly greater DNA synthesis was usually not encountered. In a single case where initial DNA synthesis was very high (chromophobe adenoma, Table 1) this high mitotic rate was maintained after a long period (20 days) of "in vivo culture." The individual DNA content/-cell is shown in Fig. 24 for this tissue sample. Freshly dispersed cells appear to be mitotically synchronized (Fig. 24A). Although the high mitotic rate in these cells has been maintained after 20 days of intracranial implantation, synchrony appears to have dissipated (Fig. 24B). The higher DNA values in some cells in this latter preparation are also noteworthy. In summary, these data show that some of the human pituitary cells in these preparations divide after

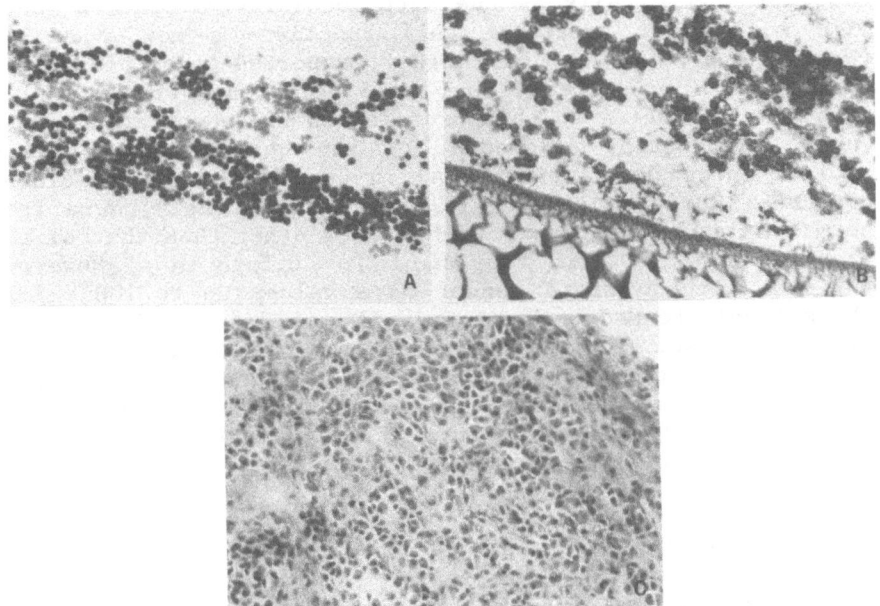

Figure 23. Morphology of human pituitary cells pre (panels A, B) and post (panel C) implantation (66 days). Patient = 23 females, 310 ng PRL/ml. Cells show good viability (H & E, panel A) with PRL immunoreactivity (panel B). After 66 days post implantation, cells have aggregated and appear in cord-like structures reminiscent of the normal gland (panel C).

encapsulation and implantation. The issue of whether or not division is greater in cells from individuals with pituitary tumors than those without obviously requires more work.

5.   Function of Other Types of Cells Using Hollow Fiber
        Technology

5.1.   Donor: Human Prostate Cells

        Recipient: Rats

5.1.1. Rationale

        Positive evidence for the maintenance of human pituitary cells in hollow fibers prompted us to look into other

cell systems for use in transplantation studies. We chose
human prostatic cells as one such model system since a specific marker for prostatic cell function is now available
(Wang et al., 1979). This marker, reported to be present in
normal human prostate tissue, is a 34,000 mol.wt. glycoprotein. An antiserum to this protein has been generated and an
enzyme immunoassay developed for the quantitation of this
antigen (prostatic antigen, PA) in sera of normal and cancer
patients (Kuriyama et al., 1980). Interestingly, sera from
normal males and patients with cancer other than that of the
prostate have similar ranges of PA (0.5 ng/ml). However,
patients with prostate cancer have values up to 100 ng/ml;
these levels tended to be positively correlated with the stage
of the disease. The results presented in this section, while
still in preliminary stage, suggest that human prostate carcinoma cells are sustained in hollow fibers on implantation
in the rat and release PA into the rats bloodstream when it
can be detected by immunoassay.

5.1.2. Materials and Methods

Surgical samples of human prostate tissue were minced
into ~ 1 mm^3 cubes and placed into explant culture. Good cell
outgrowths were obtained from $\sim 80\%$ of the pieces after 14 -
28 days in culture. These cells were harvested by washing in
0.05% trypsin - 0.5 mM EDTA, suspended in serum containing
medium, encapsulated into XM-50 fibers at densities of
100,000 - 200,000 cells/capsule, and implanted into Fischer-
Copenhagen male rats at different sites. At various times
post-implantation the animals were bled to obtain sera for
estimation of PA levels (Kuriyama et al., 1980).

5.1.3. Results and Discussion

Sections through a hollow fiber removed from the brain
of a rat seven days post-implantation show that the dissociated cells have aggregated and reorganized into recognizable
prostatic tissue (Fig. 25). In this case, it is possible to
differentiate ductal epithelium from the stromal component.
Fibers removed from other sites (subcutaneous, intraperitoneal, or testis) ofter revealed prostatic cell aggregates, but
usually not to the extent shown in Fig. 25. In these latter
cases, the cytoplasms were ofter vacuolated. The degree
of inflammatory cell infiltration into the fiber wall
was much greater in capsules removed from the subcutaneous and

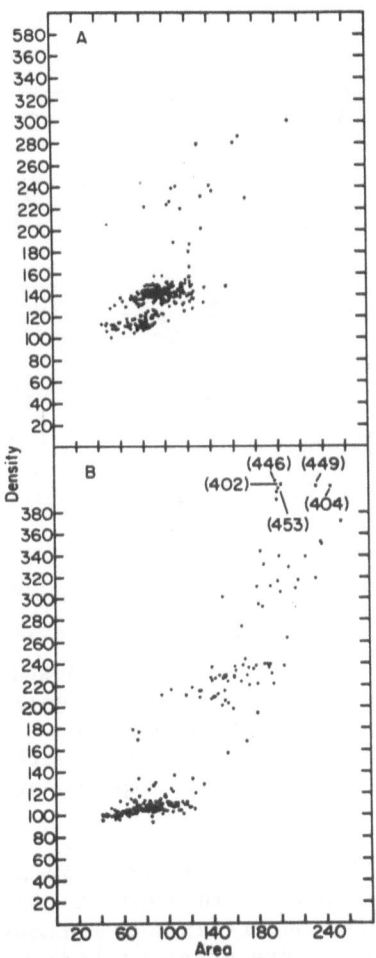

Figure 24. Nuclear DNA contents of cells prepared from a 72 male with chromophobe adenoma pre (panel A) and post (panel B) implantation (20 days). Data represent fuelgen DNA contents/cell (n = 300/sample) as determined using a scanning integrating microdensitometer.

intraperitoneal sites than the intracranial site. While these morphological data would tend to implicate the brain as the preferred implantation site, critical analysis of serially sectioned fibers remains to be done.

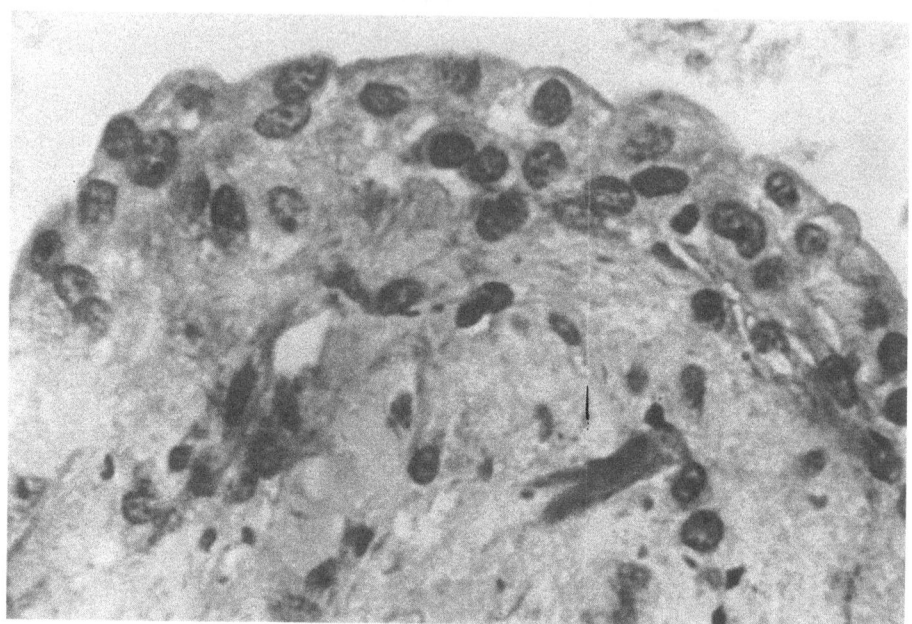

Figure 25. Light micrograph of encapsulated and implanted
(intracranial) human prostatic cancer cells (72 male) - 7 days
post implantation. Cells were implanted into Fischer-Copen-
hagen male rats (intracranial site). Note extensive reorganization into ductal and stromal compartments.

      In another experiment, tissue from a 66 male with pros-
tate carcinoma was placed in explant culture for 11 and 21
days as described in Materials and Methods. Cells harvested
from the culture dish were encapsulated in hollow fibers ($\bar{x}$ =
50,000/fiber) and implanted at various sites in the rat for
1 - 2 weeks. The data in Fig. 26 describe the levels of PA
detected in the recipient sera. Note (a) that the media derived from explants prior to implantation contained low levels
of PA (1 - 8 ng/ml), (b) that levels of PA in the rat serum
tended to rise as the implant interval increased, (c) that
cells prepared from the earlier explant period tended to
release more PA than those from the later period, and finally
(d) that culture of capsules after removal from the rat
reduced release of PA from the encapsulated cells. It is
interesting that there was no obvious correlation between
implant site and serum PA. It is also interesting that the

highest levels detected in this experiment (22 ng/ml) are well within the average reported for cancer patients (25 ng/ml [Kuriyama et al., 1980]). Taken together, these data offer positive evidence for human prostatic cell function in the rat. More experiments are obviously required to validate this system. Its potential for use as a model system to study human prostatic cancer appears considerable.

5.2. Donor: Mouse Fibroblasts

Recipient: Rat

5.2.1. Rationale

In the field of tumor biology, mouse fibroblasts are commonly used to study transformation. We have begun to use these cells in hollow fibers for the purpose of testing their transformation characteristics _in vitro_ after maintenance in the rat for various times.

5.2.2. Materials and Methods

BALB/c (clone A31) or C_3H 10T½ mouse fibroblasts, maintained in culture by standard procedures, were recovered from the culture flask by trypsinization. In most experiments, 100,000 - 200,000 cells/fiber were used. Recipients have been of the F-344 strain (female) with the leg being the most common implant site. In some cases the animals have received estrogen supplementation via silastic capsules containing ~ 8 mg DES subcutaneously. After various implant periods, capsules were removed so that cells could be recovered for subsequent culture _in vitro_. Two methods were used in attempting to recover encapsulated cells. In the first, capsules were cut longitudinally with a sterile scapel. This was done in a hanging drop plate (0.2 ml) with the aid of a dissecting microscope. Cells spilling out from the capsule were then transferred to conventional culture flasks and maintained for several months. In the second method, the hollow fiber was minced into ~ 1 mm slices in a sterile culture dish containing trypsin-EDTA. After 15', serum containing medium was added and cells allowed to grow out from the capsule slice.

5.2.3. Results and Discussion

BALB/c fibroblasts, which are normal (non-transformed) cells, were maintained in the rat for 68 days by the procedures described. Cells removed from the capsule grew and were subsequently cloned. At quiescence, these cells had a labeling index (^{3}H-TdR) of 1.6% vs 1.9% for the parent stock. Karyotypic analysis of these cells showed that they had a mode number of 77 chromosomes, the same number as the parent stock. This later result confirms that the cells recovered from the fiber were indeed mouse cells rather than primary rat cells carried over from the capsule wall. In sum, these results establish that a line of normal mouse cells were maintained in the rat, survived for > 2 months, and retained their "normal" characteristics during this period.

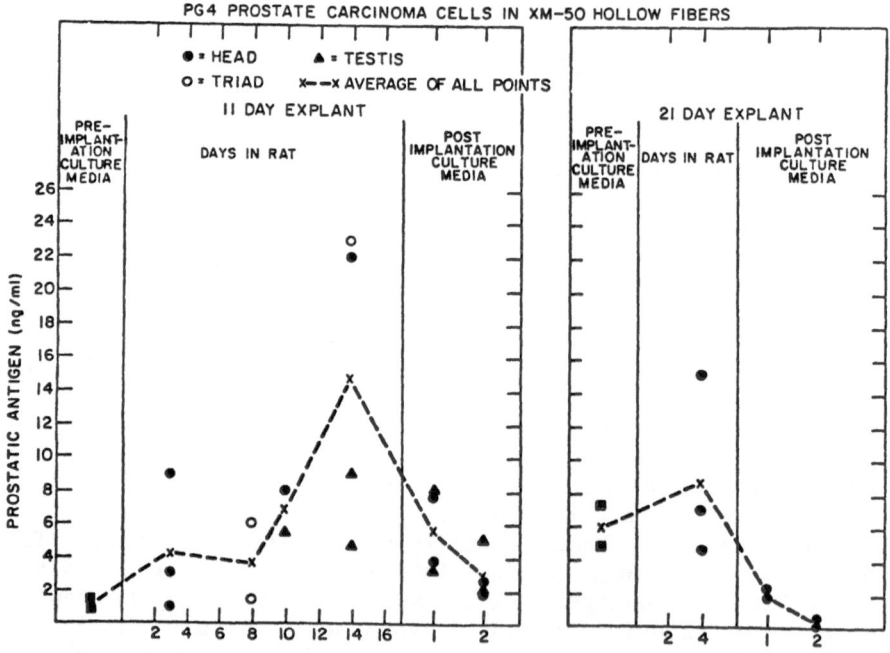

Figure 26. Human prostatic antigen in the serum of rats implanted with hollow fibers containing human prostatic cancer cells (50,000/fiber). Cells were prepared from tissue in explant culture for 11 (left) and 21 (right) days prior to encapsulation.

We were interested to find out if C_3H 10T½ mouse fibroblasts could be transformed in vivo. It has already been shown that transformation in vitro can be accomplished by a protocol involving a short exposure to UV irradiation followed by culture in medium containing the tumor promotor TPA (Terzaghi and Little, 1976). Since prolactin has been involved as a natural tumor promotor in the two stage carcinogenesis model proposed by Furth some years ago, we were interested to test that hypothesis that UV-treated 10T½ cells implanted into a DES treated F-344 rat (a condition known to result in pituitary prolactinomas (Wiklund et al., 1981) would show transformation characteristics when subsequently cultured in vivo. Preliminary results from such an experiment show that transformation does indeed occur in this experimental protocol (Fig. 27). Whether the extent of transformation is greater after DES exposure requires quantitation which we have not yet done. Nevertheless, the results are sufficiently encouraging to suggest that the hollow fiber technology will prove useful in studying mechanisms of cellular transformation.

5.3.   Donor: Chick Embryo Retinal and Optic Tectal Cells

        Recipient: Post-hatch Chicks

5.3.1. Rationale

        The question arises as to what extent the morphology of cells within the implanted hollow fiber correlates with that of cells either in vivo or in conventional cell culture. Two common methods have been to culture cells either as a monolayer on a stationary substrate, or aggregated in suspension, as developed by Moscona (1961). The hollow fibers offer a culture system combining the features of both suspension and stationary cultures; they provide a stable substrate as well as a three dimensional space in which aggregates may form.

        The reaggregation pattern in vitro is to a significant degree dependent on chemistry of the culture system (Aronowitz, 1981). The extracellular fluid of neural tissue, freely diffusible with cerebrospinal fluid, differs from the serum which is generally included in the nutrient medium in which cells are cultured (Bradbury, 1979). The purpose of our experiments was to determine the effects of neural extracellular fluid on the cells encapsulated in hollow fibers and implanted into the brain. The reaggregation and morphology of retinal and optic tectal cells within the hollow fibers was followed using the scanning electron microscope (SEM) and light microscopy of stained sections.

5.3.2. Materials and Methods

The neural retina (NR), pigmented retina (PR), and optic tectum (OT) of 7-day old chick embryos were removed and separately dissociated with trypsin. The cells were suspended in MEM and loaded into 1 cm lengths of thick XM-50 fibers. The fibers were then implanted into the borebrain of post-hatch chicks. At various post-implantation times the capsules were removed and either processed for the SEM, or embedded in paraffin, sectioned and stained by the Bodian technique for neural fibers.

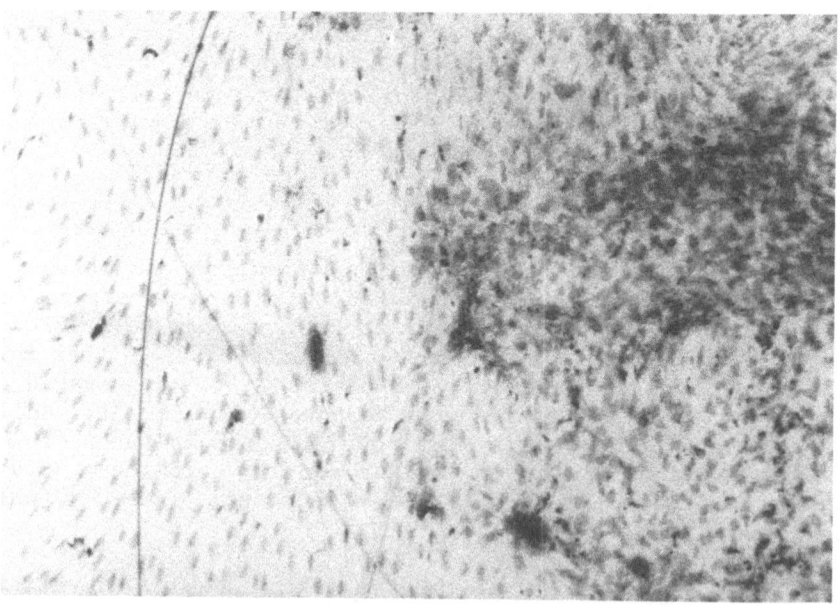

Figure 27. Photomicrograph of C_3H 10T½ cells recovered from XM-50 hollow fibers previously implanted in the triad of a Fischer 344 rat for two months. The cells were grown for six weeks in MEM containing 10% FBS and antibiotics. Note areas of normal growth adjacent to the edge of transformed colony.

5.3.3. Results and Discussion

In the first half day following dissociation, the cells remained spherical with little sign of flattening onto the fiber substrate. By 24 hrs cells from both tissues had developed processes and had begun migrating. The processes fasciculated and the cells formed small aggregates with their nearest neighbors. During the first week cells from the optic tectum continued to migrate extensively and formed large spherical aggregates connected by bundles of cell processes (Fig. 28A). Many cell bodies were found on these connectives, which appeared to provide paths along which the cells migrated. Bodian stained sections indicated that at least some of the processes within the connectives were neural fibers. During the latter half of the second week flat cells migrated out of the aggregates and formed an underlying cohesive monolayer. These flat cells have been identified as glial cells by others (Lin et al., 1977). Cultures of NR cells alone were very similar to those of OT cells. The major difference was a less extensive migration of cells, resulting in smaller aggregates. Fiber bundles were much thinner and seldom connected adjacent aggregates. As in OT cultures, flat cells migrated out of the aggregates during the second week and formed an underlying monolayer.

When PR cells were included in the cell suspension, the subsequent development was quite different. Flat cells were apparent by the second day and rapidly formed a monolayer. Spherical cells generally spread as sheets or cords on the monolayer with only localized condensations of cells. By the middle of the second week the pattern was typically a flat monolayer of cells underlying aggregates of spherical cells, with fibers and bundles of fibers spread over the monolayer (Fig. 28B).

The internal structure of the aggregates had a layered pattern resembling the layers of cells and fibers in the intact tissues. The aggregates of the different cell types varied from each other in a manner which could be related to the tissue in vivo.

Cultures of cells with the hollow fibers showed many characteristics of both suspension and stationary cultures. As in suspension cultures, the cells aggregate, sort out in an organotypic manner, differentiate and form neural fibers. In addition they resemble stationary cultures

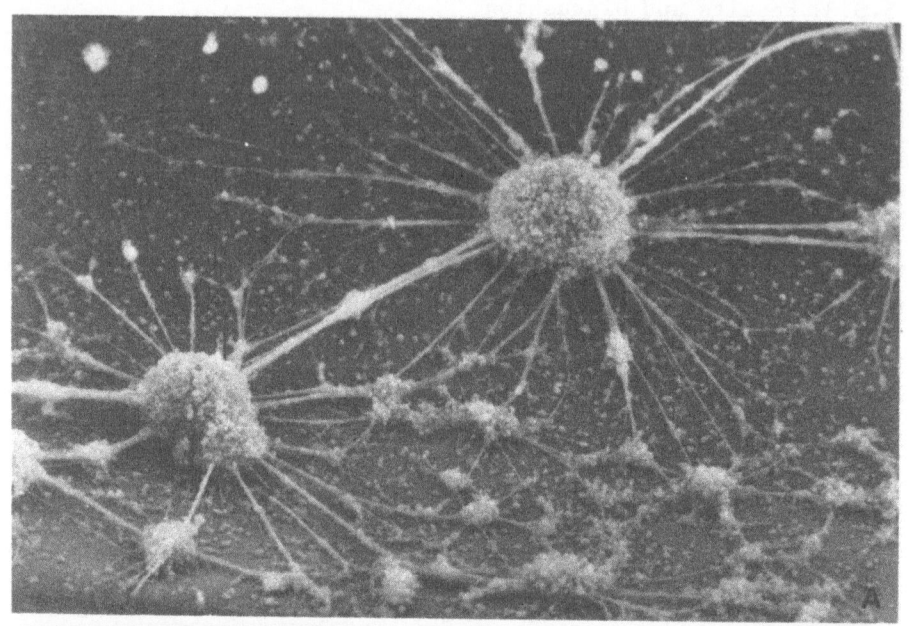

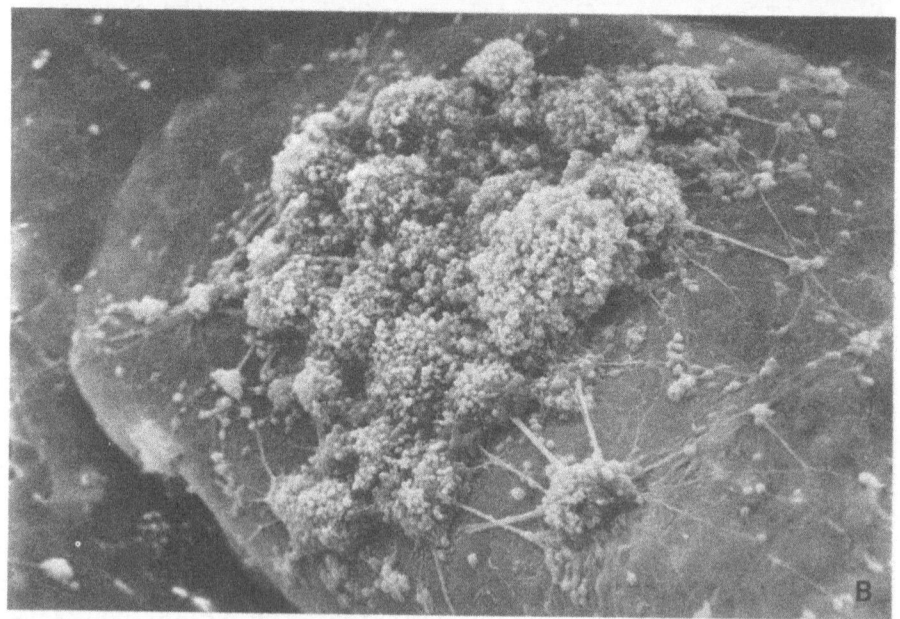

in that a monolayer of flat (glial) cells develop, underneath clumps of neuron-like cells and fibers.

The time course of appearance of the flat cells likewise had features of both culture techniques. In NR and OT cultures, flat cells migrated out of the aggregates, as they did in stationary cultures (Meller, 1979), but, as in suspension, their appearance was delayed until the latter half of the second week (Suburo and Adler, 1977). However, there were patterns unique to this system. In NR + PR cultures, the early appearance of flat cells, concurrent with the migration of the spherical cells, is clearly at variance with the flat cell development shown by NR cells cultured alone. The identity of these early forming flat cells is uncertain. They may be PR cells, or they may be glial cells which have been induced to form an initial monolayer by the presence of the PR cells. Factors responsible for this difference in behavior between NR and NR + PR cultures have not been identified.

6. Summary

In this chapter we have tried to show that the hollow fiber technology can be used in a variety of ways to study mammalian cell function. In a very real sense, these fibers provide an alternative to conventional cell culture technology in that the living animal serves as the "culture vessel". Well known variables in cell culture brought about through the use of serum, smooth plastic substrates, pH control, medium changes and the like are eliminated by using hollow fibers.

There are obviously a large number of questions about cell behavior in hollow fibers which will require further study. For example, characteristics and kinetics of cell division; details of metabolism including preferred substrate utilization; extent of capsule vascularization and correlation

---

Figure 28. (a) Aggregated cells from seven day old chick embryo optic tectum cultured for five days in implanted hollow fibers. × 200. (b) Cells from seven day old chick embryo neural retina cultured in an implanted hollow fiber for 11 days. × 280.

with cell function; extent of inflammatory cell infiltration into the capsule wall and effects of low molecular weight lymphokines on encapsulated cell functions; behavior of cells in hollow fibers with different molecular weight sieving pores; etc. Obviously, a great deal more needs to be done, but a start has been made. The future looks exciting indeed, for the clinical and commercial applications of these fibers in the biomedical sciences appears to be great.

ACKNOWLEDGMENTS

The reader will have noticed the large number of authors on this report. Each co-author, in his own way, has made significant contributions to this new technology. The senior author expresses his sincere gratitude to each of them. The capable technical assistance of Vicki Jones and Donna Bubeck is acknowledged, as is the superb secretarial assistance of Mrs. Judy Pressler. Finally, the generous gift of hollow fibers from Mr. Tony Testa, Romicon Corporation, Woburn, MA is acknowledged.

This work was supported in part by USPHS Grant CA 23248, NASA 9-15566, NASA NCA 2-OR 589-101, Lyndhurst Foundation (Chattanooga, TN), the Agricultural Experiment Station of The Pennsylvania State University and has been authorized as paper #6515 in the journal series of the Pennsylvania Agricultural Experiment station.

Aronowitz, J. L., 1981, How pure is "pure"? in: "The Growth Requirements of Vertebrate Cells in vitro", C. Waymouth, R. C. Ham, and P. J. Chapple, eds., p. 82, Cambridge University Press, Cambridge.

Bartke, A., 1965, The response of two types of dwarf mice to growth hormone thyrotropin and thyroxin, Gen. Comp. Endocrinol. 5:418.

Bartke, A., 1979, Genetic models in the study of anterior pituitary hormones, in: "Genetic Variations in Hormone Systems", Vol. I, J. G. M. Shire, ed., p. 113, CTC Press, Boca Raton.

Bradbury, M., 1979, in: "The Concept of a Blood-Brain Barrier", p. 32, John Wiley and Sons, Chichester.

Carsner, R. L., and Reynolds, E. G., 1960, Primary site of gene action in anterior pituitary dwarf mice, Science 113:829.

Chick, W. L., Like, A. A., and Lauris, V., 1975, Beta cell culture on synthetic capillaries: An artificial endocrine pancreas, Science 187:847.

Chick, W. L., Perna, J. J., Lauris, V., Lon, D., Galletti, P. M., Panol, G., Whittemore, A. D., Like, A. A., Colton, C. K., and Lysaught, M. J., 1977, Artificial pancreas using living beta cells: Effects on glucose homeostatis in diabetic rats, Science 197:780.

Dogerom, J., van Wimersam-Greidanus, T. B., and Swaab, D. F., 1977, Evidence for the release of vasopressin and oxytoxin into cerebrospinal fluid. Measurements in plasma and CSF of intact and hypophysectomized rats, Neuroendocrinology 24:108.

Faglia, G., Moriondo, P., Beck-Peccoz, P., Travaglini, P., Ambrosi, B., Spada, A., and Missim, M., 1980, Use of neuroactive drugs and hypothalamic regulatory hormones in the diagnosis of hyperprolactinemic states, in: "Neuroactive drugs in Endocrinology, Developments in Endocrinology", Vol. 9, E. E. Muller, ed., p. 263, Elsevier North Holland, Amsterdam.

Giannattasio, G., Zanini, A., Panerai, A. E., Meldolesi, J., and Müller, E. E., 1979, Studies on rat pituitary homografts, II, Effects of thyrotropin-releasing hormone on in vitro biosynthesis and release of growth hormone and prolactin, Endocrinology 104:237.

Halasz, B., Pupp, L., Uhlarik, S., and Tima, L., 1963, Growth of hypophysectomized rats bearing pituitary transplant in the hypothalamus, Acta Physiol. Hung. 23:287.

Halasz, B., Pupp, L., Uhlarik, S., and Tima, L., 1965, Further studies on hormone secretion of anterior pituitary transplanted into hypophysiotrophic area of rat hypothalamus, Endocrinology 77:343.

Hoffman, D. L., and Baker, B. L., 1977, Effect of treatment with growth hormone on somatostatin in median-eminence of hypophysectomized rats, Proc. Soc. Exp. Biol. Med. 156:265.

Hymer, W. C., Evans, W. H., Kraicer, J., Mastro, A., Davis, Jr., and Griswold, E., 1973, Enrichment of cell types from the rat adenohypophysis by sedimentation at unit gravity, Endocrinology 92:275.

Hymer, W. C., Wilbur, D. L., Page, R., Hibbard, E., Kelsey, R. C., and Hatfield, J. M., 1981a, Pituitary hollow fiber units in vivo and in vitro, Neuroendocrinology 32:339.

Hymer, W. C., Harkness, J., Bartke, A., Wilbur, D., Hatfield, J. M., Page, R., and Hibbard, E., 1981b, Pituitary hollow fiber units in the dwarf mouse, Neuroendocrinology 32:350.

Kelsey, R. C., Hymer, W. C., and Page, R., 1981, Pituitary cell transplants to the cerebral ventricle suppress the pituitary of the recipient host, Neuroendocrinology 33:312.

Knazek, R. A., 1974, Solid tissue masses formed in vitro from cells cultured on artificial capillaries, Fed. Proc., 33:1978.

Knazek, R. A., and Skylar, J. S., 1976, Secretion of human prolactin in vitro, Proc. Soc. Exp. Biol. Med. 151:561.

Knazek, R. A., Gullino, P. M., Kohler, P. O., and Dedrick, R. L., 1972, Cell culture on artificial capillaries: an approach to tissue growth in vitro, Science 178:65.

Knigge, K. M., 1980, Relationship of intracerebral pituitary grafts to central neuropeptide systems, Amer. J. Anat. 158:549.

Knigge, K. M., and Joseph, S. A., 1974, Thyrotropin releasing factor (TRF) in cerebrospinal fluid of the 3rd ventricle of rat, Acta. Endocrinol. (Copenh.) 76:209.

Kuriyama, M., Wang, M., Papsidero, L., Kiuan, C., Snimand, T., Vanenzuela, L., Nishiura, T., Murphy, G., and Chu, M., 1980, Quantitation of prostate-specific antigen in serum by a sensitive enzyme immunoassay, Cancer Res. 40:4568.

Lim, R., Turriff, D. E., Troy S. S., and Kato, T., 1977, Differentiation of glioblasts under the influence of glia maturation factor, in: "Cell, Tissue and Organ Culture in Neurobiology", S. Federoff and L. Hertz, ed., p. 223, Academic Press, NY.

Lister, R. C., 1977, Hypopituitarism in children, in: "The Pituitary: A Current Review", B. Marshall, J. R. Allen, and V. Mahesh, eds., p. 467, Academic Press, NY.

Meller, K., 1979, Scanning electron microscope studies on the development of the nervous system in vivo and in vitro, Int. Rev. Cytol. 56:23.

Mittra, I., 1980, A novel "cleaved prolactin" in the rat pituitary: Part I, Biosynthesis, characterization and regulatory control, Biochem. Biophys. Res. Comms. 95:1750.

Moscana, A. A., 1961, Rotation-mediated histogenetic aggregation of dissociated cells: a quantifiable approach to cell interactions in vitro, Exp. Cell Res., 22:455.

Phillips, J., Beamer, W., and Bartke, A., 1982, Analysis of growth hormone genes in mice with genetic defects of growth hormone expression, J. Endocrinol. 92:405.

Schroeder, L. L., Johnson, J. C., and Malarkey, W. B., 1976, Cerebrospinal fluid prolactin a reflection of abnormal prolactin secretion in patients with pituitary tumor, J. Clin. Endocrinol. 43:1255.

Suburo, A. M., and Adler, R., 1977, Neuronal and glial differentiation in reaggregation cultures, Cell Tiss. Res. 176:407.

Sun, A. M., Parisius, W., Healy, G. M., Vacek, I., and Macmorine, H. G., 1977, The use, in diabetic rats and monkeys, of artificial capillary units containing cultured islets of Langerhans (artificial endocrine pancreas), Diabetes 26:1136.

Tanaka, T., Shiv, R., Gout, P., Beer, C., Noble, R., and Friesen H., 1980, A new sensitive and specific bioassay for lactogenic hormones: measurement of prolactin and growth hormone in human serum, J. Clin. Endocrinol. Met. 51:1058.

Terzaghi, M., and Little, J., 1976, X-radiation-induced transformation in a C_3H mouse embryo derived cell line, Cancer Res., 36:1367.

Turakulov, Y. K., Gagel'gans, A. I., Salakhova, N. S., Mirakhmedov, A. K., Gol'ber, L. M., Kandrokor, V. I., and Gaidina, G. A., 1975, Thyroid hormones, biosynthesis, physiological effects, and mechanisms of action, in: "Studies in Soviet Science", Y. K. Turakulov, ed., p. 186, Consultants Bureau, NY.

Tze, W. J., Wong, F. C., Chen, L. M., and O'Young, S., 1976, Implantable artificial endocrine pancreas unit used to restore normoglycaemia in the diabetic rat, Nature 264:466.

Wang, M. C., Valenzuela, L. A., Murphy, G. P., and Chu, T. M., 1979, Purification of a human prostate specific antigen, Invest. Urol. 17:159.

Weiss, S., Bergland, R., Page, R., Turpen, C., and Hymer, W. C., 1978, Pituitary cell transplants to the cerebral ventricles promote growth of hypophysectomized rats, Proc. Soc. Exp. Biol. Med. 159:409.

Wiklund, J., Wertz, N., and Gorski, J., 1981, A comparison of estrogen effects on uterine and pituitary growth hormone and prolactin synthesis in F-344 and Hotzman rats, Endocrinology 109:1700.

Wilfinger, W. W., Davis, J. A., Augustine, E. C., and Hymer, W. C., 1979, The effects of culture conditions on prolactin and growth hormone production by rat anterior pituitary cells, Endocrinology 105:530.

DISCUSSION

CHRISTOFFERSEN: Can you point out the major advantages of the hollow fiber technique as compared to the conventionally used implantation of diffusion chambers with e.g. Millipore membranes?

HYMER: It is my understanding that the sieving properties of the Millipore membranes are not comparable to those of the hollow fibers. That is, hollow fibers have finer exclusion limits. The other advantage which comes to mind is that the hollow fiber is smaller. As such, it can be placed in more sites in vivo and is readily handled when transferred to in vitro situations.

NICHOLSON: Did the prostatic cells in the hollow fibers retain hormone-dependency and regress in castrate animals?

HYMER: This would be an interesting experiment to do. We have not done it.

PECK: I may have drifted off and missed this but how do you plug up the ends of the hollow fibers?

HYMER: No, you didn't drift - I didn't say. In fact, we take a heated forceps and seal the ends by heat fusion, followed by dipping the ends in a hot-melt wax to ensure no leakage.

GOLDFINE: Can you use this system to put beta cells into diabetic animals and then correct the hyperglycemia?

HYMER: We have not done this. Others (Tze et al.) have used this approach, but the cells were placed outside the fiber.

SCHRADER: Do the hollow fiber devices themselves evoke an inflammatory response if implanted in locations other than the brain or kidney capsule?

HYMER: If one implants an empty fiber intracranically or subcutaneously, there will be lymphocytes penetrating the capsule wall. Our distinct impression is that this response is greater in capsules placed in subcutaneous sites as opposed to the brain. It may be possible to diminish tis inflammatory response by using a "double membrane" hollow fiber; i.e. one which has the limiting membrane on the outside of the fiber as well as in its normal position lining the lumen.

PECK: To return to Schrader's question of inflammatory response, how long can you keep the capsules in a place like the peritoneal cavity or subcutaneous? We tried to do this naively with the uterus years ago and got too much scar tissue.

HYMER: We assess scar tissue histologically. As explained before, the concentration of scar tissue is certainly greater in a subcutaneous placement than in an intracranial one. In some experiments with human prolactinoma cells, we do find hormone being released from cells in the subcutaneous site.

LABRIE: What is the responsiveness of GH- and PRL-secreting cells to stimulatory and inhibitory agents in vivo? How permeable are these fibers under chronic conditions?

HYMER: Our protocols usually do not address the issue of responsiveness of the cells in vivo. However, the data in Fig. 16 do show that estrogen activated the PRL cells in vivo. Hypophysectomized rats bearing encapsulated GH cells obviously grow, but GH levels in the sera of these animals is low to undetectable. Our experiments therefore usually call for removal of the capsule from the animal followed by analysis in vitro. To our way of thinking, the ability to compare function of the group cells maintained in vivo vs. in vitro is a key advantage to the technique.

The issue of fiber permeability with advancing implantation tissue is important. We have no information on this point, but our histological findings would suggest that at no time is the outer capsule wall completely blocked.

KALRA: Did you insert these hollow fibers with the pituitary cells in the third ventricle, this may promote better secretory function?

HYMER: We have not done so because of the size of the fiber relative to the rat ventricle. However, a few laboratories are trying this experiment in the monkey.

REGULATION OF GRANULOSA CELL RESPONSIVENESS TO GONADOTROPINS:

ACTIONS OF EPIDERMAL AND PLATELET-DERIVED GROWTH FACTORS

Judith S. Mondschein and David W. Schomberg

Departments of Obstetrics and Gynecology and
Physiology, Duke University Medical Center
Durham, NC 27710

Introduction

The concept of pituitary gonadotropins as regulators of follicular and luteal development and function is central to our understanding of ovarian physiology. Patterns of gonadotropin secretion are superimposed upon patterns of target cell gonadotropin receptor levels (Richards and Midgley, 1976). The result of this well-coordinated series of events is a normal estrus or menstrual cycle. Steroid hormones provide a second level of regulation of these processes. As early as 1940 it was observed that estrogen enhanced ovarian responsiveness to gonadotropins (Pencharz, 1940). More recent studies have suggested roles for estrogens, androgens, and progestins in various aspects of ovarian physiology and pathophysiology (McNatty et al., 1979; Louvet et al., 1975; Schomberg, 1979; Schreiber and Hsueh, 1979; and references therein). The observation that growth factors can modulate follicle-stimulating hormone (FSH)-dependent luteinizing hormone (LH) receptor induction in vitro (Mondschein and Schomberg, 1981a) introduced the possibility of a third level of regulation: the growth factors, known primarily for their mitogenic effects on cultured cells, may represent a broad class of compounds which interact with more classic gonadotropic and steroidal mechanisms to determine the course of follicular and luteal development and function. Epidermal growth factor (EGF) and platelet-derived growth factor (PDGF) are examples of negative and positive modulators, respectively, of FSH-dependent LH receptor induction in granulosa cell cultures, and are the subject of this review.

2.   Epidermal Growth Factor

2.1. Effects of EGF on LH Receptor Induction

FSH has a primary role in the development and differentiation of ovarian follicular granulosa cells (Richards and
Midgley, 1976; Richards, 1980). FSH-dependent granulosa
cell LH receptor induction has been well documented in vivo
(Zeleznik et al., 1974; Richards et al., 1976) as well as in
vitro under chemically defined culture conditions (Erickson
et al., 1979). In 1981 we reported that EGF inhibits the
induction of LH receptors by FSH in serum-free cultures of
rat granulosa cells (Mondschein and Schomberg, 1981a). Our
findings appeared virtually simultaneously with the results
of Ascoli (1981) demonstrating a reduction in LH receptor
number in a Leydig tumor cell line cultured in the presence
of EGF. In both studies it was shown that EGF does not
compete with ^{125}I-hCG for LH receptor binding sites.
Scatchard analyses revealed changes in receptor number, with
no changes in affinity.

The effect of EGF on FSH-dependent LH receptor induction
is shown in Fig. 1. Treatment with FSH increases LH receptor
binding nearly 15-fold. EGF alone has no effect on LH receptor binding, but it blocks the FSH-induced increase. The
inhibitory effect of EGF is related to the doses of both EGF
and FSH (Fig. 2). Inhibition is virtually complete at 10
ng/ml EGF, while 1 ng/ml EGF partially inhibits. The inhibitory effect of 1 ng/ml is much more pronounced at higher
doses of FSH.

While serum has also been shown to inhibit FSH-dependent
LH receptor induction in rat granulosa cell cultures (Erickson
et al., 1979), its pattern of inhibition (Fig. 3) clearly
differs from that of EGF. The tendency of EGF to be more
inhibitory at higher doses of FSH suggests that EGF may be
acting, in part, to enhance the down-regulatory effect of FSH
on newly-induced LH receptor (Rao et al., 1977). This does
not appear to be the case for serum inhibition; serum does
not tend to be more inhibitory at higher doses of FSH. While
EGF is known to be present in serum, these differing patterns
suggest that serum inhibition does not result from its EGF
content. It has been suggested that the inhibitory action of
serum may result from the presence of FSH binding inhibitors

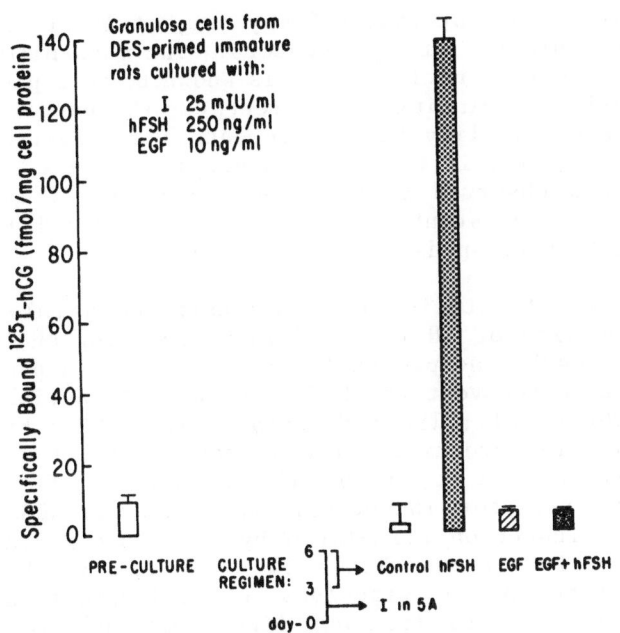

Figure 1. Effect of EGF on FSH-dependent LH receptor induction. Specific binding of ^{125}I-hCG was determined for freshly harvested cells ("pre-culture") and after 6 days of culture. Granulosa cells were cultured in serum-free McCoy's 5A nutrient medium in fibronectin-coated culture wells as previously described (Mondschein and Schomberg, 1981a). Treatments listed in the bottom line of the "culture regimen" were carried out for the entire 6-day culture period. Treatments listed in the top line were added at the 3-day medium change. Highly purified hFSH (LER 1577) was kindly provided by Dr. L. E. Reichert, Jr. Data bars represent $\bar{x}$ ± S.E.M., n = 3.

(Reichert et al., 1979). However, the multiplicity of factors present in serum hints that its action may be complex.

If EGF is added to cultures of rat granulosa cells in which significant LH receptor levels have been induced, the decline in receptor levels which occurs with time in culture is accelerated (Fig. 4). Similar results were obtained using porcine granulosa cells, which possess significant LH receptor binding levels prior to culture (Mondschein et al., 1981).

These findings suggest that EGF may act, at least in part, to enhance the turnover of LH receptors. The mechanism by which this might occur is unclear. EGF is known to be rapidly internalized following binding to its receptor (Carpenter and Cohen 1976). The possibility that LH receptors are co-internalized with EGF receptors is unlikely, since the time course of LH receptor loss observed in the presence of EGF is much longer than would be consistent with rates reported for EGF receptor internalization (Gospodarowicz et al., 1978).

Several laboratories have demonstrated a role for cAMP in the induction of LH receptor in vitro using cholera toxin (CTX), 8-Br-cAMP, and prostaglandin E_2 (PGE_2) as phamacological tools to circumvent the FSH-receptor interaction (Nimrod, 1981; Knecht et al., 1981; Sanders et al., 1981; Erickson et al., 1982). To investigate the mechanism of EGF inhibition, it was of interest to study the effects of EGF on cAMP-mediated LH receptor induction. We found that EGF inhibits LH receptor induction stimulated by CTX and 8-Br-cAMP in rat granulosa cell cultures (Table I). EGF also inhibits induction by CTX in porcine granulosa cell cultures (Schomberg et al., 1983a). Results from our laboratory indicate that EGF does not attenuate FSH-dependent cAMP production in rat or porcine granulosa cell cultures (Gunn and May, unpublished observations). Our data suggest that EGF acts at a site(s) distal to the generation of cAMP. Results from the laboratory of Knecht and Ranta (1982) are not totally in agreement. While these workers found that EGF prevents the stimulatory effects of 8-Br-cAMP and CTX on LH receptor induction, they also found that EGF inhibits FSH-stimulated cAMP production by inhibiting FSH-dependent cAMP synthesis and stimulating cAMP catabolism.*

---

[*] Differences in the experimental protocol for assessing cAMP accumulation employed by Gunn and May and by Knecht and Ranta may account for the disparate results. Our laboratory measures intracellular and extracellular cAMP produced in response to short-term FSH stimulation following the culture period. Knecht and Ranta measure extracellular cAMP produced during culture. Differences in the animal models and the culture regimens may also be involved. Resolution of this dilemma must await further study.

2.2. Effects of EGF on Steroidogenesis

The actions of EGF on another aspect of granulosa cell function, steroidogenesis, is currently an area of active investigation by several laboratories.

Hsueh et al. (1981) have shown that EGF inhibits estrogen production stimulated by FSH, dibutyryl cAMP, CTX, and PGE_2 in cultured rat granulosa cells. The inhibitory effect on estrogen production has also been demonstrated in porcine granulosa cell cultures where EGF depresses unstimulated aromatase activity (Schomberg et al., 1983b).

Table I. Effect of EGF on LH Receptor Binding Induced by
CTX and 8-Br-cAMP

Culture Conditions[a]	Specifically bound ^{125}I-hCG[b]	
	no EGF	EGF, 10 ng/ml
Control		1.2 ± 0.5
CTX, 10^{-11}M		3.1 ± 1.2[c]
10^{-10}M	86.9 ± 9.2	9.0 ± 0.4[c]
10^{-9}M	135 ± 18	12.9 ± 0.4[d]
8-Br-cAMP, 0.1mM	1.8 ± 0.8	0.3 ± 0.3[e]
1.0mM	1.6 ± 0.9	4.6 ± 0.4[e]
5.0mM	106 ± 9	1.3 ± 0.2[c]

[a]Granulosa cells from DES-primed, immature rats were cultured in serum-free DMEM:Ham's F12 (1:1) nutrient medium with insulin (25 mIU/ml) in serum-coated culture wells as previously described (Mondschein and Schomberg, 1981b). After 3 days, cultures received fresh medium, insulin, and CTX or 8-Br-cAMP as indicated. After 6 days, LH receptor levels were assessed by the specific binding of ^{125}I-hCG.
[b]fmol/mg cell protein, $\bar{x}$ ± S.E.M., n = 3.
[c]$p < 0.001$ vs. no EGF.
[d]$p < 0.005$ vs. no EGF.
[e]$p < 0.05$ vs. no EGF.

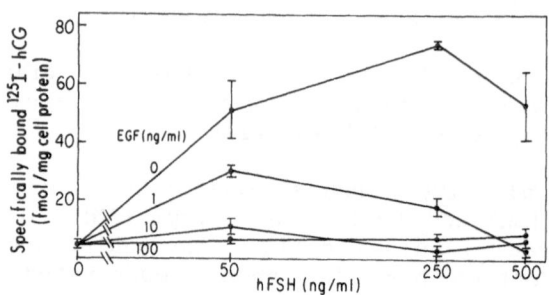

Figure 2. FSH-dependent LH receptor induction and its inhibition by EGF: dose-response relationships for EGF and FSH.
Granulosa cells from DES-primed, immature rats were cultured
in serum-free McCoy's 5A nutrient medium with insulin
(25 mIU/ml) in fibronectin-coated culture wells. After 3
days, cultures received fresh 5A and insulin, with EGF and/or
hFSH as indicated. After 6 days, LH receptor levels were
assessed by the specific binding of ^{125}I-hCG. Data points
represent x ± S.E.M., n = 3. Reproduced with permission from
Mondschein and Schomberg (1981a), copyright 1981 by the
American Association for the Advancement of Science.

EGF inhibits LH-dependent androgen synthesis in differentiating rat ovarian theca/interstitial cells (Erickson and
Case, 1982). Similarly, cultured rat Leydig cells are sensitive to EGF inhibition of testosterone production stimulated
by human chorionic gonadotropin (hCG), dibutyryl cAMP, and
CTX (Hsueh et al., 1981).

The effect of EGF on progestin production is not as
clear as the effect on estrogen and androgen production.
For cultured rat granulosa cells, we found that EGF could
be both inhibitory and stimulatory to FSH-mediated 20α-
dihydroprogesterone (20α-OHP) secretion, depending upon
the doses of EGF and FSH employed (Fig. 5). However,
none of the changes observed are marked. Knecht and Ranta
(1982) found that EGF depresses FSH-stimulated progesterone
(P) production. Jones et al. (1983) found that EGF stimulates pregnenolone (Pe), P, and 20α-OHP production and
synergizes with FSH in stimulating Pe and 20α-OHP production.
Enhancement of progestin biosynthesis is related to increases

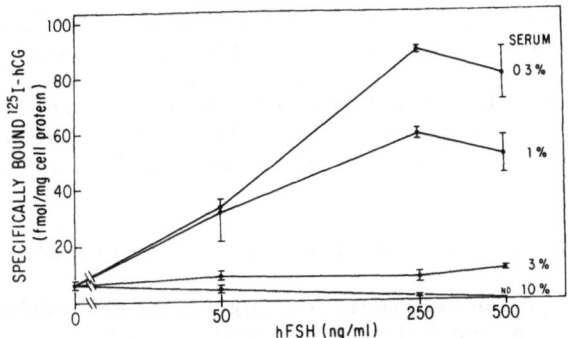

Figure 3. Dose-response effect of serum on FSH-dependent LH receptor induction. Granulosa cells from DES-primed, immature rats were cultured in McCoy's 5A nutrient medium with insulin (25 mIU/ml) and fetal calf serum as indicated. After 3 days, cultures received fresh 5A, insulin, serum as indicated, with or without hFSH as indicated. After 6 days, LH receptor levels were assessed by the specific binding of ^{125}I-hCG. Data points represent $\bar{x} \pm$ S.E.M., n = 3, ND, non-detectable.

in 3β-hydroxysteroid dehydrogenase (3β-HSD) and 20α-hydroxy-steroid dehydrogenase (20α-HSD) activities.*

---

*In our laboratory we find 20α-OHP accumulation during a 3-day culture period to represent greater than 92% of the total of P and 20α-OHP production (Pe accumulation is low relative to P and 20α-OHP in the absence of an inhibitor of Pe conversion to P). This percentage is not reduced by FSH or EGF treatments. We feel that the measurement of 20α-OHP only is a reasonable approximation of net progestin synthesis over a 3 day period. Jones et al. determined P and 20α-OHP over a 2 day culture period and find a larger percentage of P due to a less complete conversion of P to 20α-OHP (Nimrod and Lindner, 1976). The fact that we did not observe a pronounced increase in progestin production as Jones et al. did, is not that we have failed to include the contribution of P. Other differences in the experimental models may be responsible.

In porcine granulosa cell cultures, we found that EGF depresses basal P secretion and that stimulated by hCG, FSH, androstenedione, and the combination of androstenedione plus FSH, although the effect is not always marked (Schomberg et al., 1983b). Garrett et al. (1983) also observed moderate inhibition of P secretion in porcine granulosa cell cultures.

2.3. Comparison of EGF and GnRH Effects on Granulosa Cells

Since gonadotropin-releasing hormone (GnRH) is also known to be an inhibitor of granulosa cell function, it may be a useful excercise to compare its action to that of EGF. Both peptides inhibit FSH-dependent LH receptor induction as well as that stimulated by cAMP analogs and CTX (Mondschein and Schomberg, 1981a, Schomberg et al., 1983a, Knecht et al., 1981, and Knecht and Ranta, 1983). GnRH does not acutely inhibit FSH-stimulated adenylate cyclase activity during culture of granulosa cells (Knecht and Catt, 1981). The effect of EGF on cAMP formation is currently in debate (Knecht and Ranta, 1982). GnRH has been reported to stimulate phosphodiesterase activity, as has EGF (Knecht et al., 1981, and Knecht and Ranta, 1982). Other loci of action for GnRH include inhibition of aromatase activity (Hsueh and Erickson, 1979), stimulation of 20α-HSD activity (Jones and Hsueh, 1981), inhibition of FSH-stimulated 3β-HSD and side chain cleavage enzyme activities, and inhibition of cholesterol substrate availability (Hsueh and Jones, 1982). These effects on steroidogenic enzymes lead to a decrease in estrogen and P production. EGF also inhibits aromatase activity (Hsueh et al., 1981) and stimulates 20α-HSD activity, but in contrast to GnRH, EGF appears to stimulate 3β-HSD and Pe biosynthesis in rat granulosa cells. Thus EGF inhibits estrogen secretion, but, at least in one report (Jones et al., 1983), increases progestin secretion. Finally, specific binding sites for GnRH and EGF have been detected in rat granulosa cells, suggesting that their effects on granulosa cell function may be mediated by receptor-dependent mechanisms (Jones et al., 1980; Jones et al., 1983; St. Arnaud et al., 1983).

3.   Platelet-Derived Growth Factor

3.1. Effects of PDGF on LH Receptor Induction

Granulosa cell differentiation can also be enhanced by a growth factor. PDGF is a cationic peptide released from

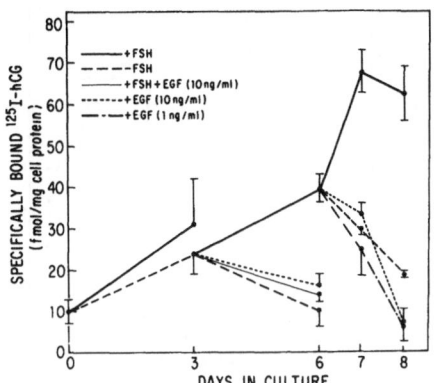

Figure 4. Effect of EGF on LH receptor binding during mono-layer culture. Granulosa cells from DES-primed, immature rats were cultured in serum-free McCoys 5A nutrient medium in fibronectin-coated culture wells. Cultures received insulin (25 mIU/ml) and the treatments indicated. Highly purified hFSH was administered at a dose of 250 ng/ml. Specific binding of ^{125}I-hCG was determined on the days indicated. Data points represent $\bar{x} \pm$ S.E.M., n = 3.

platelets during clot formation and is thought to be involved in wound healing in vivo (Ross, 1981). We were able to show that PDGF enhances FSH-dependent LH receptor induction in serum-free cultures of granulosa cells. PDGF has no effect on LH receptor induction in the absence of FSH (Mondschein and Schomberg, 1981a). Scatchard analysis of LH receptor binding following treatment with FSH plus PDGF indicates an increase in binding capacity relative to that following treatment with FSH alone, and no change in affinity. The stimulatory effect of PDGF can overcome the inhibitory action of serum (Mondschein and Schomberg, 1981b). Furthermore, a stimulatory effect of serum on FSH-dependent LH receptor induction can be demonstrated in the presence of PDGF. Thus, serum may be a source of factors which promote, as well as those which attenuate LH receptor induction. Whether the stimulatory or the inhibitory influence predominates depends on other conditions, such as the presence or absence of PDGF.

Our original studies were performed using commercially available PDGF. While some PDGF preparations significantly enhanced LH receptor induction at concentrations which stimulated DNA synthesis in fibroblast cultures, other

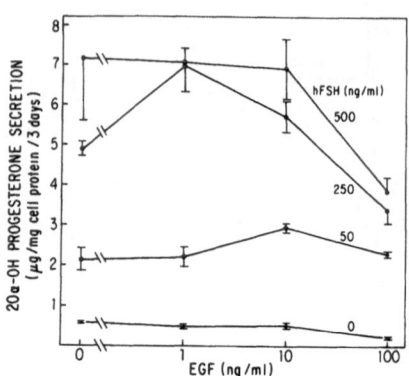

Figure 5. Effect of EGF on basal and FSH-stimulated progestin secretion. Granulosa cells from DES-primed, immature rats were cultured in serum-free McCoy's 5A nutrient medium with insulin (25 mIU/ml) in fibronectin-coated culture wells. After 3 days, cultures received fresh 5A and insulin, with EGF and/or hFSH as indicated. Radioimmunoassayable 20α-dihy-droprogesterone secreted during the second 3 days of culture was normalized on the basis of cell protein determined after 6 days. Data points represent x̄ ± S.E.M., n = 3.

preparations had no effect on receptor induction in our granulosa cell cultures. This inconsistency led us to an alternative source of PDGF; we thank Dr. W. J. Pledger for generous gifts of partially purified and highly purified PDGF. Partially purified PDGF is prepared by heat treatment of platelet lysates followed by CM-sephadex chromatography (Antoniades et al., 1979). Highly purified PDGF is prepared by further chromatography on Blue-sepharose (Deuel et al., 1981). One unit (U) of PDGF is defined as that amount which induces 50% of confluent BALB/3T3 cells to synthesize DNA (Antoniades et al., 1979).

Results obtained with partially purified PDGF are similar to those we observed with the better commercially available preparations (Table II). Partially purified PDGF enhances FSH-dependent LH receptor induction in serum-free medium, and significantly higher levels of LH receptor binding are achieved in serum-containing medium (Mondschein and Schomberg, manuscript in review). However, the levels of PDGF which must be employed are much higher than those which stimulate DNA synthesis in fibroblast cultures. Highly purified PDGF is active at levels comparable to those which stimulate DNA synthesis (Table II). While highly purified PDGF does overcome the inhibitory effect of serum, it does not appear to bring out the stimulatory effect of serum (Table II). These results suggest that PDGF activity is complex and may represent actions of several components present in differing amounts in various PDGF preparations. It is possible that the component(s) which enhances LH receptor induction in our system is(are) distinct from the component which enhances DNA synthesis in fibroblast cultures. Alternatively, the receptor-inducing and DNA synthetic activities may reside in the same molecule, with the receptor inducing activity selectively antagonized by factors present in less pure PDGF preparations. Studies using PDGF purified to homogeneity may answer this question, and are underway.

To begin to elucidate the mechanism of action of PDGF, we studied the effect of (partially and highly purified) PDGF on induction. PDGF does not enhance GC responsiveness to CTX in serum-free medium. PDGF potentiates CTX-dependent LH receptor induction in serum-containing medium, but to a significantly lesser degree than for FSH-dependent induction (Table II) (Mondschein and Schomberg, manuscript in review). Knecht and Ranta (1982) reported that PDGF enhances LH receptor induction stimulated by CTX or 8-Br-cAMP in serum-free culture. PDGF was found to increase FSH-dependent cAMP accumulation. These workers suggested that PDGF does not affect adenylate cyclase activity, but reduces phosphodiesterase activity.

The hypothesis that PDGF enhances FSH responsiveness secondary to increased cAMP accumulation is challenged, however, by the observation that there appears to be a limit to the level of LH receptor induction which can be achieved with CTX; further stimulation with higher doses of CTX impairs induction by pushing the system beyond the optimum (Mondschein and Schomberg, manuscript in review). These observations suggest the existence of a component of FSH action, a component which interacts with PDGF, which is independent of cAMP. Erickson et al. (1982) also suggest the involvement of non-cAMP actions in the mechanism of LH receptor control by FSH, since pharmacological agents (CTX, PGE_2, 8-Br-cAMP) are less effective than FSH as inducers of LH receptor binding.

While PDGF has been shown to overcome the inhibitory action of serum, it does not appear to overcome the inhibitory action of EGF in serum-free or in serum-containing medium (Fig. 6).

3.2. Effects of PDGF on Steroidogenesis

The effects of PDGF on steroidogenesis have not been studied in detail. We found that PDGF enhances FSH-stimulated progestin secretion in some but not all experiments. PDGF alone has no effect on progestin secretion (Mondschein and Schomberg, 1981b). Knecht and Ranta (1982) similarly found that PDGF enhances FSH-stimulated but not basal progesterone production. The effects of PDGF on estrogen and androgen production have not been addressed, but are certainly worthy of investigation.

4. Granulosa Cell Growth

Growth factor effects on rat granulosa cell function occur in the absence of a marked effect on cell growth as assessed by the DNA content of cell cultures. Hsueh et al. (1981) noted no difference in the DNA content of serum-free granulosa cell cultures treated with EGF and/or FSH relative to controls. We observed that neither EGF nor PDGF significantly increases DNA content relative to that of cultures which do not receive growth factors (Table III). While some cultures treated with combinations of FSH and/or growth factors appear to contain more DNA than controls on culture day 6, few contain significantly more DNA than 3 day cultures (levels for FSH and for FSH plus PDGF in 3% serum are statistically greater than day 3 levels, but increases represent much less than one cell doubling). The results suggest that certain combinations of FSH and/or growth factors may help maintain cell viability (rather than stimulate DNA synthesis), at least over a 3 day culture period. Cell counts and tritiated thymidine incorporation studies would provide more definitive results. At this point in our understanding, there is no evidence to support the hypothesis that the apparent inhibitory or stimulatory effects of growth factors on LH receptor induction are secondary to a selective growth of non-receptor-bearing or receptor-bearing cell populations, respectively.

Gospodarowicz and Bialecki (1979) observed that, despite a significant mitogenic effect on granulosa cells of the rabbit, pig, and human, EGF is not mitogenic for granulosa cells of normal rats or hypophysectomized, estrogen-treated animals. The basis for the lack of a mitogenic effect is

Table II.   Effect of PDGF on LH Receptor Induction by FSH, and CTX in Serum-Free and Serum-Contining Medium.

Experiment[a]	PDGF preparation	Culture conditions[b]	Specifically bound ^{125}I-hCG[c]	
			Serum-free	Serum
A	commercially available	control	3.5 ± 0.7	non-detectable
		FSH, 250 ng/ml	89.3 ± 2.1	4.1 ± 0.9
		PDGF, 1 U/ml	3.7 ± 2.3	1.1 ± 0.3[e]
		PDGF + FSH	178 ± 18[d]	537 ± 45[f]
B	partially purified	control	5.4 ± 0.4	2.9 ± 0.4
		FSH, 50 ng/ml	39.4 ± 7.3	5.0 ± 0.8
		PDGF, 60 U/ml	3.5 ± 0.7	1.7 ± 0.4[f]
		PDGF + FSH	167 ± 41[g]	345 ± 16[f]
C	partially purified	control		2.8 ± 0.1
		FSH, 50 ng/ml		6.4 ± 0.9
		CTX, 10^{-10}M		74.3 ± 6.5
		PDGF, 60 U/ml		2.6 ± 0.9[f]
		PDGF + FSH		416 ± 27
		PDGF + CTX		130 ± 15[e]
D	highly purified	control	6.2 ± 1.1	2.9 ± 0.3
		FSH, 50 ng/ml	135 ± 16	12.4 ± 2.0
		CTX, 10^{-10}M	170 ± 7	92.6 ± 9.3
		PDGF, 0.6 U/ml	9.1 ± 0.8[d]	4.1 ± 0.4[f]
		PDGF + FSH	269 ± 21	226 ± 12
		PDGF + CTX	161 ± 25	158 ± 1[h]

[a]Granulosa cells brom DES-primed, immature rats were cultured in serum-free McCoy's 5A nutrient medium (A) or in serum-free DMEM:Ham's F12 (1:1) nutrient medium (B, C, and D) with insulin (25 mIU/ml) in serum-coated culture wells, or in medium containing insulin and 3% fetal calf serum. After 3 days, cultures received fresh medium and insulin, with serum, hFSH, PDGF, and/or CTX as indicated. After 6 days, LH receptor levels were assessed by the specific binding of ^{125}I-hCG.
[b]Doses of FSH, CTX, and PDGF indicated are those which gave optimal LH receptor induction in each experiment. Dose-response curves for each of these agents do not exhibit a plateau, but rather a dose optimum; doses in excess of the optimum are virtually always less effective.
[c]fmol/mg cell protein $\bar{x} \pm$ S.E.M., n = 3.
[d]p < 0.01 vs. no PDGF.
[e]p < 0.025 vs. no PDGF.
[f]p < 0.001 vs. no PDGF.
[g]p < 0.05 vs. no PDGF.
[h]p < 0.005 vs. no PDGF.

unclear since EGF does appear to promote follicle growth in
rats when administered in vivo (Gospodarowicz et al., 1978a).
EGF receptors have been demonstrated on rat granulosa cells
(Jones et al., 1983; St. Arnaud et al., 1983), although the
presence of EGF receptors does not guarantee a mitogenic
response to EGF. Bovine luteal cells, which possess even
greater numbers of EGF receptors than do bovine granulosa
cells, are insensitive to the mitogenic effect of EGF
(Gospodarowicz et al., 1978b). The important thing to note
is that growth factor effects on cellular differentiation are
not obligatorily coupled to mitogenic effects (Johnson et
al., 1980).

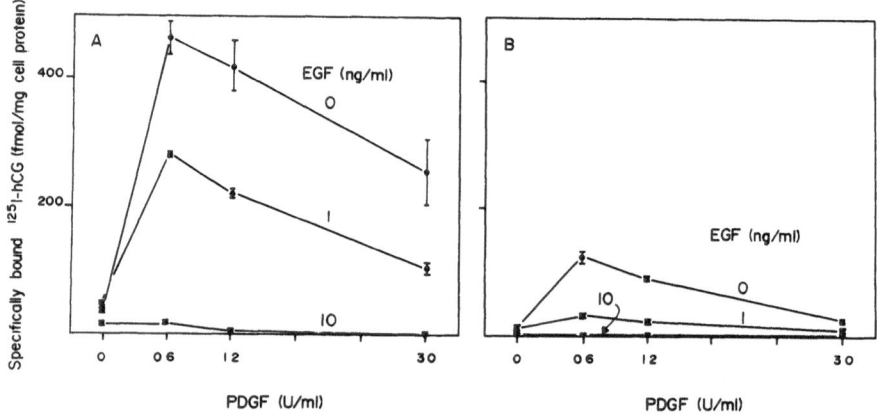

Figure 6. FSH-dependent LH induction: effect of EGF on PDGF
in combination. Granulosa cells from DES-primed immature
rats were cultured (A) in serum free DMEM:Hams F11 (1:1)
nutrient medium with insulin (25 mIU/ml) in serum-coated
culture wells as previously described (Mondschein and
Schomberg, 1981b) and (B) in medium containing insulin and 3%
fetal calf serum. After 3 days, cultures received fresh
medium, insulin, and hFSH (50 ng/ml) with or without serum.
Cultures also received EGF and/or highly purified PDGF as
indicated. After 6 days, LH receptor levels were assessed by
the specific binding of ^{125}I-hCG. Data points represent $\bar{x}$ ±
S.E.M., n = 3.

The effects of growth factors on cell growth, assessed
by the protein content of cell cultures, have been observed
during the investigation of LH receptor regulation. Although

Table III. DNA Content of Granulosa Cells Before
and During Culture

Day of culture	Culture conditions[a]	DNA content (μg/culture)[b]	
0	pre-culture	19.6 ± 0.4	
		serum-free	serum
1	control	11.5 ± 0.3	10.8 ± 0.7
3	control	11.8 ± 0.3	8.5 ± 0.1[d]
6	control	8.3 ± 1.3[d]	7.7 ± 0.2[c,d]
	FSH, 50 ng/ml	12.8 ± 0.6[c]	9.0 ± 0.1[c,d]
	EGF, 10 ng/ml	10.0 ± 1.3[c]	8.2 ± 0.2
	EGF + FSH	13.5 ± 1.0[d]	8.2 ± 0.4[d]
	PDGF, 0.6 U/ml	7.8 ± 0.7[c]	7.7 ± 0.2[c,d]
	PDGF + FSH	14.5 ± 1.3[c]	10.5 ± 0.1[d]
	PDGF + EGF	11.3 ± 0.7[c]	8.0 ± 0.1
	PDGF + EGF + FSH	13.2 ± 1.1[c]	8.5 ± 0.3

[a]Granulosa cells were isolated from DES-primed, immature rats. Aliquots of approximately 10^6 cells were assayed for DNA content (day 0) or placed in culture. Cells were cultured in serum-free DMEM:Ham's F12 (1:1) nutrient medium with insulin (25 mIU/ml) in serum-coated culture wells or in medium containing insulin and 3% fetal calf serum. DNA content was determined following 1 and 3 days of culture. After 3 days, some cultures received fresh medium and insulin, with serum, hFSH, EGF, and/or highly purified PDGF as indicated. After 6 days, DNA content was assessed.
[b]DNA was determined by the method of Erwin et al. (1981). Data represent x̄ S.E.M., n = 3. DNA determinations for freshly isolated cells include the contribution of approximately 60% non-viable cells, as assessed by trypan blue exclusion. DNA determinations for cultured cells reflect only the contributions of cells attached to the substratum, consisting of < 95% viable cells.
[c]p > 0.05 or better vs. control.
[d]p > 0.05 or better vs. day 3.

exhaustive studies of hormones, growth factors, serum, and doses and combinations thereof have not been completed, a few generalizations have emerged. EGF, FSH, and serum increase the protein content of granulosa cell cultures over a three day culture period. The increased levels are usually less than double the protein content of cultures maintained in the absence of these agents; when administered in combination they may more than double cell protein content. PDGF does not generally increase cell protein when administered alone, nor does it potentiate the effects of FSH and serum. A significant stimulatory effect of PDGF is observed in the presence of FSH plus EGF (Fig. 7).

A most interesting observation was made during studies of the functionability of LH receptor sites induced with PDGF plus FSH (Mondschein and Schomberg, 1981b). Levels of LH receptor binding achieved appeared to be related to the ability of hCG to increase the protein content of cell cultures (Table IV). Cultures treated with PDGF plus FSH plus serum exhibited the highest levels of binding, and more than doubled their protein content in one day in response to hCG. In these cells, hCG also stimulated 20α-OHP secretion and induced morphological changes characteristic of luteinization (Channing, 1969). Thus, while direct effects on granulosa cell growth may not be remarkable, growth factors may indirectly affect growth as part of their role in granulosa cell differentiation.

5.   Discussion and Conclusions

Is there scope for growth factor involvement in reproductive function? In the case of EGF, the evidence is encouraging. EGF synthesis in the mouse submaxillary gland has been shown to be stimulated by androgens (Byyny et al., 1974). Erickson and Case (1982) have speculated that a negative feed-back mechanism may exist between the sites of EGF synthesis and ovarian (and presumably testicular) androgen production. EGF receptor sites have been identified for granulosa cells of bovine, porcine (Gospodarowicz et al., 1978b), and rodent (Jones et al., 1983; St. Arnaud et al., 1983) species and for a Leydig cell tumor line (Ascoli, 1981). Porcine and bovine granulosa cell EGF receptors internalize and degrade like the EGF receptors of other cell types (Gospodarowicz et al., 1978b). Luteal cells,

Table IV. Functional Assessment of Newly Induced LH
Receptor Sites: Protein Synthetic Response to hCG

Culture contitions[a]	Protein content (day 7)[b]		^{125}I-hCG bound (day 6)[c]
	no hCG	hCG	
serum-free:			
control	37.5 ± 2.1	36.2 ± 1.5[d]	3.5 ± 0.7
FSH	45.4 ± 1.4	54.5 ± 1.6[d]	89.3 ± 2.1
PDGF	26.3 ± 1.6	24.6 ± 2.2	3.7 ± 2.3
PDGF + FSH	39.0 ± 0.8	68.0 ± 2.7[e]	178 ± 18
serum:			
control	57.3 ± 2.9	63.6 ± 0.3	non-detectable
FSH	66.6 ± 2.5	67.4 ± 3.1	4.1 ± 0.9
PDGF	41.0 ± 1.6	43.8 ± 2.1	1.1 ± 0.3
PDGF + FSH	53.9 ± 3.8	133.4 ± 3.0[e]	537 ± 45

[a]Granulosa cells from DES-primed immature rats were cultured
in serum-free McCoy's 5A nutrient medium with insulin in
serum-coated culture wells or in medium containing insulin
and 3% fetal calf serum. After 3 days, cultures received
fresh medium, insulin, with serum as indicated, hFSH
(250 ng/ml) and/or PDGF (commercially available, 1U/ml).
After 6 days, LH receptor levels were assessed by the
specific binding of ^{125}I-hCG in one set of cultures.
Another set of cultures received fresh serum-free medium
with insulin with or without hCG (100 ng/ml) for one
additional day of culture. Protein content of these cultures
was determined after 7 days.

[b]μg/protein/culture, $\bar{x}$ ± S.E.M., n = 3.

[c]fmol/mg cell protein, $\bar{x}$ ± S.E.M., n = 3.

[d]$p < 0.01$ vs. no hCG.

[e]$p < 0.001$ vs. no hCG.

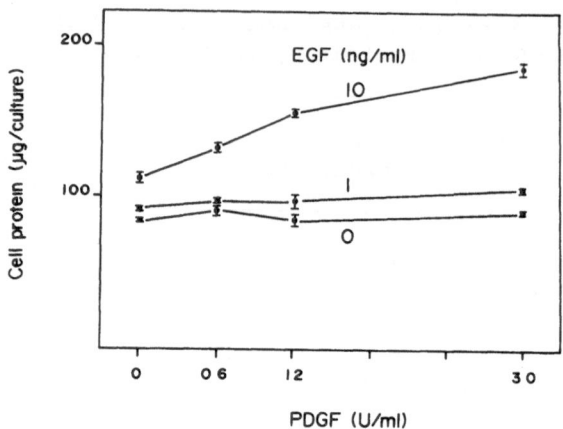

Figure 7. Effects of EGF and PDGF on protein content of granulosa cell cultures. Granulosa cells from DES-primed, immature rats were cultured in serum-free DMEM:Ham's F12 (1:1) nutrient medium with insulin (25 mIU/ml) in serum-coated culture wells. After 3 days, cultures received fresh medium, insulin, hFSH (50 ng/ml), with EGF and/or highly purified PDGF as indicated. Monolayer protein content was determined after 6 days (following LH receptor binding determinations). Data points represent x̄ ± S.E.M., n = 3. Similar results were obtained in serum-containing medium (data not shown).

developmentally derived from granulosa cells, possess even greater numbers of EGF receptors than do granulosa cells (Gospodarowicz et al., 1978b). Rat ovarian cell EGF receptor binding appears to be increased by hCG and FSH, and decreased by GnRH and androgens (St. Arnaud et al., 1983).

In the case of PDGF, the evidence for a role in gonadal function is limited, but the speculation is great. We have suggested that the formation of the corpus hemorrhagicum may provide a local concentration of PDGF to granulosa cells at a relatively late stage in their development, and thus may be involved in the differentiation of granulosa cells to luteal cells (Mondschein and Schomberg, 1981a). PDGF has only recently been purified to homogeneity (Heldin et al., 1979) and only limited amounts have been available for radioiodination and receptor binding studies (Heldin et al., 1981). We are anxiously awaiting the opportunity to apply these new technologies to determine whether granulosa cells possess

PDGF receptors, and whether these putative PDGF receptors can be regulated by gonadotropins, steroids, GnRH, etc. A word of caution is in order here since a platelet factor (or factors) other than "the" PDGF may be the agent which is active in granulosa cell cultures. If this is found to be the case, identification and purification of the new factor must preceed receptor studies.

We believe that modulation of granulosa cell function by growth factors in vitro may represent a physiologically relevent control system which operates in vivo. PDGF and EGF may be actual physiological effectors, or they may be analogs of other molecules, perhaps species which are produced locally within the ovary (or testis), which regulate gonadal function.

Studies in vitro utilizing granulosa cells and other culture models contribute greatly to our understanding of reproductive endocrinology. Results of growth factor studies broaden our concepts of gonadal control mechanisms, and may be of potential clinical importance, especially in the area of fertility control.

ACKNOWLEDGEMENTS: Supported in part by Grant No. HD 11827, from the NICHHD, NIH, USPHS. We gratefully acknowledge the secretarial assistance of Ms. Lynn Browning.

REFERENCES

Antoniades, H. N., Scher, C. D., and Stiles, C. D., 1979, Purification of human platelet-derived growth factor, Proc. Natl. Acad. Sci. USA 76:1809.

Ascoli, M., 1981, Regulation of gonadotropin receptors and gonadotropin responsiveness in a clonal strain of Leydig tumor cells by epidermal growth factor, J. Biol. Chem. 256:179.

Byyny, R. L., Orth, D. N., Cohen, S., and Doyne, E. S., 1974, Epidermal growth factor: effects of androgens and adrenergic agents, Endocrinology 95:776.

Carpenter, G., and Cohen, S., 1976, ^{125}I-labeled human epidermal growth factor: binding, internalization, and degradation in human fibroblasts, J. Cell Biol. 79:159.

Channing, C. P., 1969, The use of tissue culture of granulosa

cells as a method of studying the mechanism of luteinization, in: "The Gonads", K. W. McKerns, ed., pp. 245-275,
Appleton-Century Crofts, New York.

Deuel, T. F., Huang, J. S., Proffitt, R. T., Baenziger, J. U.,
Chang, D., and Kennedy, B. B., 1981, Human platelet-derived
growth factor: purification and resolution into two active
protein fractions, J. Biol. Chem. 256:8896.

Erickson, G. F., and Case, E., 1982, Epidermal growth factor
inhibits LH-dependent theca/interstitial cell differentiation in serum-free culture, Endocrinology 110 (Supplement): 237 (Abstract #773).

Erickson, G. F., Wang, C., and Hsueh, A. J. W., 1979, FSH
induction of functional LH receptors in granulosa cells
cultured in chemically defined medium, Nature 279:336.

Erickson, G. F., Wang, C., and Casper, R., 1982, Studies on the
mechanism of LH receptor control by FSH, Proceedings of the
29th Annual Meeting of the Society for Gynecological
Investigation, Abstract #281, p. 162.

Erwin, B. G., Stoschek, C. M., and Florini, J. R., 1981, A
rapid fluorometric method for the estimation of DNA in
cultured cells, Anal. Biochem. 110:291.

Garrett, R., Kroman, N., Conn, T., and Channing, C. P., 1983,
Ability of EGF and FGF to enhance growth of porcine granulosa cells in culture while they lead to a decrease in
progesterone secretion: changes in responsiveness throughout follicular maturation, in: "Factors Regulating Ovarian
Function", P. Terranova and G. S. Greenwald, eds., Raven
Press, New York. (In press.)

Gospodarowicz, D., and Bialecki, H., 1979, Fibroblast and
epidermal growth factors are mitogenic agents for cultured
granulosa cells of rodent, porcine, and human origin,
Endocrinology 104:757.

Gospodarowicz, D., Mescher, A. L., and Birdwell, C. R., 1978a,
Control of cellular proliferation by the fibroblast and
epidermal growth factors, Natl. Cancer Inst. Monogr.
48:109.

Gospodarowicz, D., Vlodavsky, I., Bialecki, H., and Brown,
K. D., 1978b, The control of proliferation of ovarian cells
by the epidermal and fibroblast growth factors, in: "Novel
Aspects of Reproductive Physiology", C. H. Spilman and J.
W. Wilks, eds., pp. 107-108, Spectrum Publications, New
York.

Heldin, C.-H., Wasteson, Å., and Westermark, B., 1981, Specific
binding of ^{125}I-labeled platelet-derived growth factor to
cultured cells, in: "The Biology of Normal Human Growth",

M. Ritźen, ed., pp. 23-31, Raven Press, New York.

Hseuh, A. J. W., and Erickson, G. F., 1979, Extrapituitary action of gonadotropin-releasing hormone: direct inhibition of ovarian steroidogenesis, Science, 204:854.

Hsueh, A. J. W., and Ling, N. C., 1979, Effect of an antagonistic analog of gonadotropin-releasing hormone upon ovarian granulosa cell function, Life Sci. 25:1223.

Hsueh, A. J. W., and Jones, P. B. C., 1982, Direct hormonal modulation of ovarian granulosa cell maturation: effect of gonadotropin-releasing hormone, in: "Follicular Maturation and Ovulation", International Congress Series #506, R. Roland, E. V. Van Hall, S. G., Hillier, K. P., McNatty, and J. Schoemaker, eds., pp. 19-33, Exerpta Medica, Amsterdam.

Hsueh, A. J. W., Welsh, T. H., and Jones, P. B. C., 1981, Inhibition of ovarian and testicular steroidogenesis by epidermal growth factor, Endocrinology 108:2002.

Johnson, L. K., Baxter, J. D., Vlodavsky, I., and Gospodarowicz, D., 1980, Epidermal growth factor and expression of specific genes: effects on cultured rat pituitary cells are dissociable from the mitogenic response, Proc. Natl. Acad. Sci. USA 77:394.

Jones, P. B. C., and Hsueh, A. J. W., 1981, Regulation of ovarian 20α-hydroxysteroid dehydrogenase by gonadotropin-releasing hormone and its antagonist in vitro and in vivo, J. Steroid Biochem. 14:1169.

Jones, P. B. C., Conn, P. M., Marian, J., and Hsueh, A. J. W., 1980, Binding of gonadotropin-releasing hormone agonist to rat ovarian granulosa cells, Life Sci. 27:2125.

Jones, P. B. C., Welsh, T. H., and Hsueh, A. J. W., 1983, Regulation of ovarian progestin production by epidermal growth factor in cultured granulosa cells, in: "Factors Regulating Ovarian Function", P. Terranova and G. S. Greenwald, eds., Raven Press, New York (in press).

Knecht, M., and Catt, K. J., 1981, Gonadotropin-releasing hormone: regulation of adenosine 3',5'-monophosphate in ovarian granulosa cells, Science 214:1346.

Knecht, M., and Ranta, T., 1982, Growth factors modify granulosa cell function through alterations in FSH-induced cAMP accumulation, Endocrinology 110 (Supplement):290 (Abstract #841).

Knecht, M., Amsterdam, A., and Catt, K. J., 1981, The regulatory role of cAMP in hormone-induced granulosa cell differentiation, J. Biol. Chem. 256:10628.

Louvet, J.-P., Harman, S. M., Schreiber, J. R., and Ross, G. T.,

1975, Evidence for a role of androgens in follicular maturation, Endocrinology 97:366.

McNatty, K. P., Smith, D. M., Makris, A., Osathanondh, R., and
Ryan, K., 1979, The microenvironment of the human antral
follicle: interrelationships among steroid levels in
antral fluid, the population of granulosa cells, and the
status of the oocyte in vivo and in vitro, J. Clin.
Endocrinol. Metab. 49:851.

Mondschein, J. S., and Schomberg, D. W., 1981a, Growth factors
modulate gonadotropin receptor induction in granulosa cell
cultures, Science 211:1179.

Mondschein, J. S., and Schomberg, D. W., 1981b, Platelet-derived
growth factor enhances granulosa cell luteinizing hormone
receptor induction by follicle-stimulating hormone and
serum, Endocrinology 109:325.

Mondschein, J. S., May, J. V., Gunn, E. B., and Schomberg, D.
W., 1981, Modulation by epidermal growth factor of LH/hCG
receptor binding in porcine granulosa cell cultures:
implications for follicle development and atresia, in:
"Dynamics of Ovarian Function", N. B. Schwartz and
M. Hunzicker-Dunn, eds., pp. 83-88, Raven Press, New
York.

Nimrod, A., 1981, The induction of ovarian LH-receptors by
FSH is mediated by cAMP, F. E. B. S. Letters 131:31.

Nimrod, A., and Lindner, H. R., 1976, A synergistic effect of
androgen on the stimulation of progesterone secretion by
FSH in cultured rat granulosa cells, Mol. Cell. Endocrinol.
5:315.

Pencharz, R. I., 1940, Effects of estrogen and androgens alone
and in combination with chorionic gonadotropin on the ovary
of the hypophysectomized rat, Science 91:554.

Rao, M. C., Richards, J. S., and Midgley, A. R., Jr., 1977,
Regulation of gonadotropin receptors by luteinizing hormone
in granulosa cells, Endocrinology 101:512.

Reichert, L. E., Jr., Sanzo, M. A., and Darga, N. S., 1979,
Studies on a low molecular weight follicle-stimulating
hormone binding inhibitor from human serum, J. Clin.
Endocrinol. Metab. 49:866.

Richards, J. S., 1980, Maturation of ovarian follicles: actions
and interactions of pituitary and ovarian hormones on
follicular cell differentiation, Physiol. Rev. 60:51.

Richards, J. S., and Midgley, A. R., Jr., 1976, Protein hormone
action: a key to understanding ovarian follicular and
luteal cell development, Biol. Reprod. 14:1562.

Richards, J. S., Ireland, J. J., Rao, M. C., Bernath, G. A.,

Midgley, A. R., Jr., and Reichert, L. E., Jr., 1976, Ovarian follicular development in the rat: hormone receptor regulation by estradiol, follicle-stimulating hormone, and luteinizing hormone, Endocrinology 99:1563.

Ross, R., 1981, The platelet-derived growth factor, in: "Tissue Growth Factors", R. Baserga, ed., pp. 133-159, Springer-Verlag, Berlin.

Sanders, M. M., and Midgley, A. R., Jr., 1981, Cyclic nucleotides can induce LH/hCG receptors in cultured rat granulosa cells, Endocrinology 108 (Supplement):165 (Abstract #332).

Schomberg, D. W., 1979, Steroidal modulation of steroid secretion in vitro: an experimental approach to intra-follicular regulation mechanisms, in: "Ovarian Follicular and Corpus Luteum Function", C. P. Channing, J. M. Marsh, and W. A. Sadler, eds., pp. 155-168, Plenum Press, New York.

Schomberg, D. W., Stouffer, R. L., and Tyrey, L., 1976, Modulation of progestin secretion in ovarian cells by 17β-hydroxy-5α-androstan-3-one (dihydrotestosterone): a direct demonstration in monolayer culture, Biochem. Biophys. Res. Comm. 68:77.

Schomberg, D. W., May, J. V., and Mondschein, J. S., 1983a, Epidermal growth factor attenuates FSH-, cAMP-, or cholera toxin-mediated LH receptor induction in granulosa cell cultures, in: "Factors Regulating Ovarian Function", P. Terranova and G. S. Greenwald, eds., Raven Press, New York (in press).

Schomberg, D. W., May, J. V., and Mondschein, J. S., 1983b, Interactions between hormones and growth factors in the regulation of granulosa cell differentiation in vitro, J. Steroid Biochem. (in press).

Schreiber, J. R., and Hsueh, A. J. W., 1979, Progesterone "receptor" in rat ovary, Endocrinology 105:915.

St-Arnaud, R., Kelly, P. A., Walker, P., and Labrie, F., 1983, Characterization and hormonal control of epidermal growth factor (EGF) receptors in the rat ovary, in: "Factors Regulating Ovarian Function", P. Terranova and G. S. Greenwald, eds., Raven Press, New York (in press).

Vlodavsky, I., Brown, K. D., and Gospodarowicz, D., 1978, A comparison of the binding of epidermal growth factor to cultured granulosa and luteal cells, J. Biol. Chem. 253:3744.

Zeleznik, A. J., Midgley, A. R., Jr., and Reichert, L. E., 1974, Granulosa cell maturation in the rat: increased binding of hCG following treatment with FSH in vivo, Endocrinology 95:818.

REGULATION OF GONADOTROPIN RECEPTORS AND STEROIDOGENIC

RESPONSES IN CULTURED LEYDIG TUMOR CELLS

Mario Ascoli[abc] and Dale A. Freeman[ab]

[a]Division of Endocrinology
[b]Departments of Medicine and [c]Biochemistry
Vanderbilt Medical School
Nashville, TN 37232

1. Introduction

The regulation of cell surface receptors for polypeptide hormones is now recognized as an important mechanism in the regulation of target cell responsiveness (reviewed by Hazum, 1982; King and Cuatrecasas, 1981; Kaplan, 1981; Tell et al., 1978; Catt et al., 1979). Thus, changes in target cell responsiveness associated with several physiological or pathological conditions can be explained in terms of changes in the number of surface receptors (Olefsky and Ciaraldi, 1981; Archer et al., 1975; Purvis et al., 1978; Briefel et al., 1982; Klemcke and Bartke, 1981).

The number of cell surface receptors for a given polypeptide hormone can theoretically be regulated by the homologous hormone, as well as by heterologous hormones. The homologous down-regulation of receptors is a well documented and rather common phenomenon (Hazum, 1982; Kaplan, 1981; King and Cuatrecasas, 1981; Tell et al., 1978; Catt et al., 1979). Heterologous regulation (up or down), however, is not as common and has not been explored in great detail. Some examples include the up-regulation of LH/hCG receptors in granulosa cells by FSH (Zeleznik et al., 1974; Erickson et al., 1979); the down-regulation of somatostatin receptors in pituitary tumor cells by TRH and glucocorticoids (Schonbrum and Tashjian, 1980; Schonbrum, 1981); the up-regulation of insulin receptors in 3T3 cells and IM-9 lymphocytes by glucocorticoids (Fantus et al., 1982; Knutson et al., 1982); the down-regulation of EGF receptors by nerve growth factor in PC12 cells (Huff and Guroff, 1979); and the down-regulation of LH/hCG receptors in granulosa cells and Leydig tumor cells by mEGF (Ascoli, 1981b; Mondschein and Schomberg, 1981).

The normal responsiveness of target cells can also be regulated by changes in the specific metabolic pathways that are involved in the cellular response (henceforth referred to as effector system). The best examples of this kind of regulation are perhaps provided by mutant cell lines that have relatively normal numbers of hormone receptors, but do not respond to the hormone with the expected alterations of cell function (Rae et al., 1979; Johnson et al., 1980). Some pathological states have now been explained on this basis (Briefel et al., 1982; Farfel et al., 1980; Chait et al., 1982).

The data reviewed in this chapter deals with the regulation of LH/hCG receptors and responses in cultured Leydig tumor cells. Where appropriate, the results obtained in this system are compared with the results of other investigators in normal Leydig cells and/or granulosa/luteal cells. A more detailed description of these systems can be found in several recent reviews (Catt et al., 1979, 1980; Nozu et al., 1982; Harwood et al., 1978).

2.   Cultured Leydig Tumor Cells as a Model to Study the Regulation of LH/hCG Receptors and Responses

The MA-10 cells are a clonal strain of Leydig tumor cells adapted to continuous culture in this laboratory (Ascoli, 1981a). The cells originated from a transplantable tumor - designated M5480P - of the C57BL/6 mouse (Ascoli and Puett, 1978a). The transplanted tumor was shown to have functional LH/hCG receptors, and the major steroid produced by the cells was identified as progesterone (Ascoli and Puett, 1978a; Lacroix et al., 1979). Upon culturing and cloning, the number of hCG receptors increased about 2-fold, and the steroid pathway remained essentially unchanged, except for an apparent increase in 20α-hydroxylase activity (Ascoli, 1981a). Thus, the major steroid synthesized by the MA-10 cells is progesterone, but some of it is eventually metabolized to 20α-dihydroprogesterone (Ascoli, 1981a,b). Increased production of this steroid is a rather common phenomenon that also occurs upon culturing other steroidogenic cells (reviewed by Ascoli, 1982a). This is one of the two major differences between the differentiated function of the

MA-10 cells and normal Leydig cells. The inability of the
MA-10 cells to synthesize testosterone from endogenous precursors (Fig. 1) is apparently due to a decrease in the activity
of 17α-hydroxylase, which occurred during transplantation
(Moyle and Greep, 1974; Lacroix et al., 1980). The apparent
loss of 17α-hydroxylase activity does not seem too surprising
in view of recent data that suggest that in normal Leydig
cells this enzyme is regulated by several hormones (Nozu et
al., 1982; Rommerts and Brinkman, 1981; Welsh and Hsueh,
1982; Adashi and Hsueh, 1982; Bambino et al., 1980). Because
of these changes, the final products of the steroidogenic
pathway of the MA-10 cells resemble the final products of
normal granulosa/luteal cells, and other steroid producing
cells of malignant origin (Ascoli, 1982a), more than the
final products of normal Leydig cells.

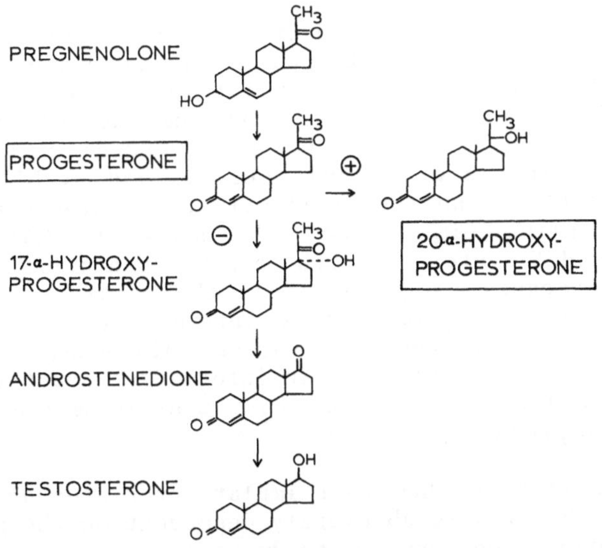

Figure 1. Pathway for steroid biosynthesis in normal mouse
Leydig cells and the MA-10 cells. Normal mouse Leydig cells
synthesize testosterone primarily via the Δ4 pathway. The
MA-10 cells synthesize progesterone and 20α-dihydroprogester-
one presumably because of reduced levels of 17α-hydroxylase
(indicated by-) and elevated levels of 20α-hydroxylase
(indicated by +) activities. Data taken from Lacroix et al.
(1979) and Ascoli (1981a).

The other major difference between normal Leydig cells and the MA-10 cells is in the coupling between hCG binding and steroid production. Thus, while maximal stimulation of testosterone production in normal rat Leydig cells occurs when only about 1% of the hCG receptors are occupied (Mendelson et al., 1975), maximal stimulation of progesterone production in the MA-10 cells occurs when 60-70% of the hCG receptors are occupied (Fig. 2). Since normal rat Leydig cells (Tsuruhara et al., 1977; Catt et al., 1980) and the MA-10 cells (Ascoli, 1981a,b; Freeman and Ascoli, 1981) have 10-20,000 hCG receptors/cell, the difference in coupling does not appear to be due to changes in the number of hCG receptors. Therefore, one must consider other factors such as species variability (see Mendelson et al., 1975; Schumacher et al., 1979), different experimental protocols, the hetero-geneity of rat Leydig cells (Payne et al., 1982), and the efficiency of translation of hormone binding into a metabolic response (Strickland and Loeb, 1981). Nevertheless, the main aspect of the differentiated function of normal Leydig cells (i.e., the presence of LH/hCG receptors "coupled" to the steroidogenic pathway) has been retained by the MA-10 cells. This characteristic, together with the ease of experimental manipulation inherent in anchorage dependent cultured cells, the homogeneity (i.e., clonal strain) and stability of the cell population, and the availability of large quantities of cells (doubling time $\cong$ 20 hr), makes the MA-10 cells a suitable model system in which to study gonadotropin actions. Moreover, because progesterone is the major steroid product and since it is an obligatory intermediate in all steroid producing cells (adrenals, ovaries, placenta, and testes), one may argue that any specific information about the factors controlling the synthesis of this steroid may be common to all steroid producing tissues.

The ability of hCG to stimulate progesterone production in the MA-10 cells is absolutely dependent on the presence of hCG receptors and appears to be mediated by the adenylate cyclase/protein kinase pathway. Evidence for the absolute requirement of the hCG receptors is nicely illustrated by studies on three other clonal lines (designated MA-14, MA-16 and MA-19) derived from the same culture used to establish the MA-10 cells (Ascoli, 1981a). These clonal lines bind little or no hCG and do not respond to the hormone with increased steroid production. Their effector system, however, is intact, as judged by the ability of cholera toxin and cAMP to stimulate steroid production (Ascoli, 1981a). The binding

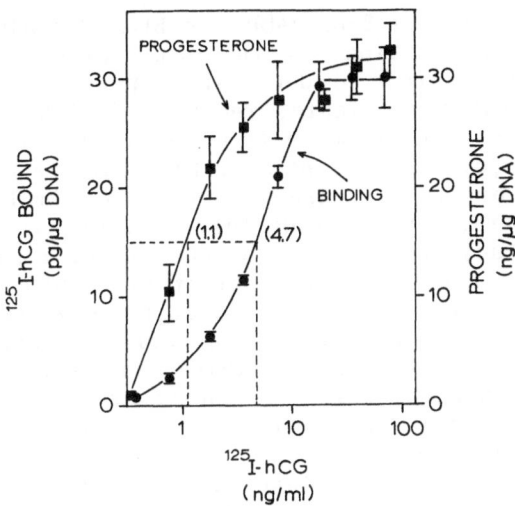

Figure 2. Relationship between ^{125}I-hCG binding (black circles) and progesterone production (black squares) in the MA-10 cells. Hormone binding and progesterone accumulation were measured after a 2 hr incubation at 37° in serum-free medium.

of hCG to its cell surface receptors is followed by the internalization and degradation of the hormone. It is important to note that these steps do not appear to be required for the stimulation of cAMP or steroid production (Ascoli and Puett, 1978b,c; Ascoli, 1978, 1979, 1982b,c; Segaloff and Ascoli, 1981) but seem to be required for the down-regulation of receptors (see Section 3).

The involvement of cAMP in the stimulation of progesterone biosynthesis by hCG has not been rigorously established in the MA-10 cells. Its role is inferred by analogy with other steroid producing cells (Ascoli, 1982a) and by the finding that hCG increases the intracellular levels of cAMP in a dose-dependent manner prior to increasing progesterone biosynthesis (Segaloff and Ascoli, 1981). Moreover, when the surface-bound hCG is released from the cells, the elevated intracellular levels of cAMP and the elevated rate of progesterone production fall in a parallel fashion (Segaloff and Ascoli, 1981). The involvement of cAMP is also supported by the ability of cholera toxin and cAMP analogues to stimulate progesterone production (Fig. 3). During short-term (4 hr) incubations, hCG and 8-Br-cAMP (or Bt_2cAMP) always stimulate progesterone production to the same extent. The maximal amount of progesterone produced in response to cholera toxin, however, is rather variable, reaching 60-100% of the maximal amounts produced in response to hCG or cAMP analogues (Ascoli, 1978; 1981a,b,c; Segaloff et al., 1981a,b; Freeman and Ascoli, 1981). The ability of these compounds to stimulate progesterone biosynthesis offers a useful experimental tool that can be used to study the activity of the effector system independently of the hCG receptor (Catt et al., 1980; Ascoli, 1978, 1981a,b,c; Segaloff et al., 1981a,b; Freeman and Ascoli, 1981). Cholera toxin binds to a surface receptor different than the hCG receptor (Ascoli, 1978) and presumably stimulates progesterone biosynthesis by increasing adenylate cyclase activity, the step most proximal to hCG binding. On the other hand, the addition of a cAMP analogue bypasses this step and presumably stimulates progesterone biosynthesis by increasing the activity of cAMP-dependent protein kinases.

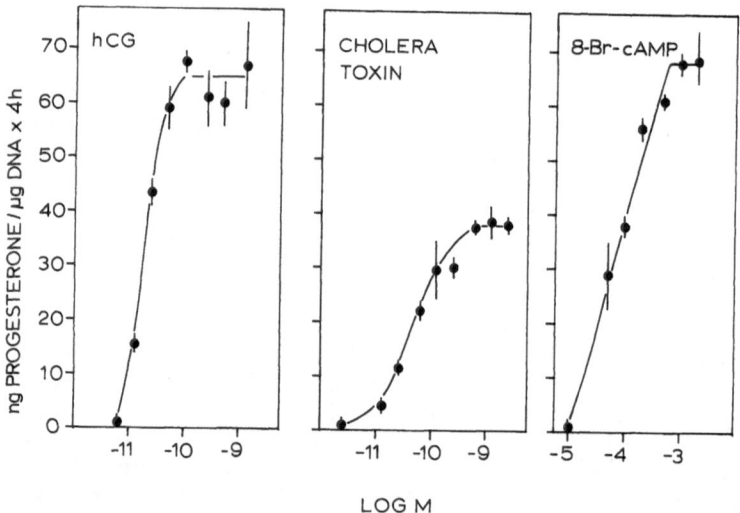

Figure 3. Effects of hCG, cholera toxin and 8-Br-cAMP on progesterone production by the MA-10 cells. Cells were incubated in serum-free medium with the indicated concentrations of each stimuli for 4 hr at 37° prior to the determination of progesterone.

The hormonal message that is initiated by the binding of hCG to the cell surface and translated by the adenylate cyclase/protein kinase pathway eventually leads to increased mobilization of cholesterol into the mitochondria and increased conversion of cholesterol to pregnenolone. The conversion of pregnenolone to progesterone does not appear to be affected by hCG (Ascoli, 1982a).

As will be discussed below (see Section 5), the supply of cholesterol is an important factor in the regulation of progesterone production in the MA-10 cells. Like other cells, the MA-10 cells have three sources of cholesterol: intracellular stores, newly synthesized cholesterol, and lipoprotein-derived cholesterol. Recent studies from this laboratory show that when progesterone biosynthesis is stimulated with hCG the MA-10 cells utilize all of these sources to different extents, depending on their availability and on the duration of hormonal stimulation (Ascoli, 1981c; Freeman and Ascoli, 1982a,b). These results can be summarized as follows (Fig. 4). Under basal conditions (Fig. 4A), the cells have 2-4 times more free than esterified cholesterol (Albert et al., 1980; Segaloff et al., 1981b; Ascoli, 1981c; Freeman and Ascoli, 1982a,b), and progesterone biosynthesis is very low. The intracellular levels of cholesterol appeared to be derived primarily from a relatively high level of de novo synthesis, rather than from the uptake of lipoproteins (Morris and Chaikoff, 1959; Andersen and Dietschy, 1978; Ascoli, 1981c; Freeman and Ascoli, 1982a,b). When the cells are stimulated with hCG (Fig. 4B), most (~70%) of the progesterone synthesized in the first four hours is derived from intracellular stores. Kinetic studies indicate that the esterified cholesterol is used more rapidly than the free cholesterol. In the absence of LDL in the medium, the decline in intracellular levels of esterified and free cholesterol is dramatic: 70 and 50% reduction, respectively. In the presence of LDL, these declines are not as pronounced (Freeman and Ascoli, 1982a,b). During this time, the activity of HMG-CoA reductase increases 2-3 fold, and cholesterol esterification declines to 10-20% of control levels. The presence of LDL does not affect these events. Upon prolonged stimulation (Fig. 4C), the binding, uptake and degradation of LDL increase about 30% (Freeman and Ascoli, 1982a,b), and the activity of HMG-CoA reductase and cholesterol esterification return toward control levels. If LDL is present, it provides most (~65%) of the cholesterol

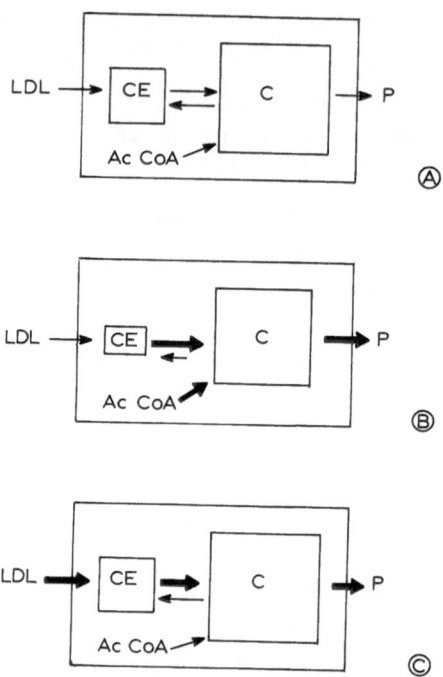

Figure 4. Model for the effects of hCG on cholesterol metabolism and steroid biosynthesis in the MA-10 cells. In the
absence of hCG (Panel A), the intracellular levels of cholesterol (C) and cholesterol esters (CE) are maintained by the
uptake of LDL, de novo synthesis of cholesterol, and the
hydrolysis and formation of cholesterol esters. Under these
conditions the rate of progesterone (P) biosynthesis is low,
and the cells have 2-4 times more free than esterified
cholesterol. Upon addition of hCG (Panel B), the rate of
progesterone biosynthesis increases and the intracellular
stores of free and esterified cholesterol decline. As a
consequence of this, the rate of de novo synthesis of
cholesterol increases and the rate of cholesterol esterification declines. Upon prolonged stimulation (Panel C), the
rates of de novo synthesis of cholesterol and of cholesterol
esterification return toward non-stimulated levels and the
binding, uptake and degradation of LDL increase. The
cholesterol so derived is used to replenish the intracellular
pools and to maintain an elevated rate of progesterone biosynthesis. After Freeman and Ascoli (1982a,b).

needed for progesterone biosynthesis apparently via the classic LDL pathway (Brown and Goldstein, 1979; Brown et al., 1979), and the rate of progesterone biosynthesis remains elevated. If LDL is not present, most (∿95%) of the cholesterol needed for steroid biosynthesis is derived from de novo synthesis. Under these conditions, the rate of progesterone biosynthesis falls because it is limited by the supply of cholesterol (Freeman and Ascoli, 1982a,b).

In the following sections, we review our data on the mechanisms by which two hormones, mEGF and hCG, regulate the hCG receptors and steroidogenic responses of the MA-10 cells. The results show that (a) both hormones down-regulate the number of surface hCG receptors, albeit by different mechanisms, and (b) hCG, but not mEGF, reduce the activity of the effector system by depleting the intracellular levels of cholesterol.

3.   Down-Regulation of hCG Receptors by mEGF and hCG

3.1. General Properties of hCG Receptor Regulation

The MA-10 cells have separate receptors for mEGF and hCG (Ascoli, 1981b). Evidence for the specificity of these receptors is provided by the finding that a high concentration of mEGF does not prevent the binding of ^{125}I-hCG, and a high concentration of hCG does not prevent the binding of ^{125}I-mEGF. Moreover, the number of mEGF receptors present in the MA-10 and MA-14 cells are nearly identical, while the numbers of hCG receptors differ by a factor of at least 50.

During preliminary studies on the effects of mEGF on the multiplication of the cultured Leydig tumor cells, we noticed that mEGF had little or no effect on cell multiplication, but reduced the ^{125}I-hCG binding activity in all the clonal lines of Leydig tumor cells (Ascoli, 1981a,b). In more detailed studies on the effects of mEGF on the ^{125}I-hCG binding activity of the MA-10 cells, it was shown that prolonged exposure (48 hr) to mEGF reduced ^{125}I-hCG binding by 70-90% (Ascoli, 1981b). Because of previous studies on the effects of hCG on the ^{125}I-hCG binding activity of normal rat Leydig cells (Catt et al., 1979), normal rat granulosa/luteal cells (Harwood et al., 1978), and freshly isolated Leydig tumor

cells (Ascoli and Puett, 1978b), we also tested the ability
of hCG to reduce ^{125}I-hCG binding activity in the MA-10
cells. As expected, a reduction, which cannot be accounted
for by receptor occupancy, was observed (Freeman and Ascoli,
1981). The results presented in Table I summarize our data
and show that prolonged exposure of the MA-10 cells to hCG
results in a reduction in ^{125}I-hCG binding (homologous down-
regulation) and little or no change in ^{125}I-mEGF binding;
prolonged exposure to mEGF results in a reduction in ^{125}I-mEGF
binding (homologous down-regulation) and ^{125}I-hCG binding
(heterologous down-regulation).

Table I. Effects of Prolonged Exposure to mEGF or hCG on
^{125}I-mEGF and ^{125}I-hCG Binding in the MA-10 Cells

Pretreatment	^{125}I-Hormone Bound (pg/µg DNA)	
	^{125}I-mEGF	^{125}I-hCG
None	5.24	21.40
mEGF	0.14	5.30
hCG	4.50	0.30

Cells were incubated at 37° for 48 hr with 5 ng/ml mEGF or
for 24 hr with 40 ng/ml hCG. The binding of ^{125}I-mEGF and
^{125}I-hCG was determined at 4° as described elsewhere (Ascoli,
1982b).

The time courses required for the homologous and heterologous down-regulation of ^{125}I-hCG binding are different
(Figure 5). Homologous down-regulation occurs rapidly.
Half maximal and maximal reduction were observed about 2 hr
and 14 hr, respectively, after addition of hCG. Heterologous

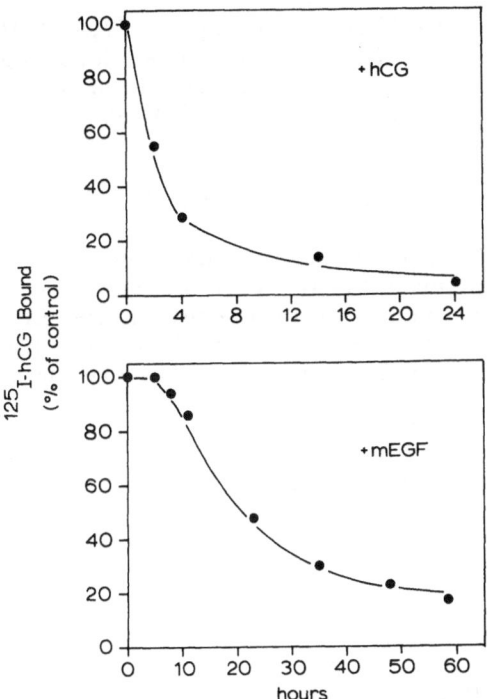

Figure 5. Time course of homologous and heterologous down-regulation of ^{125}I-hCG binding activity. Cells were incubated with 40 ng/ml hCG (top panel) or 5 ng/ml mEGF (bottom panel) at 37°. ^{125}I-hCG binding was determined (after washing) at different times after addition of the hormones. In the experiment shown in the top panel, the surface-bound hCG was released prior to determining ^{125}I-hCG binding. Reproduced (by permission) from Ascoli (1981b) and Freeman and Ascoli (1981).

down-regulation is not detectable for at least 5 hr following addition of mEGF. Half maximal and maximal reduction were observed 15-18 hr and 36-48 hr, respectively, after addition of mEGF.

The concentrations of mEGF and hCG required to reduce ^{125}I-hCG binding are shown in Fig. 6. For the homologous down-regulation, half maximal and maximal effects were obtained with

1 ng/ml (2.6 × 10^{-11}M) and 10 ng/ml (2.6 × 10^{-10}M) of hCG, respectively. For the heterologous down-regulation, half maximal and maximal effects were observed with 0.5 ng/ml (8 × 10^{-11}M) and 2 ng/ml (3.2 × 10^{-10}M) of mEGF, respectively. These hormone concentrations are well within the range of those required for the expression of other biologic actions (cf. Fig. 2, and Carpenter and Cohen, 1979).

Further experiments were done in which ^{125}I-hCG binding activity was assayed by analysis of the binding of ^{125}I-hCG under conditions where binding equilibrium occurs and all of the hormone is localized at the cell surface (Ascoli, 1982b,c; Lloyd and Ascoli, 1983). These results are summarized in

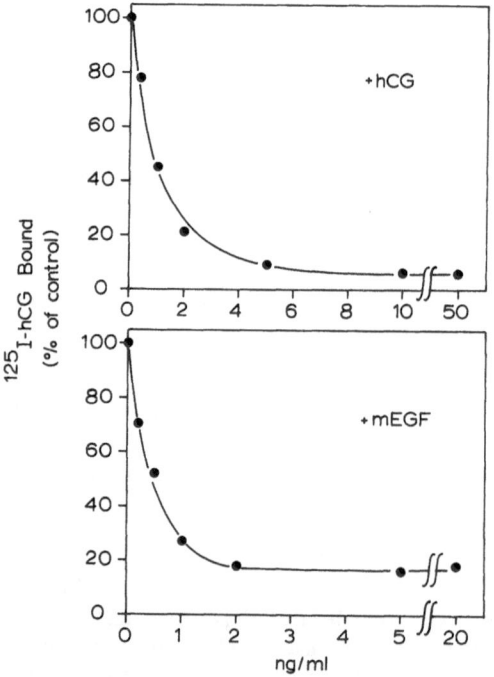

Figure 6. Dose-responses for the homologous and heterologous down-regulation of ^{125}I-hCG binding activity. Cells were incubated with the indicated concentrations of hCG (top panel) or mEGF (bottom panel) for 14 hr or 48 hr, respectively. ^{125}h-CG binding was determined after washing. Bottom panel is reproduced (by permission) from Ascoli (1981b).

Table II and show that both hormones reduce the number of surface hCG receptors. hCG has no effect on the affinity of the hCG receptor, but mEGF increases it about 50%. It should also be noted that the maximal reduction in the number of surface hCG receptors observed with mEGF and hCG are somewhat different. With mEGF, the surface hCG receptors can be maximally reduced by 70-90% (Ascoli, 1981b; Lloyd and Ascoli, 1983). With hCG, the maximal reduction is at least 90% (Freeman and Ascoli, 1981).

Table II. Effects of mEGF and hCG on the Equilibrium Binding Constants of ^{125}I-hCG binding to the Surface of the MA-10 Cells

Pretreatment	Kd ($M \times 10^{-10}$)	R_S^0 (Receptors/cell)
None	5.0	12,075
mEGF	7.4	2,593
hCG	5.0	604

Cells were incubated at 37° for 48 hr with 5 ng/ml mEGF or for 14 hr with 40 ng/ml hCG. Equilibrium binding of ^{125}I-hCG was analyzed at 4° as described elsewhere (Ascoli, 1982b,c; Lloyd and Ascoli, 1983).

These results suggested to us that the mechanisms involved in the homologous and heterologous down-regulation of the surface hCG receptors may be different. Further support for this hypothesis came from studies on the time courses required for the receptors to recover from the down-regulated state. The results presented in Fig. 7 show that following homologous down-regulation the surface hCG receptors begin to recover as soon as hCG is removed. Following heterologous down-regulation, the surface hCG receptors do not begin to recover until about 8 hr after removal of mEGF.

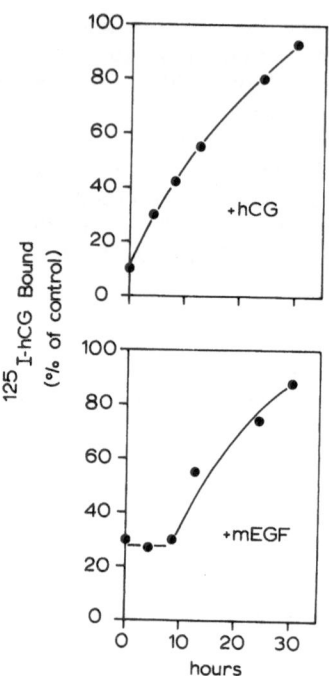

Figure 7. Time course of recovery of ^{125}I-hCG binding activity from the down-regulated state. Cells were preincubated with 40 ng/ml hCG (top panel) or 5 ng/ml mEGF (bottom panel) for 16 hr or 48 hr (37°), respectively. The cells were washed (t = 0) to remove the free hormones and incubated further (37°) in hormone-free medium. ^{125}I-hCG binding was determined at the indicated times following hormone removal.

3.2. mEGF and hCG Down-Regulate hCG Receptors by Different Mechanisms

We have recently begun to study the mechanisms by which mEGF and hCG down-regulate the surface hCG receptors (Lloyd and Ascoli, 1983). In order to study these phenomena, we started with the assumption that at any given steady state the number of surface hCG receptors (R_S) is given by:

$$[R]_S = V_R/kt \qquad (1)$$

where V_R = rate of insertion of receptors into the membrane, and kt = rate constant for internalization of the surface receptors (Wiley and Cunningham, 1981). It follows, then, that $[R]_S$ can be altered by changes in V_R and/or kt. Thus, if one could determine these constants in cells pretreated with mEGF or hCG, the mechanisms involved in the regulation of surface hCG receptors could be assessed. One way to approach this problem is to use a model recently described by Wiley and Cunningham (1981, 1982) to study the interaction of polypeptide ligands with their target cells. This model is based on the observation that, upon binding to their cell surface receptors, some polypeptide ligands are internalized and degraded, and that these processes eventually reach a steady state. By analyzing the surface binding, internalization, and degradation of the ligand at the steady state, it is possible to calculate V_R and kt (see above), as well as the rate constant for internalization of the ligand-receptor complex (ke) and the rate constant for degradation of the internalized ligand (kh) (Wiley and Cunningham, 1981, 1982). This model was easily applied to the study of the interaction of hCG with the MA-10 cells because we had previously characterized the binding, internalization, and degradation of hCG in some detail (Ascoli, 1982b,c). Thus, by measuring these processes in control and mEGF-treated cells, it was possible to show (Table III) that hCG down-regulates its surface receptors because the rate of internalization of the occupied receptor (ke) is 24 times faster than the rate of internalization of the unoccupied receptor (kt). On the other hand, mEGF down-regulates the hCG receptor because it decreases the rate of receptor insertion into the membrane (V_R) five-fold. mEGF has little or no effect on the rate constants for internalization of the unoccupied (kt) or occupied hCG receptors (ke), or the rate constant for degradation of the internalized hCG (kh) (Lloyd and Ascoli, 1983).

Our current thinking about the interaction of hCG with the MA-10 cells and the mechanisms involved in the regulation of hCG receptors is presented in Fig. 8. In this model, the number of surface hCG receptors, R_S, is balanced by the rate of insertion of receptors into the surface (V_R) and the rate constant for receptor internalization (kt). V_R may be defined as the product of the number of intracellular receptors (Ri) times a rate constant for insertion (ki). Alternatively, V_R may be viewed as being directly proportional to the rate of receptor synthesis (Z).

The heterologous down-regulation of surface hCG receptor by mEGF occurs because V_R is reduced. It is not known if this

is due to reduction in receptor synthesis (Z), the number
of intracellular receptors (Ri), or the rate constant
for insertion of receptors into the surface (ki).

When hCG (H) is added to the cells it binds to the cell
surface receptor, presumably in a reversible fashion, dictated
by an association (ka) and a dissociation (kd) rate constant.
Our studies have shown that upon binding of hCG, the receptor-
bound hormone $(HR)_s$ is internalized $((H-R)_i)$ and eventually
degraded (Ascoli and Puett, 1978b,c; Ascoli, 1979, 1980,
1982b,c). The homologous down-regulation of the surface hCG
receptors occurs because the rate constant for internalization
of the occupied receptor (ke) is faster than the rate constant
for internalization of the free hCG receptor (kt). Also note
that in order for internalization of $(H-R)_s$ to occur, the
rate constant for internalization (ke) must be faster than
the rate constant for dissociation of the hormone from the
surface receptor (kd). Although we have not measured kd,
other investigators have determined it to be in the order of
10^{-3}-10^{-4} min^{-1} in normal rat target membranes (Lee and Ryan,
1973; Ketelslegers et al., 1975). These constants are 40-400
times slower than our estimates of ke (cf. Table III).

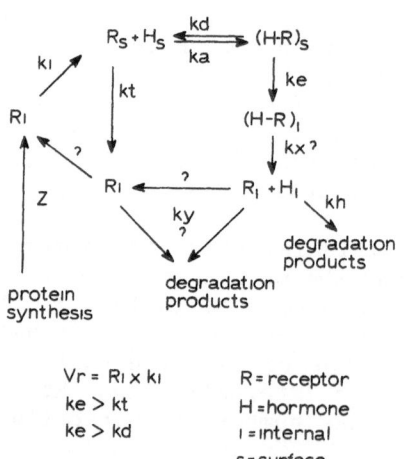

Figure 8. A model for the metabolic fate of the receptor-
bound hCG and the regulation of surface hCG receptors. See
text for details.

Table III. Cellular Constants for the Turnover of Free and Occupied hCG Receptors in Control and mEGF-Treated MA-10 Cells

	Control	mEGF
V_R (Receptors/cell $\times$ min)	21	4
kt (min^{-1})	1.7×10^{-3}	1.5×10^{-3}
ke (min^{-1})	4.0×10^{-2}	3.7×10^{-2}
kh (min^{-1})	5.5×10^{-3}	6.1×10^{-3}

Cells were incubated with or without mEGF (5 ng/ml) for 48 hr prior to analysis. The different constants shown were measured as described by Wiley and Cunningham (1982).

     In our model, we presume that hCG is internalized while bound to its receptor $(H-R)_i$. The fate of the internalized hormone (Hi) has been studied in detail. Our studies have shown that it reaches its place of degradation (presumably the lysosomes) in the intact form (i.e., without dissociating into subunits). The pathway of degradation is complex and involves partial degradation of the intact hormone, followed by subunit dissociation and further degradation of the free subunits (Ascoli, 1980, 1982b,c). In Fig. 8, this process occurs at a rate dictated by kh. The fate of the receptor is not known. We propose that the internalized hCG (Hi) dissociates from the internalized complex - $(H-R)_i$ - before degradation of the hormone occurs. This pathway is proposed because we have shown that the hCG-receptor complex dissociates rapidly under acidic conditions (Ascoli, 1982b,c), and the internalized complex should be exposed to an acidic environment, either in endocytotic vesicles (Tycko and Maxfield, 1982) or in the lysosomes (Ohkuma and Poole, 1978). The rate constant that determines this dissociation (kx) is probably faster than ke, since the dissociation of the hormone-receptor complex at pH 3 is almost complete (or complete) in 2 min

(Ascoli, 1982b,c). The fate of the receptor (Ri) is not known. It may be degraded or recycled back to the cell surface (pathways indicated by ? in Fig. 8).

4.   Regulation of Steroidogenic Responses by mEGF and hCG

4.1. Regulation of hCG Stimulated Steroidogenesis

The results presented in Figures 9 and 10 show that, when the surface hCG receptors of the MA-10 are down-regulated with mEGF (Fig. 9) or hCG (Fig. 10), there is a parallel loss of hCG-stimulated progesterone production. This loss is observed mainly as a reduction in the maximal amount of progesterone produced in response to high concentrations of hCG. Further analysis of the data (Table IV) confirmed (cf. Table II) that hCG reduces the maximal binding of ^{125}I-hCG without changing the affinity of the cells for the hormone, and that mEGF, in addition to reducing the maximal binding of ^{125}I-hCG, increases the affinity of the cells to the hormone. The progesterone responses to hCG are similarly affected by both hormones: the maximal amount of progesterone

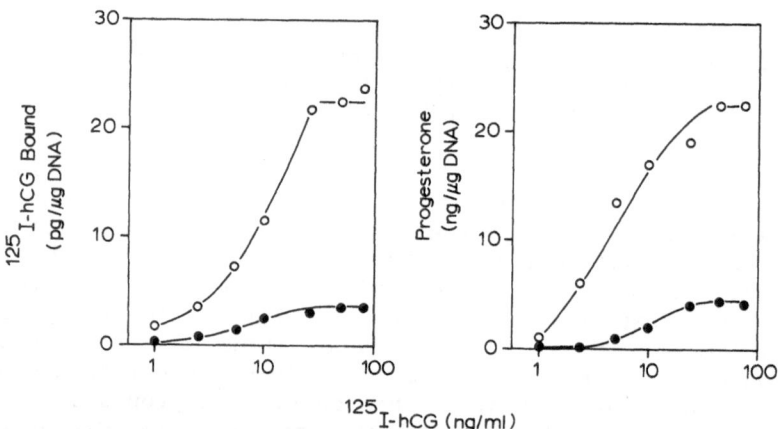

Figure 9. Relationship between ^{125}I-hCG binding (left panel) and progesterone production (right panel) in mEGF-treated cells. Cells were incubated without (open circle) or with (black circle) 5 ng/ml mEGF for 48 hr at 37°. The cells were washed, and ^{125}I-hCG binding and ^{125}I-hCG stimulated progesterone production were measured after a further 2 hr incubation in serum-free medium at 37°. Redrawn (by permission) from Ascoli (1981b).

produced is reduced to a similar extent as the reduction in hormone binding and the amount of hCG required for half-maximal increase in progesterone production is increased 2-3 fold (Table IV). As a result of these changes, the coupling between hCG binding and progesterone production increases. Thus, the ratio of the ED_{50} for hCG binding to the ED_{50} for progesterone production decreases from 2-4 in the control cells to 0.7 - 1.3 in the mEGF or hCG-treated cells (Table IV). These results are expected, since the MA-10 cells have only a few "spare" receptors (cf. Fig. 2). It is worth noting that in another cell type with few spare receptors (3T3-L1 cells) down-regulation of insulin receptors is associated with tighter coupling between insulin binding and action (Ronnet et al., 1982; Karlsson et al., 1979). On the other hand, cells that have a large excess of "spare" gonadotropin receptors, such as normal rat Leydig cells, do not show a reduction in the maximal response to the hormone when the receptors are reduced. They do, however, show an increase in ED_{50} greater in magnitude than that observed in the MA-10 cells (Cigorraga et al., 1978).

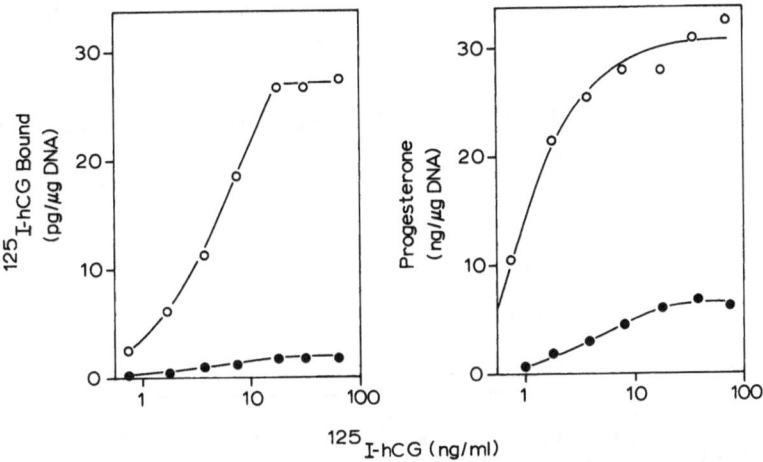

Figure 10. Relationship between ^{125}I-hCG binding (left panel) and progesterone production (right panel) in hCG-treated cells. Cells were incubated without (open circles) or with (black circles) 40 ng/ml hCG for 14 hr at 37°. The cells were washed, and ^{125}I-hCG binding and ^{125}I-hCG stimulated progesterone production were measured after a further 2 hr incubation in serum-free medium at 37°. Data reproduced (by permission) from Freeman and Ascoli (1981).

Table IV. Effects of mEGF and hCG on ^{125}I-hCG Binding and ^{125}I-hCG Stimulated Progesterone Production

Expt. No.	Pretreatment	Binding	
		Maximum (Molecules/cell)	ED_{50} (M × 10^{-10})
1	None	10,440 (100)	1.3 (100)
	hCG	596 (5.7)	1.2 (92)
2	None	8,799 (100)	2.1 (100)
	mEGF	1,285 (15)	1.7 (81)

Expt. No.	Pretreatment	Progesterone	
		Maximum (ng/µg DNA)	ED_{50} (M × 10^{-10})
1	None	29.4 (100)	0.34 (100)
	hCG	6.5 (22)	0.90 (289)
2	None	28 (100)	1.1 (100)
	mEGF	6 (21)	2.3 (209)

Cells were preincubated with hCG (40 ng/ml) or mEGF (5 ng/ml) for 14 or 48 hr, respectively. After washing, ^{125}I-hCG binding and ^{125}I-hCG progesterone production were measured during a 2 hr incubation at 37°. Reproduced (by permission) from Ascoli (1981b) and Freeman and Ascoli (1981).

4.2 Regulation of Cholera Toxin and cAMP Stimulated Steroidogenesis

The results discussed above clearly show that in the MA-10 cells the down regulation of hCG receptors leads to a decrease in hormonal responsiveness. Because of previous work done by other investigators in normal cells (Catt et al., 1979, 1980; Harwood et al., 1978) and by us in freshly isolated Leydig tumor cells (Segaloff et al., 1981a,b), it was of interest to determine the effects of mEGF and hCG on the activity of the effector system of the MA-10 cells. As outlined above, this can easily be tested by measuring the ability of cholera toxin and cAMP analogues to stimulate progesterone production. The results presented in Fig. 11 show that the steroidogenic response to these stimuli is reduced (by about 50%) in the hCG-treated cells but unchanged in the mEGF-treated cells. The hCG-induced loss of steroido-genic responses to cholera toxin and cAMP has been called

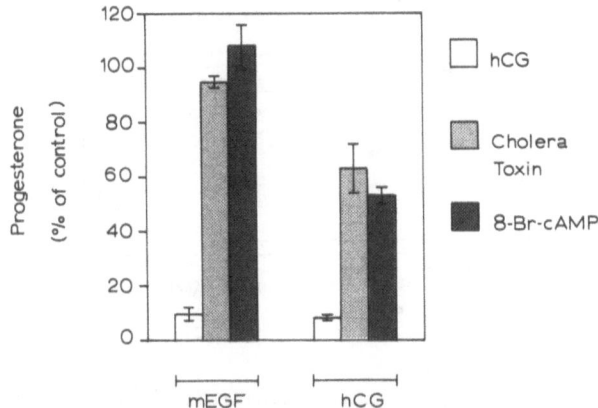

Figure 11. Effects of hCG, cholera toxin and 8-Br-cAMP on progesterone production by hCG and mEGF-treated cells. Cells were incubated (37°) with the indicated concentration of mEGF or hCG for 48 hr or 14 hr, respectively. The cells were washed, and progesterone production was determined after a further incubation (4 hr, 37°) in serum-free medium containing hCG (1 nM), cholera toxin (1.2 nM), or 8-Br-cAMP (1 mM). Redrawn (by permission) from Ascoli (1981b) and Freeman and Ascoli (1981).

"desensitization" (Freeman and Ascoli, 1981). These results suggested to us that the effects of mEGF on the hormonal response of the MA-10 cells was confined to the hCG receptors, while the effects of hCG appeared to be expressed at two loci: the receptor and the effector system. Inasmuch as the loss of steroidogenic responses in the hCG-treated cells is not as pronounced when the cells are restimulated with cholera toxin or 8-Br-cAMP as when they are restimulated with hCG, it can be concluded that the receptor defect is limiting.

The finding that both hormones down-regulate hCG receptors but only one (hCG) desensitizes the cells suggests that these phenomena occur independently. Further support for this hypothesis was provided by examining the time courses required for the loss of steroidogenic responses to occur

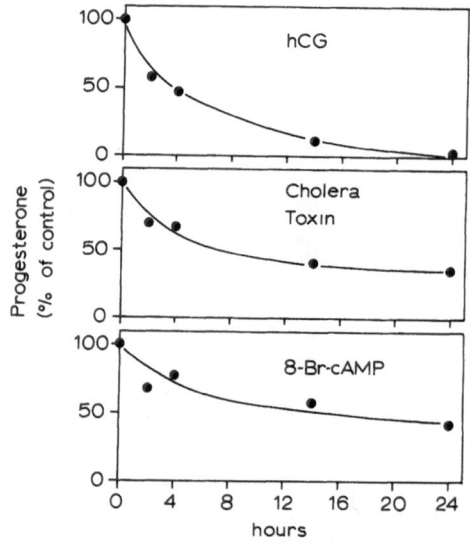

Figure 12. Time course of hCG-induced desensitization of steroidogenic response. Cells were incubated (37°) with 40 ng/ml hCG. At the times indicated, the cells were washed and incubated (37°, 4 hr) in serum-free medium containing hCG (1 nM), cholera toxin (1.2 nM), or 8-Br-cAMP (1 mM). Progesterone production was measured and compared to that of cells incubated without hCG. Reproduced (by permission) from Freeman and Ascoli (1981).

(Freeman and Ascoli, 1981). The results presented in Fig. 12 show that the loss of steroidogenic responses to cholera toxin and 8-Br-cAMP are nearly maximal 4 hr after addition of hCG, while the loss of steroidogenic response to hCG is not maximally expressed until about 14 hr after addition of hCG. Also note that the time course of loss of response to hCG parallels the loss of hCG receptors (cf. Fig. 5A).

An obvious difference between the effects of mEGF and hCG on the MA-10 cells is that, while hCG has pronounced stimulatory effects on cAMP and steroid biosynthesis, mEGF has little or no effect on these processes (Ascoli, 1981b, and unpublished observations). Thus, it was of interest to expose the cells to other compounds that stimulate steroidogenesis (such as cholera toxin or cAMP analogues) and test for desensitization. In order to do this experiment, we first chose concentrations of cholera toxin and 8-Br-cAMP that stimulate progesterone biosynthesis to the same extent as obtained with 40 ng/ml hCG (the concentration used in the experiments shown in Fig. 10, 11 and 12). The time course involved in the stimulation of progesterone production by the concentrations of stimuli chosen are shown in Fig. 13. The data show that although the time courses involved in the stimulation of this process are different, the final levels of progesterone accumulated in the medium are the same. Cells treated with these concentrations of cholera toxin or 8-Br-cAMP

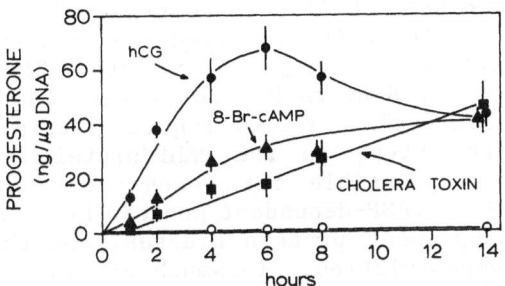

Figure 13. Time course of the effects of hCG, cholera toxin and 8-Br-cAMP on progesterone production. Cells were incubated (37°) with 1 nM hCG (black circles), 24 pM cholera toxin (black squares), 70 μM 8-Br-cAMP (black triangles), or buffer only (open circles). Progesterone accumulation was determined at the times indicated.

accumulated 100-150 times more progesterone in the medium than control cells, and bound as much ^{125}I-hCG as control cells (Freeman and Ascoli, 1981). When these cells were incubated with freshly added hCG cholera toxin, or 8-BR-cAMP, their steroidogenic response was reduced to about 50% of control (Fig. 14). It is important to note that under these conditions the loss of steroidogenic responses to all three stimuli is very similar. This is in contrast to the effects of hCG treatment (cf. Fig. 11), which results in a more drastic reduction in hCG responses than in cholera toxin or cAMP responses.

These results, together with the inability of mEGF to induce densensitization, lead us to conclude that the hCG-induced lesion(s) in the effector system are due to its ability to stimulate progesterone biosynthesis, and that this lesion(s) is independent of the hCG-induced down-regulation of the hCG receptor (Ascoli, 1981; Segaloff et al., 1981a,b; Freeman and Ascoli, 1981). In this respect, the MA-10 cells behave similarly to normal rat leydig cells and granulosa/-luteal cells. In both of these sytems, hCG has been shown to induce lesion(s) in the receptor and effector systems (Catt et al., 1979, 1980; Harwood et al., 1978).

5.   Regulation of the Effector System

The finding that the steroidogenic responsiveness of the MA-10 cells to 8-Br-cAMP is densensitized after hCG treatment suggests that the lesion(s) involved are localized beyond the hormonal activation of adenylate cyclase. The induction of densensitization by 8-Br-cAMP also suggest that the stimulation of adenylate cyclase is not required for desensitization to occur. Other steps in the cAMP/protein kinase pathway that could be responsible for desensitization include the binding of cAMP to cAMP-dependent protein kinases, the activation of cAMP-dependent protein kinases, and the stimulation of protein phosphorylation. Inasmuch as some of these steps have been examined and found to be normal in densensitized rat Leydig cells and granulosa/luteal cells (Tsuruhara et al., 1977; Sen et al., 1979), we did not investigate them further. Our efforts toward understanding the mechanisms involved in densnsitization were thus directed to the steroidogenic pathway.

Our studies of the sources of cholesterol used for steroidogenesis had shown that cellular stores supplied the bulk of substrate for steroidogenesis during short-term stimulation (Freeman and Ascoli, 1982a), and that the time course for the induction of desensitization (Fig. 12) correlated well with the time course for depletion of cellular cholesterol stores. In our earlier studies (cf. Fig. 11, 12, and 14), desensitization had been assessed in media devoid of lipoproteins (Ascoli, 1981b; Segaloff et al., 1981a,b; Freeman and Ascoli, 1981). Since under these conditions cells desensitized by hCG would be dependent on newly synthesized cholesterol for subsequent steroid production, their steroidogenic response is limited by the absence of lipoproteins (Freeman and Ascoli, 1982a,b). Thus, it seemed possible that in the absence of lipoproteins, the hCG-induced depletion of cellular cholesterol was responsible for desensitization. This contention was also supported by the finding that hCG, but not mEGF, depleted the intracellular cholesterol stores of the MA-10 cells (Table V).

Since we had previously shown that under prolonged hCG stimulation (when the intracellular stores of cholesterol are depleted) LDL provides most of the colesterol needed for steroid biosynthesis, we tested the effects for this lipoprotein on desensitization.

Table V. Effects of mEGF and hCG on the Cholesterol
Content of the MA-10 Cells

| Additions | Cellular cholesterol content (ng/µg DNA) | |
	Free	Esterified
None	209 ± 14 (100)	103 ± 4 (100)
mEGF (5 ng/ml)	226 ± 15 (108)	113 ± 6 (110)
hCG (49 ng/ml)	107 ± 5 (51)	31 ± 2 (30)

Cells were incubated (37°) for 24 hr in lipoprotein-deficient medium containing the indicated concentrations of mEGF or hCG, prior to the determination of cholesterol.

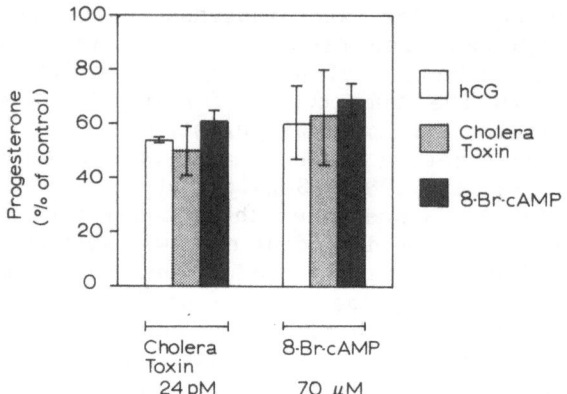

Figure 14. Effects of hCG, cholera toxin and 8-Br-cAMP on progesterone production by cholera toxin and 8-Br-cAMP treated cells. Cells were incubated with the indicated concentrations of cholera toxin or 8-Br-cAMP for 14 hr at 37°. After washing the cells were incubated (37°, 4 hr) in serum-free medium containing hCG (1 nM), cholera toxin (1.2 nM), or 8-Br-cAMP (1 mM). Progesterone production was determined and compared to that of control cells. Reproduced (by permission) from Freeman and Ascoli (1981).

The results presented in Figure 15 (top panel) show that when cells are first incubated with hCG in lipoprotein-deficient medium, and subsequently incubated with Bt_2cAMP, their steroidogenic response is reduced to 17% of control if LDL is not present. The addition of increasing concentrations of LDL stimulated progesterone production 6.5 fold and restored the steroidogenic response to 90% of control. In contrast, the addition of LDL to control or mEGF-treated cells increased Bt_2cAMP-stimulated progesterone production only 1.6 fold. As expected, the steroidogenic response of these two groups of cells was very similar, either in the absence or presence of LDL.

The data presented in Figure 15 (bottom panel) show the results of a similar experiment, in which control, mEGF-treated, or hCG-treated cells were restimulated with hCG. The addition of LDL increased progesterone production 1.9, 2.5, and 13 fold, respectively, in the control, mEGF-, and hCG-treated cells. Thus, LDL again had a greater effect in the hCG-treated cells than in the other two groups. The steroidogenic response of the mEGF or hCG-treated cells, however, remained well below control, even at high concentrations of LDL. Thus, it is concluded that the reduction in hCG receptors induced by mEGF or hCG limits the subsequent biological response to hCG even in the presence of LDL.

The finding that LDL could largely overcome the effector lesion(s) of densensitized cells is consistent with the hypothesis that cholesterol depletion is responsible for desensitization. If the effect of LDL is mediated by increasing cellular cholesterol stores, it should be possible to show

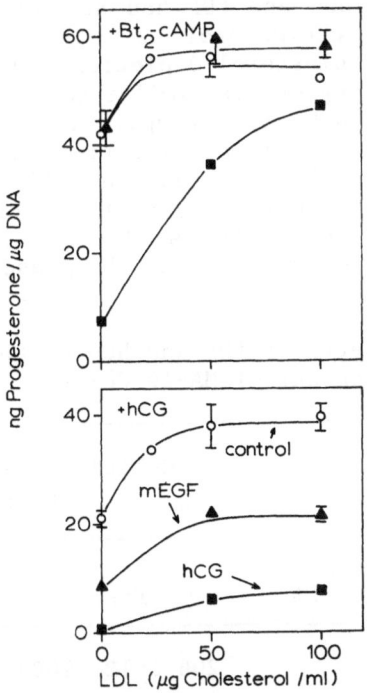

Figure 15. Effects of LDL on the steroidogenic responses of hCG on mEGF-treated cells. Cells were preincubated (24 hr, 37°) in lipoprotein-deficient medium containing buffer only (open circles), 5 ng/ml mEGF (black triangles), or 40 ng/ml hCG (black squares). After washing the cells were incubated (37°) in lipoprotein-deficient medium containing the indicated concentrations of LDL and 1 mM Bt$_2$-cAMP (top panel) or 40 ng/ml hCG (bottom panel). The amount of progesterone produced was determined at the end of an 8 hr incubation.

that cells treated with hCG in the presence of LDL have greater cholesterol stores than cells treated with hCG in the absence of LDL. Moreover, the intracellular levels of cholesterol should correlate with the ability of cAMP to stimulate progesterone production.

The data in Table VI show the effect of hCG treatment on cellular cholesterol stores of cells incubated in the absence or presence of LDL. Cells treated with hCG in the absence of LDL had 52% as much free and 34% as much esterified cholesterol as cells incubated in the absence of hCG and LDL. Cells treated with hCG and LDL had 86% as much free and 59% as much esterified cholesterol as cells incubated with LDL alone. The total cholesterol depletion induced by hCG in the absence of LDL (160 ng/μg) is similar to the depletion induced in the presence of LDL (154 ng/μg). However, levels of free and esterified cholesterol in cells treated with both hCG and LDL were higher than those present in cells incubated without LDL and hCG, or without LDL and with hCG (Table VI). Therefore, the addition of LDL to MA-10 cells increases cellular stores of cholesterol regardless of the presence of hCG.

Table VI.   Effects of LDL and hCG on Cholesterol
Content of MA-10 Cells

Additions		Cellular cholesterol content (ng/μg DNA)	
hCG (40 ng/ml)	LDL (50 μg/ml)	Free	Esterified
-	-	206 ± 12 (100)	92 ± 3 (100)
+	-	107 ± 5 (52)	31 ± 3 (34)
-	+	270 ± 6 (100)	286 ± 39 (100)
+	+	233 ± 22 (86)	169 ± 10 (59)

Cells were incubated (37°) in lipoprotein-deficient medium containing the indicated additions for 24 hr prior to the determination of cholesterol.

The data depicted in Fig. 16 shows the ability of Bt_2cAMP to restimulate progesterone production in these four groups of cells. When the cells were preincubated with hCG in the absence of LDL, and subsequently exposed to Bt_2cAMP in the absence of LDL, their steroidogenic response was reduced to 16% of control (i.e., cells preincubated without hCG or LDL). On the other hand, when cells were preincubated with hCG in the presence of LDL, and subsequently exposed to Bt_2cAMP in the presence of LDL, their steroidogenic response was reduced only to 86% of control (i.e., cells preincubated without hCG in the presence of LDL).

The insert in Fig. 16 correlates the cellular total cholesterol levels at the beginning of the second incubation with the production of progesterone in response to cAMP. The data show that the correlation coefficient between cholesterol stores and the production of progesterone is 0.978. The same plot performed against esterified cholesterol or free cholesterol gives correlation coefficients of 0.959 and 0.953, respectively. These data show that the steroidogenic response of the MA-10 cells is dictated by the levels of intracellular cholesterol and by the presence of LDL.

The results of these series of experiments indicate: (a) hCG, but not mEGF, causes depletion of cholesterol stores and induction of desensitization; (b) suppling adequate cholesterol via LDL largely corrects desensitization; and (c) cholesterol stores correlate closely with the quantity of steroid produced in response to stimulation. Taken together, these results indicate that hCG induces desensitization by causing depletion of cellular cholesterol stores.

6.   Relevance to the Function of Normal Gonadal Cells

Although early observations on the biology of mEGF suggested a relationship between gonadal tissues and mEGF (Byyny et al., 1974; Barthe et al., 1974; Stastny and Cohen, 1972), its effects on normal gonadal tissues are just beginning to be explored in detail. Thus, mEGF appears to be required for the multiplication and/or maintenance of cultures of normal mouse and pig Leydig cells in serum-free medium (Mather et al., 1982a,b). mEGF receptors have been identified in primary cultures of normal rat testicular cells (Welsch and Hsueh, 1982), but the effects of mEGF on hCG receptors in normal Leydig cells have not been investigated. It has been

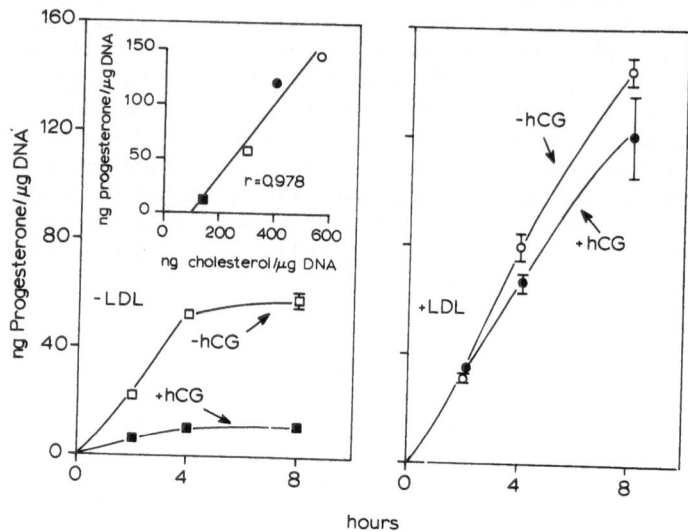

hours

Figure 16. Effects of LDL and Bt$_2$cAMP on steroid production by hCG-treated cells. Cells were preincubated (24 hr, 37°) in lipoprotein-deficient medium without (left panel) or with (right panel) 50 μg/ml of LDL cholesterol in the absence (open circles, open squares) or presence (black circles, black squares) of 40 ng/ml hCG. After washing, the cells were incubated (37°) in lipoprotein-deficient medium containing 1 mM Bt$_2$cAMP without (left panel) or with (right panel) 50 μg/ml of LDL cholesterol. The accumulation of progesterone in the medium was measured at the times indicated.

reported that in cultures of normal rat testicular cells mEGF inhibits the ability of hCG, cholera toxin and cAMP to stimulate testosterone production (Hsueh et al., 1981; Welsch and Hsueh, 1982). This effect appears to be mediated by an inhibition of 17α-hydroxylase and 17,20-lyase activities. On the other hand, Murphy and Moger (1982) have recently reported that mEGF enhances LH-stimulated androgen biosynthesis in primary cultures of mouse testicular cells. mEGF receptors have also been identified in cultured bovine granulosa/luteal, and its effects on cell multiplication have been studied (Gospodarowicz et al., 1977a,b, 1978; Wlodavsky et al., 1978). Because of the results summarized here, it is of interest to note that mEGF inhibits the ability of FSH to induce

LH/hCG receptors in cultures of normal rat granulosa cells (Mondschein and Schomberg, 1981) and the normal development of ovarian follicles in the neonatal mouse (Lintern-Moore et al., 1981). Thus, it is possible that a mechanism similar to that proposed here for the mEGF-induced down-regulation of hCG receptors is responsible for these phenomena.

The hCG-induced down-regulation of LH/hCG receptors and desensitization of steroidogenic responses have been extensively studied in normal gonadal cells (reviewed by Harwood et al., 1978; Catt et al., 1979, 1980; and Nozu et al., 1982). There is general agreement between our results and those obtained in normal gonadal cells, since in both experimental systems hCG has been shown to down-regulate its receptors and to reduce the activity of the effector system. The relative importance of these two lesions to the steroidogenic potential of the cells and the mechanisms involved in the regulation of the activity of the effector system, however, show some important differences. Thus, although hCG induced a drastic reduction in the number of HL/hCG receptors in normal gonadal cells in vivo, the associated reduction in steroidogenic responses to hCG is most readily explained in terms of a reduction in the activity of the effector system (Catt et al., 1979, 1980).

The hCG-induced desensitization of testosterone responses in normal rat Leydig cells appears to be due to (a) an estrogen-induced reduction in 17α-hydroxylase and 17,20-desmolase activities (called late steroidogenic lesion), and (b) other unidentified lesion(s) localized prior to the formation of pregnenolone (called early steroidogenic lesion(s)). The late steroidogenic lesion could not be expressed in the MA-10 cells or granulosa/luteal cells simply because it is localized beyond the formation of progesterone. On the other hand, the early steroidogenic lesion(s) could be similar (or identical) in normal rat Leydig cells and the MA-10 cells. In fact, recent observations on the effects of lipoproteins on the steroidogenic responses of desensitized rat Leydig cells suggest that the depletion of intracellular cholesterol is responsible (at least in part) for the early steroidogenic lesion(s) (Quinn et al., 1981, Charreau et al., 1981).

In terms of the kind of steroids produced (i.e., progesterone), the MA-10 cells more closely resemble normal granulosa/luteal cells than normal Leydig cells. Since hCG-induced desensitization of the progesterone responses in granulosa/luteal cells have only been measured in the absence of lipoproteins (Harwood et al., 1978), we suggest that cholesterol depletion is also responsible for this phenomenon in granulosa/luteal cells.

ACKNOWLEDGMENTS. We wish to thank Carolyn Lloyd and Dr. Deborah Segaloff for their contribution to some of the studies presented here, and Professor Stanley Cohen for his generous gift of mEGF. We are also grateful to Dr. David Rabin for his continuous guidance and encouragement. This research was supported by research grants from the National Cancer Institute (CA-23603) and the American Cancer Society (BC-343). D. A. Freeman has been supported by a training grant (HD-07043) and a National Research Service Award (HD-06297) from the National Institute of Child Health and Human Development.

FOOTNOTES. Abbreviations used in this chapter: (LH) lutropin; (hCG) human choriogonadotropin; (mEGF) mouse Epidermal Growth Factor; (LDL) human low density lipoprotein; (cAMP) Adenosine 3',5'-monophosphate; (8-Br-cAMP) 8-Bromo Adenosine 3',5'-monophosphate; (Bt$_2$cAMP) N^6,0^2-Dibutyryl Adenosine 3',5;-monophosphate.

REFERENCES

Adashi, E. Y., and Hsueh, A. J. W., 1982, Direct inhibition of rat testicular androgen biosynthesis by Arginine-Vasotocin, J. Biol. Chem. 257:1301.
Albert, D. A., Ascoli, M., Puett, D., and Coniglio, J. G., 1980, Lipid composition and gonadotropin-mediated lipid metabolism of the M5480 murine Leydig cell tumor, J. Lipid Res. 21:862.
Andersen, J. M., and Dietschy, J. M., 1978, Relative importance of high and low density lipoproteins in the regulation of cholesterol synthesis in the adrenal gland, ovary, and testis of the rat, J. Biol. Chem. 253:9024.
Archer, J. A., Gorden, P., and Roth, J., 1975, Defect in insulin binding to receptors in obese man. Amelioration with calorie restriction, J. Clin. Invest. 55:166.

Ascoli, M., 1978, Demonstration of a direct effect of inhibition of the degradation of receptor-bound human choriogonadotropin on the steroidogenic pathway, J. Biol. Chem. 253:7839.

Ascoli, M., 1979, Inhibition of the degradation of receptor-bound human choriogonadotropin by leupeptin, Biochim. Biophys. Acta 586:608.

Ascoli, M., 1980, Degradation of the subunits of receptor-bound human choriogonadotropin by Leydig tumor cells, Biochim. Biophys. Acta 629:409.

Ascoli, M., 1981a, Characterization of several clonal lines of cultured Leydig tumor cells: Gonadotropin receptors and steroidogenic responses, Endocrinology 108:88.

Ascoli, M., 1981b, Regulation of gonadotropin receptors and gonadotropin responses in a clonal strain of Leydig tumor cells by Epiderman Growth Factor, J. Biol. Chem. 256:179.

Ascoli, M., 1981c, Effects of hypocholesterolemia and chronic hormonal stimulation of sterol and steroid metabolism in a Leydig cell tumor, J. Lipid Res. 22:1247.

Ascoli, M., 1982a, Regulation of steroid production in gonadal, adrenal, and placental tumor cells, in: "Cellular Regulation of Secretion and Release," P. M. Conn, ed., Academic Press, New York. p. 409.

Ascoli, M., 1982b, Receptor-mediated uptake and degradation of human choriogonadotropin: Fate of the hormone subunits, Ann. N. Y. Acad. Sci. 383:151.

Ascoli, M., 1982c, Internalization and degradation of receptor-bound human choriogonadotropin in Leydig tumor cells: Fate of the hormone subunits, J Biol. Chem., 257:13306.

Ascoli, M., and Puett, D., 1978a, Gonadotropin binding and stimulation of steroidogenesis in Leydig tumor cells, Proc. Natl. Acad. Sci. USA 75:99.

Ascoli, M., and Puett, D., 1978b, Degradation of receptor-bound human choriogonadotropin by murine Leydig tumor cells, J. Biol. Chem. 253:4892.

Ascoli, M., and Puett, D., 1978c, Inhibition of the degradation of receptor-bound human choriogonadotropin by lysosomotropic agents, protease inhibitors, and metabolic inhibitors, J. Biol. Chem. 253:7832.

Bambino, T. H., Schreiber, J. R., and Hsueh, A. J. M., 1980, Gonadotropin-releasing hormone and its agonist inhibit testicular luteinizing hormone receptor and steroidogenesis in immature and adult hypophysectomized rats, Endocrinology 107:908.

Barthe, P. L., Bullock, L. P., Mowszowicz, I., Bardin, C. W., and Orth, D. N., 1974, Submaxillary gland Epidermal Growth Factor: A sensitive index of biologic androgen activity, Endocrinology 95:1019.

Briefel, G. R., Panajiotis, D., Tsitouras, D., Kowatch, M. A., Harman, S. M., and Blackman, M. R., 1982, Decreased in vitro testosterone production by isolated Leydig cells from uremic rats, Endocrinology 110:976.

Brown, M. S., and Goldstein, J. L., 1979, Receptor-mediated endocytosis: insights from the lipoprotein receptor system, Proc. Natl. Acad. Sci. USA 76:3330.

Brown, M. S., Kovanen, P. T., and Goldstein, J. L., 1979, Receptor-mediated uptake of lipoprotein-cholesterol and its utilization for steroid biosynthesis in the adrenal cortex, Recent Prog. Horm. Res. 35:215.

Byyny, R. L., Orth, D. N., Cohen, S., and Doyne, E. S., 1974, Epidermal Growth Factor: effects of androgens and adrenergic agents, Endocrinology 95:776.

Carpenter, G., and Cohen, S., 1979, Epidermal growth factor, Annu. Rev. Biochem. 48:193.

Catt, K. J., Harwood, J. P., Aguilera, G., and Dufau, M. L., 1979, Hormonal regulation of peptide receptors and target cell responses, Nature 280:109.

Catt, K. J., Harwood, J. P., Clayton, R. N., Davies, T. F., Chan, V., Katikineni, M., Nozu, K., and Dufau, M. L., 1980, Regulation of peptide hormone receptors and gonadal steroidogenesis, Recent Prog. Horm. Res. 36:557.

Chait, A., Kanter, R., Green, W., and Kenny, M., 1982, Defectiv thyroid hormone action in fibroblasts cultured from subjects with the syndrome of resistance to thyroid hormones, J. Clin. Endocrinol Metab. 54:767.

Charreau, E. H., Calvo, J. C., Nozu, K., Pignataro, O., Catt, K. J., and Dufau, M. L., 1981, Hormonal modulation of 3-hydroxy-3-methylglutaryl Coenzyme A reductase activity in gonadotropin-stimulated and -desensitized testicular Leydig cells, J. Biol. Chem. 256:12719.

Cigorraga, S. B., Dufau, M. L., and Catt, K. J., 1978, Regulation of luteinizing hormone receptors and steroidogenesis in gonadotropin-desensitized Leydig cells, J. Biol. Chem. 253:4297.

Erickson, G. F., Wang, C., and Hsueh, A. J. W., 1979, FSH induction of functional LH receptors in granulosa cells cultured in a chemically defined medium, Nature 279:336.

Fantus, G. I., Saviolakis, G. A., Hedo, J. A., and Gorden, P., 1982, Mechanism of glucocorticoid-induced increase in insulin receptors of cultured human lymphocytes, J. Biol. Chem. 257:8277.

Farfel, Z., Brinckman, A. S., Kaslow, H. R., Brothers, V. M., and Bourne, H. R., 1980, Defect of receptor-cyclase coupling protein in pseudohypoparathyroidism, N. Engl. J. Med. 303:237.

Freeman, D. A., and Ascoli, M., 1981, Desensitization to gonadotropins in cultured Leydig tumor cells involves loss of gonadotropin receptors and decreased capacity for steroidogenesis, Proc. Natl. Acad. Sci. USA 78:6309.

Freeman, D. A., and Ascoli, M., 1982a, Studies on the source of cholesterol used for steroid biosynthesis in cultured Leydig cells, J. Biol. Chem., in press.

Freeman, D. A., and Ascoli, M., 1982b, Desensitization of steroidogenesis in cultured Leydig tumor cells: Role of cholesterol, Proc. Natl. Acad. Sci. USA, in press.

Harwood, J. P., Conti, M., Conn, P. M., Dufau, M. L., and Catt, K. J., 1978, Receptor regulation and target cell responses: studies in the ovarian luteal cell, Mol. Cell. Endocrinol. 11:121.

Hazum, E., 1982, Receptor regulation by hormones: Relevance to secretion and other biological functions, in: "Cellular Regulation of Secretion and Release", P. M. Conn, ed., Academic Press, New York, in press.

Hsueh, A. J. W., Welsh, T. H., and Jones, P. B. C., 1981, Inhibition of ovarian and testicular steroidogenesis by Epidermal Growth Factor, Endocrinology 108:2002.

Huff, K. R., and Guroff, G., 1979, Nerve Growth Factor reduction in Epidermal Growth Factor responsiveness and Epidermal Growth Factor receptors in PC12 cells: An aspect of cell differentiation, Biochem. Biophys. Res. Commun. 89:175.

Johnson, G., Kaslow, H. R., Farfel, Z., and Bourne, H. R., 1980, Genetic analysis of hormone-sensitive adenylate cyclase, Adv. Cyclic Nucleotide Res. 13:1.

Kaplan, J., 1981, Polypeptide-binding membrane receptors: Analysis and classification, Science 212:14.

Karlsson, S., Grumfeld, C., Kahn, C. R., and Roth, J., 1979, Regulation of insulin receptors and insulin responsiveness in 3T3-L1 fatty fibroblasts, Endocrinology 104:1383.

Ketelslegers, J. M., Knott, G. D., and Catt, K. J., 1975, Kinetics of gonadotropin binding by receptors of the rat testis. Analysis by a non-linear curve-fitting model, Biochemistry 14:3075.

King, C. A., and Cuatrecasas, P., 1981, Peptide hormone-induced receptor mobility, aggregation and internalization, N. Engl. J. Med. 305:77.

Klemcke, H. G., and Bartke, A., 1981, Effects of chronic hyper-
    prolactinemia in mice on plasma gonadotropin concentrations
    and testicular human choriogonadotropin binding sites,
    Endocrinology 108:1763.
Knutson, V. P., Ronnet, G. V., and Lane, M. D., 1982, Control
    of insulin receptor level in 3T3 cells: Effect of insulin-
    induced down-regulation and dexamethasone-induced up-regu-
    lation on rate of receptor activation, Proc. Natl. Acad.
    Sci. USA 79:2822.
Lacroix, A., Ascoli, M., Puett, D., and McKenna, T. J., 1979,
    Steroidogenesis in hCG-responsive Leydig cell tumor
    variants, J. Steroid Biochem. 10:669.
Lee, C. Y., and Ryan, R. J., 1973, Interaction of ovarian
    receptors with human luteinizing hormone and human chronic
    gonadotropin, Biochemistry 12:4609.
Lintern-Moore, S., Moore, G. P. M., Panaretto, B. A., and
    Robertson, I., 1981, Follicular development in the neonatal
    mouse ovary: Effect of Epidermal Growth Factor, Acta
    Endocrinol. 96:123.
Lloyd, C. E., and Ascoli, M., 1983, On the mechanisms involved
    in the regulation of the cell surface receptors for human
    choriogonadotropin and mouse epidermal growth factor in
    cultured Leydig tumor cells, J. Cell Biol., in press.
Mather, J. P., Saez, J. M., and Haour, F., 1982a, Regulation of
    gonadotropin receptors and steroidogenesis in cultured
    porcine Leydig cells, Endocrinology 110:933.
Mather, J. P., Zhuang, L. -Z., Perez-Infante, V., and Phillips,
    D. M., 1982b, Culture of testicular cells in hormone-
    supplemented serum-free medium, Ann. N. Y. Acad. Sci.
    383:44.
Mendelson, C., Dufau, M. L., and Catt, K. J., 1975, Gonadotropin
    binding and stimulation of cyclic adenosine 3',5'-monophos-
    phate and testosterone production in isolated Leydig cells,
    J. Biol. Chem. 250:8818.
Mondschein, J. A., and Schomberg, D. W., 1981, Growth factors
    modulate gonadotropin receptor induction in granulosa cell
    cultures, Science 211:1179.
Morris, M. D., and Chaikoff, L. L., 1959, The origin of choles-
    terol in liver, small intestine, adrenal gland, and testis
    of the rat: Dietary versus endogenous contributions, J
    Biol. Chem. 234:1095.
Moyle, W. R., and Greep, R. O., 1974, Steroid-secreting tumors
    as models in endocrinology, in: "Hormones and Cancer",
    K. W. McKerns, ed., p. 329, Academic Press, New York.

Murphy, P. R., and Moger, W. H., 1982, Short-term primary cultures of mouse interstitial cells: Effects of culture conditions on androgen production, Biol. Reprod. 27:38.

Nozu, K., Deheia, A., Zawistowich, L., Catt, K. J., and Dufau, M. L., 1982, Gonadotropin-induced desensitization of Leydig cells in vivo and in vitro: Estrogen action in the testis, Ann. N. Y. Acad. Sci. 383:212.

Ohkuma, S., and Poole, B., 1978, Fluorescent probe measurement of the intralysosomal pH in living cells and the perturbation of pH by various agents, Proc. Natl. Acad. Sci. USA 75:3327

Olefsky, J. M., and Ciaraldi, T. P., 1981, The insulin receptor: basic characteristics and its role in insulin resistant states, in "Handbook of Diabetes Mellitus" Volume 2, M. Brownlee, ed., p. 71, Garland, New York.

Payne, A. H., O'Shaughnessy, P. J., Chase, D. J., Dixon, G. E. K., and Christensen, K. A., 1982, LH receptors and steroidogenesis in distinct population of Leydig cells, Ann. N. Y. Acad. Sci. 383:174.

Purvis, K., Clansen, O. P. F., and Hansson, V., 1978, Decreased Leydig cell responsiveness in the testicular feminized male rat, Endocrinology 102:1053.

Quinn, P. G., Dombrausky, L. J., Chen, Y. -D. I., and Payne, A. H., 1981, Serum lipoprotein increase testosterone production in hCG-desensitized Leydig cells, Endocrinology 109:1790.

Rae, P. A., Gutmann, N. S., Tsao, J., and Schimmer, B. P., 1979, Mutations in cyclic AMP-dependent protein kinase and corticotropin (ACTH)-sensitive adenylate cyclase affect adrenal steroidogenesis, Proc. Natl. Acad. Sci. USA 76:1896.

Rommerts, F. F. G., and Brinkman, A. O., 1981, Modulation of steroidogenic activities in testis Leydig cells, Mol. Cell. Endocrinol. 21:15.

Ronnett, G. V., Knutson, V. P., and Lane, D. M., 1982, Insulin-induced down-regulation of insulin receptors in 3T3-LI adipocytes, J Biol. Chem. 257:4285.

Schonbrum, A., 1982, Glucocorticoids down-regulate somatostatin receptors on pituitary cells in culture, Endocrinology 110:1147.

Schonbrum, A., and Tashjian, Jr., A. H., 1980, Modulation of somatostatin receptors by thyrotropin-releasing hormone in a clonal pituitary cell strain, J. Biol. Chem. 255:190.

Schumacher, M., Schafer, G., Lichtenberg, V., and Hilz, H., 1979, Maximal steroidogenic capacity of mouse Leydig cells,

FEBS Lett. 107:398.

Segaloff, D. L., and Ascoli, M., 1981, Removal of the surface bound human choriogonadotropin results in the cessation of hormonal responses in cultured Leydig tumor cells, J. Biol. Chem. 256:11420.

Segaloff, D. L., Puett, D., and Ascoli, M., 1981a, Dynamics of the steroidogenic responses of Leydig tumor cells to ovine luteinizing hormone, human choriogonadotropin, cholera toxin, and adenosine 3',5'-monophosphate, Endocrinology 108:632.

Segaloff, D. L., Ascoli, M., and Puett, D., 1981b, Characterization of the desensitized state of Leydig tumor cells, Biochim. Biophys. Acta 675:351.

Sen, K. K., Azhar, S., and Menon, K. M. J., 1979, Receptor-mediated gonadotropin action in the ovary, J. Biol. Chem. 254:5664.

Stastny, M., and Cohen, S., 1972, The stimulation of orinthine decarboxylase activity in testes of the neonatal mouse, Biochim. Biophys. Acta 261:177.

Stricklnd, S., and Loeb, J. N., 1981, Obligatory separation of hormone binding and biological response curves in systems dependent upon secondary mediators of hormone action, Proc. Natl. Acad. Sci. USA 78:1366.

Tell, G. P., Haour, F., and Saez, J. M., 1978, Hormonal regulation of membrane receptors and cell responsiveness: A review, Metabolism 27:1566.

Tsuruhara, T., Dufau, M. L., Cigorraga, S., and Catt, K. J., 1977, Hormonal regulation of testicular luteinizing hormone receptors, J. Biol. Chem. 252:9002.

Tycko, B., and Maxfield, F. R., 1982, Rapid acidification of endocytic vesicles containing α_2-macroglobulin, Cell 28:643.

Welsh, T. H., and Hsueh, A. J. W., 1982, Mechanism of the inhibitory action of epidermal growth factor on testicular androgen biosynthesis in vitro, Endocrinology 110:1498.

Wiley, H. S., and Cunningham, D. D., 1981, A steady state model for analyzing the cellular binding, internalization and degradation of polypeptide ligands, Cell 25:433.

Wiley, H. S., and Cunningham, D. D., 1982, The endocytotic rate constant. A cellular parameter for quantitating receptor-mediated endocytosis, J. Biol. Chem. 257:4222.

Zeleznik, A. J., Midgley, A. R. Jr., and Reichert, L. E., 1974, Granulosa cell maturation in the rat: Increased binding of human choriogonadotropin following treatment with follicle-stimulating hormone in vivo, Endocrinology 95:818.

Index